AF544816

New Insights in Intracerebral Hemorrhage

Frontiers of Neurology and Neuroscience

Vol. 37

Series Editor

J. Bogousslavsky Montreux

New Insights in Intracerebral Hemorrhage

Volume Editors

Kazunori Toyoda Suita, Osaka
Craig S. Anderson Sydney, N.S.W.
Stephan A. Mayer New York, N.Y.

31 figures and 20 tables, 2016

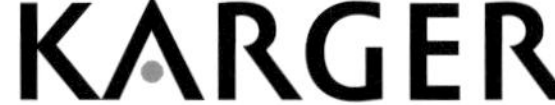

Basel · Freiburg · Paris · London · New York · Chennai · New Delhi · Bangkok · Beijing · Shanghai · Tokyo · Kuala Lumpur · Singapore · Sydney

Frontiers of Neurology and Neuroscience
Vols. 1–18 were published as Monographs in Clinical Neuroscience

Prof. Kazunori Toyoda
Department of Cerebrovascular Medicine
National Cerebral and Cardiovascular Center
Suita, Osaka 565-8565 (Japan)

Prof. Craig S. Anderson
The George Institute for Global Health
University of Sydney and Royal Prince Alfred Hospital
Sydney, NSW 2050 (Australia)

Prof. Stephan A. Mayer
Institute for Crititcal Care Medicine
The Mount Sinai Hospital
New York, NY 10029 (USA)

Library of Congress Cataloging-in-Publication Data

New insights in intracerebral hemorrhage / volume editors, Kazunori Toyoda, Craig S. Anderson, Stephan A. Mayer.
p. ; cm. -- (Frontiers of neurology and neuroscience, ISSN 1660-4431 ; vol. 37)
Includes bibliographical references and indexes.
ISBN 978-3-318-05596-2 (hard cover : alk. paper) -- ISBN 978-3-318-05597-9 (e-ISBN)
I. Toyoda, Kazunori (Physician), editor. II. Anderson, Craig S., editor.
III. Mayer, Stephan A., editor. IV. Series: Frontiers of neurology and neuroscience ; v. 37. 1660-4431
[DNLM: 1. Cerebral Hemorrhage--diagnosis. 2. Cerebral Hemorrhage--therapy. W1 MO568C v.37 2016 / WL 355]
RC388.5
616.81--dc23

2015033406

Bibliographic Indices. This publication is listed in bibliographic services, including Current Contents® and Index Medicus.

Disclaimer. The statements, opinions and data contained in this publication are solely those of the individual authors and contributors and not of the publisher and the editor(s). The appearance of advertisements in the book is not a warranty, endorsement, or approval of the products or services advertised or of their effectiveness, quality or safety. The publisher and the editor(s) disclaim responsibility for any injury to persons or property resulting from any ideas, methods, instructions or products referred to in the content or advertisements.

Drug Dosage. The authors and the publisher have exerted every effort to ensure that drug selection and dosage set forth in this text are in accord with current recommendations and practice at the time of publication. However, in view of ongoing research, changes in government regulations, and the constant flow of information relating to drug therapy and drug reactions, the reader is urged to check the package insert for each drug for any change in indications and dosage and for added warnings and precautions. This is particularly important when the recommended agent is a new and/or infrequently employed drug.

All rights reserved. No part of this publication may be translated into other languages, reproduced or utilized in any form or by any means electronic or mechanical, including photocopying, recording, microcopying, or by any information storage and retrieval system, without permission in writing from the publisher.

© Copyright 2016 by S. Karger AG, P.O. Box, CH–4009 Basel (Switzerland)
www.karger.com
Printed in Switzerland on acid-free and non-aging paper (ISO 9706) by Kraft Druck GmbH, Ettlingen
ISSN 1660–4431
e-ISSN 1662–2804
ISBN 978–3–318–05596–2
e-ISBN 978–3–318–05597–9

Contents

VII **Preface**
Toyoda, K. (Suita, Osaka); Anderson, C.S. (Sydney, N.S.W.); Mayer, S.A. (New York, N.Y.)

1 **Epidemiology of Intracerebral Haemorrhage**
Poon, M.T.C. (Oxford); Bell, S.M. (Sheffield); Al-Shahi Salman, R. (Edinburgh)

13 **Emergency Imaging of Intracerebral Haemorrhage**
Alobeidi, F.; Aviv, R.I. (Toronto, Ont.)

27 **Evidence-Based Critical Care of Intracerebral Hemorrhage: An Overview**
Küppers-Tiedt, L. (Frankfurt a.M.); Steiner, T. (Frankfurt a.M./Heidelberg)

35 **New Insights into Blood Pressure Control for Intracerebral Haemorrhage**
Manning, L.S.; Robinson, T.G. (Leicester)

51 **Emergency Reversal Strategies for Anticoagulation and Platelet Disorders**
Levi, M. (Amsterdam)

62 **Reperfusion-Related Intracerebral Hemorrhage**
Hayakawa, M. (Suita, Osaka)

78 **Cerebral Microbleeds: Detection, Associations and Clinical Implications**
Yakushiji, Y. (Saga)

93 **New Insights into Nonvitamin K Antagonist Oral Anticoagulants' Reversal of Intracerebral Hemorrhage**
Yasaka, M. (Fukuoka)

107 **Ultra-Early Hemostatic Therapy for Intracerebral Hemorrhage: Future Directions**
Wartenberg, K.E. (Halle); Mayer, S.A. (New York, N.Y.)

130 **Ventriculostomy and Lytic Therapy for Intracerebral Hemorrhage**
Ziai, W.C.; Nyquist, P.A.; Hanley, D.F. (Baltimore, Md.)

148 **Surgical Craniotomy for Intracerebral Hemorrhage**
Mendelow, A.D. (Newcastle upon Tyne)

155 **New Insights in Minimally Invasive Surgery for Intracerebral Hemorrhage**
Wang, W.-M.; Jiang, C.; Bai, H.-M. (Guangzhou)

166 **Surgical Strategies for Acutely Ruptured Arteriovenous Malformations**
Martinez, J.L.; Macdonald, R.L. (Toronto, Ont.)

182 **Prognosis and Outcome of Intracerebral Haemorrhage**
Moulin, S.; Cordonnier, C. (Lille)

193 **Author Index**

194 **Subject Index**

Preface

A new era for acute stroke care has come. Promptly visiting to a stroke center can be a key to success in dramatic recovery via acute reperfusion therapy. The therapeutic time window has been expanding with the progression of penumbral imaging, and the opportunity for stroke therapy has shifted to the prehospital setting in trials. Indeed, a new era for stroke medicine has come. However, this is the situation for ischemic stroke therapy. What is the status of intracerebral hemorrhage therapy?

Although the age-standardized mortality rate for hemorrhagic stroke (intracerebral hemorrhage and subarachnoid hemorrhage combined) has decreased worldwide in the past two decades, the incidence, number of deaths, and number of disability-adjusted life-years lost continue to increase [1]. Despite having half the incidence of ischemic stroke globally, hemorrhagic stroke causes more deaths and disability-adjusted life-years lost than ischemic stroke. In particular, intracerebral hemorrhage is relatively common in nonwhite ethnic populations. The development of a therapeutic strategy for intracerebral hemorrhage is as eagerly awaited as that for ischemic stroke. However, no established strategy for acute ICH analogous to reperfusion therapy for ischemic stroke has been established.

We encountered several milestone studies on intracerebral hemorrhage in the past decade. The Surgical Treatment for Ischemic Heart Failure (STICH) [2], involving 83 centers from 27 countries, was the largest trial on early hematoma evacuation surgery ever. That trial did not show overall benefit from surgery compared to initial medical therapy. In the Factor Seven for Acute Hemorrhagic Stroke Treatment (FAST) trial [3], emergent hemostatic therapy with recombinant activated factor VII reduced early hematoma growth. Although hemostatic therapy improved survival and functional outcomes in the initial trial, these clinical effects were not reproducible in a further trial. The hemostatic strategy is currently limited to cases of hemorrhage associated with coagulopathy or antithrombotic use; however, this strategy may be essential for the prevention of the ultra-early growth of intracerebral hemorrhage in general. The Second Intensive Blood Pressure Reduction in Acute Cerebral Haemorrhage Trial (INTERACT2) [4] significantly proved the safety and almost significantly showed the efficacy of early intensive blood pressure reduction for patients with hyperacute intracerebral hemorrhage. Several guidelines revised their recommendations for intensive antihypertensive therapy based on that trial. Thus, the initial hours after onset seem to be a golden time window for intracerebral hemorrhage as is the case for ischemic stroke.

Surprisingly, this is the first occasion in the 40-year history of 'Frontiers of Neurology and Neuroscience' in which intracerebral hemorrhage has been accepted as a main theme. It is time to thoroughly understand this devastating disease. This book covers all the recent topics related to the diagnosis and management of intracerebral hemorrhage and is written by top opinion experts. We hope that this book assists in your understanding of the current and future aspects of the optimal management of patients with intracerebral hemorrhage.

Kazunori Toyoda, Suita, Osaka, Japan
Craig S. Anderson, Sydney, N.S.W., Australia
Stephan A. Mayer, New York, N.Y., USA

References

1 Krishnamurthi RV, Feigin VL, Forouzanfar MH, et al: Global and regional burden of first-ever ischaemic and haemorrhagic stroke during 1990–2010: findings from the Global Burden of Disease Study 2010. Lancet Glob Health 2013;1:e259–e281.

2 Mendelow AD, Gregson BA, Fernandes HM, et al: Early surgery versus initial conservative treatment in patients with spontaneous supratentorial intracerebral haematomas in the International Surgical Trial in Intracerebral Haemorrhage (STICH): a randomised trial. Lancet 2005;365:387–397.

3 Mayer SA, Brun NC, Begtrup K, et al: Efficacy and safety of recombinant activated factor VII for acute intracerebral hemorrhage. N Engl J Med 2008;358:2127–2137.

4 Anderson CS, Heeley E, Huang Y, et al: Rapid blood-pressure lowering in patients with acute intracerebral hemorrhage. N Engl J Med 2013;368:2355–2365.

Toyoda K, Anderson CS, Mayer SA (eds): New Insights in Intracerebral Hemorrhage.
Front Neurol Neurosci. Basel, Karger, 2016, vol 37, pp 1–12 (DOI: 10.1159/000437109)

Epidemiology of Intracerebral Haemorrhage

Michael T.C. Poon[a] • Simon M. Bell[b] • Rustam Al-Shahi Salman[c]

[a]John Radcliffe Hospital, Oxford University Hospitals NHS Trust, Oxford, [b]The Royal Hallamshire Hospital, Sheffield Teaching Hospitals NHS Foundation Trust, Sheffield, and [c]Centre for Clinical Brain Sciences, University of Edinburgh, Edinburgh, UK

Abstract

Introduction: Intracerebral haemorrhage (ICH) has an overall incidence of 24.6 per 100,000 person-years and is associated with a high case fatality. Understanding the risk factors for ICH occurrence informs primary prevention strategies. This article provides an update on the current global patterns of ICH incidence and the common and emerging risk factors associated with ICH. ***Methods:*** We searched Ovid Medline (from 1980 to Oct 2014) for systematic reviews that addressed the epidemiology of ICH and for recent original studies that revealed new insights into the frequency of and the risk factors associated with ICH. ***Results:*** The incidence of ICH has not changed over the last 30 years, and this consistency is thought to be due to changes in the risk factor profiles of ICH patients. It appears that ICH is more common in men and during the winter months. ICH affects Asian populations more frequently than other populations. In addition to the known risk factors of hypertension and increasing age, alcohol consumption, the presence of the apolipoprotein ε2 or ε4 allele, extremes of body mass index, diabetes, and ophthalmic conditions have been suggested to be associated with ICH. Factors associated with a reduced risk of ICH include hypercholesterolaemia and a diet high in fruits and vegetables. ***Conclusions:*** The overall incidence of ICH has remained unchanged, but its regional incidence varies by race, sex, season and geographical location. In high income countries, the beneficial effect of improving blood pressure control may be counterbalanced by the increased use of antithrombotic drugs. Emerging modifiable risk factors include alcohol consumption, body mass index, diabetes, and fruit and vegetable intake, all of which may be amenable to interventions for the primary prevention of ICH (as well as many other diseases). © 2016 S. Karger AG, Basel

Introduction

Intracerebral haemorrhage (ICH) is a common cause of stroke that displays a worldwide incidence of 24.6 per 100,000 person-years [1]. The incidence of ICH is not uniform across different countries, with low to middle income countries having a rate double that of high income countries [2]. ICH is associated with a high case fatality of

40% at 1 month [1], 54% at 1 year, and 71% at 5 years [3]. Of those who survive 1 year, only about a quarter independently perform daily activities [3]. These short- and long-term outcomes have remained static over the past few decades [1, 3]. The current priority seems to be the improvement of primary prevention by lowering blood pressure and by treating other modifiable risk factors.

Understanding the epidemiology of ICH is crucial for developing a reliable risk stratification method to identify the people who are most at risk of ICH. As most published population-based studies of ICH cohorts were conducted in high income countries, there is a paucity of epidemiological data from low income regions of the world [2]. This update aims to ascertain the progress that has been made in studying risk factors for ICH in all regions of the world.

We have searched Ovid Medline from 1980 to 29 October, 2014, by combining the terms ('cerebral hemorrhage' OR 'Intracerebral hemorrhage') AND ('incidence' OR 'prevalence' OR 'risk factor') to identify systematic reviews that addressed the epidemiology of ICH and recent original studies that revealed new insights into the frequency of and the risk factors associated with ICH.

Nomenclature

Terminology slightly complicates our understanding of the epidemiology of ICH. As most readers know, ICH is just one type of intracranial haemorrhage (fig. 1). Furthermore, extradural haemorrhage and subdural haemorrhage have not been classified as sub-types of stroke; so, in most cases, 'haemorrhagic stroke' (HS) constitutes the remaining types of intracranial haemorrhage, principally non-traumatic (also known as spontaneous) ICH and subarachnoid haemorrhage (fig. 1). We have tried to restrict this chapter to the epidemiology of spontaneous ICH, although some noteworthy studies that we have included describe the epidemiology of intracranial haemorrhage or HS [4] without describing spontaneous ICH separately.

Incidence and Early Case Fatality Rate

The latest data on the frequency of HS are contained in a systematic review performed by the Global Burden of Diseases, Injuries and Risk Factors study in 2010, which included 58 studies from high income countries and 61 studies from low income countries; this study estimated that in 2010, a total of 5,324,997 people worldwide experienced a HS [4]. Additionally, 80% of all HS cases occurred in low and middle income countries, clearly indicating that the major global burden lies in these regions. The overall incidence of HS appears to vary between countries [4] and racial origins [1]. Unlike ischaemic stroke, the age-specific incidence of HS is higher in low-middle income countries than in high income countries [4].

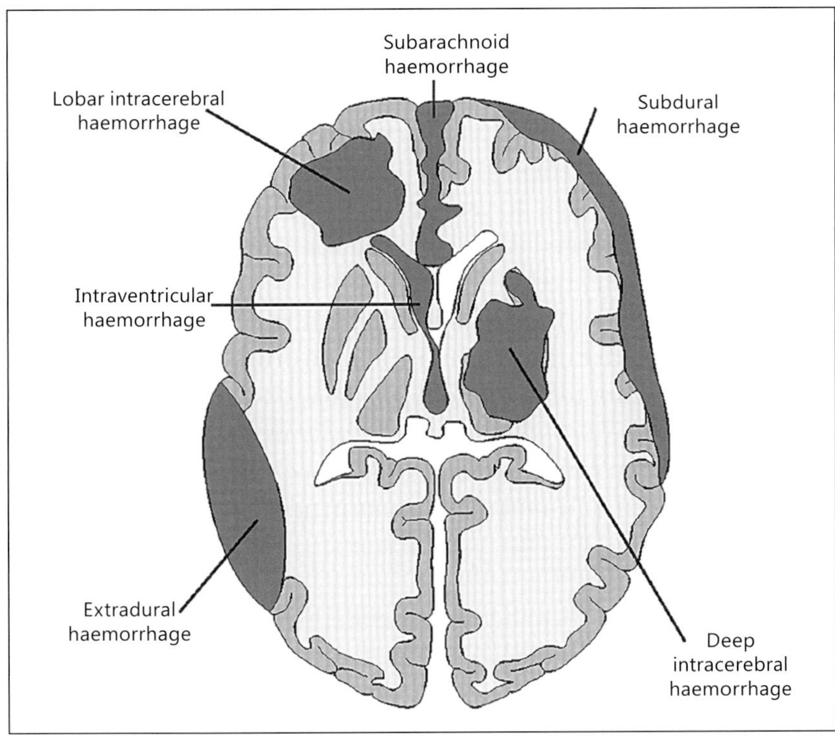

Fig. 1. Intracranial haemorrhage and its sub-types. Reproduced with permission from [42].

The rate of early fatality is high among patients who have had an ICH: The median one-month case fatality after ICH was 40.1% in a systematic review of 36 population-based studies conducted in 1983–2006 [1]. Again, low-middle income countries appear to fare worse, with a one-month case fatality rate of 30–48% compared to 15–35% in high income countries based on a systematic review of 56 population based studies [2]. Of the 5,324,997 people who experienced a HS, 3,038,763 (57%) individuals died during the study period.

Secular Trends

Whether the incidence of ICH has changed over the last few decades appears to depend on the population studied. In low-middle income countries, the ICH incidence appears to be increasing, whereas in some high income countries, the incidence appears to be falling [4]. This difference may be explained by the changing risk factors associated with ICH in high income countries. For example, this issue was studied in the Oxfordshire Community Stroke Project (OCSP) and the Oxford Vascular (OXVASC) study, which were performed 20 years apart on the same community in Oxford, UK. In this community containing 87,861 patients, although the incidence of ICH did not change over two decades, the proportion of ICH cases associated with systemic arterial hypertension decreased (relative risk [RR] 0.37, 95% confidence interval [CI] 0.21–0.67) [5]. On the other hand, the proportion of ICH cases associated with the use of oral antithrombotic drugs has increased over time. Therefore, the overall incidence of ICH may not have changed because one risk factor has been controlled whilst another has become more prevalent [5].

A static overall ICH incidence over a 30 year period (1985–2008) was also seen in Dijon, France. However, the age-related ICH incidence has changed in this community. The study reported that people aged ≥75 years had an increased incidence of ICH over time. As with the findings from the Oxford study, this result was thought to be secondary to the more prevalent use of oral antithrombotic drugs [6].

These findings have implications for low-middle income countries, where ongoing and future epidemiological transitions may result in similar changes. In these countries, effectively treating hypertension and identifying the people who are at highest risk of antithrombotic-associated ICH might reduce its incidence.

Geographical Variation

The Global Burden of Diseases, Injuries and Risk Factors 2010 study found that Asia and Southern Sub-Saharan Africa had the highest incidence of HS (101–158/100,000 person-years and 73–101/100,000 person-years, respectively) but that North America, Western Europe, Latin America and Oceania had the lowest incidence of HS in 2010 [4]. The country with the highest reported incidence of HS was China, with 159.81 cases per 100,000 person-years. The country with the lowest reported incidence of HS in 2010 was Qatar, with an incidence of 14.55 cases per 100,000 person-years [4].

There is a difference in the incidence of ICH between white populations and other racial populations around the world. People of Asian descent have a higher incidence of ICH when compared to whites and other races [1, 7].

The obvious difference in the incidence of ICH between Asian populations and white populations is not as apparent when comparing other races. A large cohort study of 14,357 people in the United States (US) (with RRs adjusted for age [≥65 years], sex, presence of hypertension, use of cholesterol-lowering drugs and smoking status) found no significant difference in the incidence of ICH between black and white ethnic groups [8]. A different study in the US reported that young black men were at higher risk of ICH than age-matched white Americans [9]. This difference in the incidence of ICH between black and white populations was also reported in a paper by Howard et al. [10]. This group stratified the age at presentation of ICH and found that black people aged <45 years had a higher risk of ICH than age-matched white people. This difference in the incidence of ICH disappeared after the age of 45 years [10], possibly explaining the discrepancy between the other 2 studies.

The incidence of ICH in Maori New Zealanders appears to be less than that in New Zealanders of European origin (9.6 per 100,000 person-years compared to 16.9 per 100,000 person-years), and being from a Maori background was significantly associated with a higher 30-day mortality rate [11].

Seasonal Effect on Intracerebral Haemorrhage Incidence

A small study in China based on hospital admissions has suggested that meteorological factors may play a role in the incidence of ICH [12]: in the summer months, the incidence of ICH was lower than in the winter months. A similar finding was reported in a population-based study in Germany, which found that the incidence of ICH was higher in the spring and winter months than in the summer months (Spring RR 2.0, 95% CI 1.24–3.22, Winter RR 1.55, 95% CI 0.94–2.55) [13]. It is unclear why these seasonal differences arise, but the lower risk in summer months has been hypothesised to be due to higher leukocyte counts and higher blood pressure at admission [13] or due to higher temperature, humidity and atmospheric pressure [12].

Gender Differences

The incidence of ICH appears to be higher in men than in women according to a systematic review and meta-analysis of 59 studies in 19 countries (RR 1.6, 95% CI 1.47–1.74) [14] and according to a North American population-based study (RR 1.5, 95% CI 1.2–1.8) [9]. However, the severity of ICH (based on the National Institutes of Health Stroke Scale [NIHSS]) is greater in women (NIHSS 10.0) than in men (NIHSS 8.2) [14]. Part of this difference in the incidence of ICH between men and women might be explained by sex differences in blood pressure. The American Heart Association guidelines for the prevention of stroke in women suggest that women over their whole life generally have a lower blood pressure than men [15]. This difference is most apparent below the age of 55 years, as after this age, the sex difference in blood pressure is eliminated; in fact, women are more likely to develop hypertension the older they become [15].

Intracerebral Haemorrhage Location

The overall incidence of ICH appears to be similar between supratentorial lobar regions (9.8 per 100,000 adults/year, 95% CI 7.7–12.4) and other locations in the brain (supratentorial deep regions, brainstem, and cerebellum: 8.6 per 100,000 adults/year, 95% CI 6.7–11.1) [16]. Some studies have found that the incidence of lobar ICH is greater than that of deep ICH with increasing age [5, 9], whereas others have not [16]. However, racial origin may influence these distributions, with supratentorial deep and brainstem locations being more common in blacks than in whites [17].

Secondary Intracerebral Haemorrhage

Establishing the underlying cause of ICH is difficult because there are almost always at least two possible causes. However, studies reporting ICH classification systems use algorithms to allocate a single cause. Furthermore, there is a surprising lack of epidemiological data on the frequency of ICH secondary to underlying structural causes that are identifiable with brain imaging, such as arterial aneurysms, arteriovenous malformations (AVM), cerebral cavernous malformations (CCM), tumours, and intracranial venous thrombosis.

A recent community-based study in Scotland found that 15% of all incident diagnoses of ICH were secondary to an underlying structural cause, excluding antithrombotic drugs [16]. 51% of the remaining patients with 'primary' ICH had taken an oral antithrombotic drug until the time of the ICH; although these drugs may have caused some of these ICHs, there were competing co-morbidities in many cases, and the vast majority of cases had underlying small vessel diseases such as arteriolosclerosis and/or cerebral amyloid angiopathy (CAA) [16].

The incidence of ICH attributable to AVM is 0.89 per 100,000 adults/year (95% CI 0.7–1.12) and to CCM is 0.24 per 100,000 adults/year (95% CI 0.15–0.38) [18]. Detecting such underlying causes is important not only because they have potential treatment implications to prevent recurrence but also because the outcome of these forms of ICH appears to be better than that of primary ICH: patients who experienced an ICH secondary to an underlying AVM exhibited better survival outcomes and functional outcome than those who experienced a spontaneous ICH [19]. Although patients with an ICH secondary to an underlying AVM or CCM may exhibit a better outcome than patients with a spontaneous ICH because the extent of bleeding tends to be smaller in volume and because these cases tend to occur at a younger age [20], the association of ICH secondary to an underlying AVM or CCM with improved outcome remained after adjusting for these known prognostic factors [19].

Risk Factors

Many recent studies have focused on developing preventative measures against ICH and risk stratification methods for its occurrence. Research studies of novel risk factors associated with ICH have generated new ideas about preventative measures and the potential reasons underlying the variation in ICH incidence discussed above. However, the association of several conventional risk factors, such as diabetes mellitus, with the ICH incidence remains uncertain, as does the additive effect of known risk factors. Table 1 summarises some reports of the strength of the associations between the risk factors discussed and ICH.

Extensively Investigated Risk Factors

Hypertension has been consistently shown to be an important risk factor for ICH. A systematic review and several large population-based studies have found hypertension to be associated with at least a twofold increase in the risk of ICH [21–24]. This risk appears to increase with increasing average blood pressure [21]. Age is an established risk factor for ICH, similar to other cerebrovascular diseases [21, 22]. The RR of developing ICH doubles with every 10 years of age. Hypercholesterolaemia may be associated with a lower risk of ICH [21–24]. Black people have been reported to have up to a fivefold higher risk of ICH than white people, but this increased risk among black people diminishes with increasing age [10, 22]. High alcohol intake is associated

Table 1. Some recently reported significant associations between risk factors and ICH based on multivariate analyses

Risk factor	Study design	Association, OR/RR/HR (95% CI)
Hypertension	Case-control [23]	OR 9.18 (6.80–12.39)
Ethnicity (black)	Population-based cohort [10]	HR 5.30 (1.41–19.91)
Retinal arteriolar wall signs	Cross-sectional [39]	OR 3.70 (1.8–7.6)
Alcohol consumption	Systematic review [21]	OR 3.36 (2.21–5.12)
CAA	Systematic review [28]	OR 2.21 (1.09–4.45)[†]
Age (per 10 years)	Population-based cohort [22]	RR 2.06 (1.76–2.51)
High BMI (<30)	Case-control [32]	OR 1.75 (1.12–2.72)[‡]
Diabetes mellitus	Systematic review [33]	HR 1.59 (1.19–2.05)
Venular calibre	Population-based cohort [38]	HR 1.53 (1.09–2.15)
APOE ε4 allele	Case-control [24]	OR 1.50 (1.17–1.93)
APOE ε2 allele	Systematic review [30]	OR 1.42 (1.21–1.67)
Hypercholesterolaemia	Population-based cohort [22]	RR 0.73 (0.52–1.03)
SSRI use	Systematic review [40]	OR 1.30 (1.02–1.67)
Fruit and vegetable intake	Systematic review [41]	RR 0.78 (0.69–0.88)[§]

CAA = Cerebral amyloid angiopathy; APOE = apolipoprotein E; BMI = body mass index; AMD = age-related macular degeneration; SSRI = selective serotonin reuptake inhibitor.
[†] Association with lobar ICH only.
[‡] Association with deep ICH only.
[§] Association with haemorrhagic stroke.

with a threefold increase in the ICH risk [21, 23, 25], perhaps because of the coagulopathy associated with alcoholic liver disease or the effect of alcohol on platelet aggregation [26].

Hypertension is a risk factor for ICH regardless of its location, although this association seems to be higher for deep ICH [24, 27], whereas CAA is associated with ICH in lobar regions but not in other regions [28]. However, the interaction between these two underlying small vessel diseases is uncertain, nor is the role of CAA when hypertensive small vessel disease is also present.

Recently Investigated Risk Factors

An international multicentre case-control study conducted by the International Stroke Genetics Consortium (ISGC) found that genetic polymorphisms account for up to 44% of the ICH risk [29]. The most studied single gene related to ICH is the apolipoprotein E *(APOE)* gene. Both the *APOE* ε2 and ε4 alleles are found to be associated with ICH (OR 1.50 [24] and 1.42 [30], respectively) in studies investigating these associations using international multicentre genetic databases [24, 30, 31]. Interestingly, this association appears to be attributable to the stronger association between lobar ICH and *APOE* variants [24, 31]. These findings suggest that ICH has a genetic basis and that risk alleles and genetic polymorphisms may influence the location of ICH. The ISGC study found that 73% and 34% of the variance in the risk of lobar and deep ICH, respectively, are accounted for by genetic risk factors [29]. Further genome-wide association studies may identify other genetic variants that influence the susceptibility for ICH.

Body mass index (BMI), a measure of obesity, was identified as a risk factor for ICH in a pooled study of 2 prospective US population-based cohorts – the Atherosclerosis Risk in Communities Study (ARIC) and the Cardiovascular Health study (CHS) [22]. However, this study compared overweight (BMI between 25 and 30) and overweight (BMI >30) individuals to normal individuals (BMI <25). A hospital-based prospective study recruiting consecutive ICH patients aged ≥55 years found that low BMI (<18.5) and high BMI (>30) are associated with deep ICH compared with normal BMI (18.5–24.9) in multivariate analyses [32]. In light of the identification of the waist-to-hip ratio as a risk factor for ICH in the INTERSTROKE study [23], it is possible that these anthropometric measures are helpful in assessing the risk of ICH.

Diabetes mellitus was associated with the occurrence of ICH in a meta-analysis of prospective observational studies (hazard ratio 1.59, 95% CI 1.19–2.05) [33], although neither insulin resistance nor the fasting insulin level was not associated with ICH in a prospective population-based study in Rotterdam, The Netherlands [34]. However, whether the type of diabetes mellitus, glycaemic control, or oral hypoglycaemic drug use affects the risk of ICH remains unclear.

Hypercholesterolaemia is a risk factor for many cardiovascular diseases but tends to be associated with a lower risk of ICH. In theory, the increasing use of medication, particularly statins, to lower the blood cholesterol levels may change the balance of cardiovascular risks. The prospective Genetic and Environmental Risk Factors for Hemorrhagic Stroke (GERFHS) study has demonstrated that statin use does not attenuate the protective effect of hypercholesterolaemia on ICH occurrence [24, 35]. This finding may represent the involvement of genetic factors affecting lipid metabolism. However, among individuals carrying the same *APOE 4/4* or *APOE 2/4* genotype, people taking statins have a higher risk of lobar ICH than those with normal cholesterol levels or with hypercholesterolaemia not treated with statins [35]. However, this association was not observed for non-lobar ICH. These findings are interesting because they suggest a possible gene-by-drug effect for lobar ICH whilst highlighting the differences in the disease mechanism between lobar and non-lobar ICH. The clinical application of this result, however, requires confirmation of findings with larger cohorts across different genetic backgrounds.

Other medical conditions may share a similar underlying pathophysiology with ICH, as revealed by their association with ICH, although there are other possible explanations for these results. For example, a systematic review and meta-analysis of 3 population-based cohort studies showed an association between early age-related macular degeneration (AMD) and ICH with a RR of 1.29 (95% CI 1.00–1.68) [36]. Moreover, there is evidence to suggest that long-term aspirin use (longer than 10 years) is associated with early AMD [37]. The association of antiplatelet therapy with an increased risk of HS (Antithrombotic Trialists' Collaboration) may confound the AMD-associated risk, as the analysis was not adjusted for antiplatelet use.

Because vascular injury is a predominant pathophysiological mechanism underlying ICH, it would be useful clinically to assess the integrity of the intracranial vasculature. Blood vessels in the retina may act as a proxy for this purpose. An increase in the venular calibre is associated with smoking, the glucose levels and atherosclerosis. A wider retinal venular calibre was found to be a risk factor for ICH (hazard ratio 1.53; 95% CI 1.09–2.15) independent of other cardiovascular risk factors in the Rotterdam population-based cohort [38]. This association was stronger for lobar ICH than for deep ICH. In a prospective multicentre hospital-based study, retinal arteriolar wall signs were found to be associated with deep ICH [39]. In the absence of retinopathy, mild hypertensive retinopathy is defined as retinal arteriolar wall signs (focal arteriolar narrowing, arteriovenous nicking, and enhancement of the arteriolar light reflex) with generalised arteriolar narrowing. Identifying these signs may be an adjunct to risk stratification. The additional risk of ICH associated with retinal arteriolar wall signs is not available because the study compared ICH patients with ischaemic stroke patients rather than a control cohort. Additionally, the effect size of these risk factors may not allow them to serve as a reliable clinical indicator of ICH risk, as they may simply be a marker of known underlying cerebral small vessel diseases.

Selective serotonin reuptake inhibitors (SSRIs) are a frequently used class of antidepressants. In addition to their effect in the brain, SSRIs can reduce the serotonin levels in platelets, and this reduction may affect platelet aggregation. A systematic review and meta-analysis of 5 observational studies (all except one of which examined population-based cohorts) found an association between SSRI exposure and ICH (RR 1.30; 95% CI 1.02–1.67; I^2 29%) [40]. Furthermore, the combination of an SSRI and an oral anticoagulant exerts an additional risk for ICH compared to the oral anticoagulant alone. It is interesting to note that this review found a stronger risk of intracranial haemorrhage (defined by authors as ICH, subarachnoid haemorrhage, and HS) among those with recent or short-term exposure to SSRIs. As suggested by the authors, this increased risk may be related to the inhibitory effect of SSRIs on platelet function after a few weeks of SSRI exposure. The lack of an association of long-term or past SSRI exposure with ICH may represent the normalisation of platelet function with time or simply the removal of the patient from the cohort at risk for ICH due to incident ICH. Whether these findings will be borne out by randomised trials remains to be seen.

A healthy lifestyle and a balanced diet are vital in promoting cardiovascular health among the general population. The consumption of fruits and vegetables is associated with many health benefits. A systematic review and meta-analysis of 20 prospective cohort studies from Europe, the US and Asia reported a protective effect of fruit and vegetable intake against HS with a RR of 0.78 (95% CI 0.69–0.88) [41]. The underlying mechanism of this protective effect is uncertain. Additionally, whether consuming fruits or vegetables (or avoiding other foodstuffs) explains this benefit is yet to be established. There may be additive or synergistic effects of the combined consumption of fruits and vegetables. Whether specific types of fruits and vegetables mediate this beneficial effect is yet to be determined.

Summary

ICH incidence has remained stable over the last 30 years, in the developed world. This is possibly explained by better hypertension management but more antithrombotic drug use. ICH is more common in men than in women, and in the winter months. ICH is more common in people from an Asian descent than people from other races. Brain vascular malformation-related ICHs seem to be associated with a better survival outcome than spontaneous ICH.

The known risk factors for ICH include hypertension and increasing age. Emerging factors are the presence of apolipoprotein ε4 and ε2 gene allele. A diet high in fruit and vegetables appears to be protective against ICH. Extremes of BMI and diabetes may increase the risk of ICH, but this relationship has not been consistently shown. Alcohol consumption has also been associated with ICH, but further work is needed to fully understand this relationship.

References

1 van Asch CJ, Luitse MJ, Rinkel GJ, van der Tweel I, Algra A, Klijn CJ: Incidence, case fatality, and functional outcome of intracerebral haemorrhage over time, according to age, sex, and ethnic origin: a systematic review and meta-analysis. Lancet Neurol 2010;9:167–176.

2 Feigin VL, Lawes CM, Bennett DA, Barker-Collo SL, Parag V: Worldwide stroke incidence and early case fatality reported in 56 population-based studies: a systematic review. Lancet Neurol 2009;8:355–369.

3 Poon MTC, Fonville AF, Al-Shahi Salman R: Long-term prognosis after intracerebral haemorrhage: systematic review and meta-analysis. J Neurol Neurosurg Psychiatry 2014;85:660–667.

4 Krishnamurthi RV, Feigin VL, Forouzanfar MH, Mensah GA, Connor M, Bennett DA, Moran AE, Sacco RL, Anderson LM, Truelsen T, O'Donnell M, Venketasubramanian N, Barker-Collo S, Lawes CM, Wang W, Shinohara Y, Witt E, Ezzati M, Naghavi M, Murray C: Global and regional burden of first-ever ischaemic and haemorrhagic stroke during 1990–2010: findings from the global burden of disease study 2010. Lancet Glob Health 2013;1:e259–e281.

5 Lovelock CE, Molyneux AJ, Rothwell PM: Change in incidence and aetiology of intracerebral haemorrhage in Oxfordshire, UK, between 1981 and 2006: a population-based study. Lancet Neurol 2007;6:487–493.

6 Bejot Y, Cordonnier C, Durier J, Aboa-Eboule C, Rouaud O, Giroud M: Intracerebral haemorrhage profiles are changing: results from the Dijon population-based study. Brain 2013;136:658–664.

7 Tsai C-F, Thomas B, Sudlow CLM: Epidemiology of stroke and its subtypes in chinese vs white populations: a systematic review. Neurology 2013;81:264–272.

8 Koton S, Schneider ALC, Rosamond WD, Shahar E, Sang Y, Gottesman RF, Coresh J: Stroke incidence and mortality trends in us communities, 1987 to 2011. JAMA 2014;312:259–268.

9 Labovitz DL, Halim A, Boden-Albala B, Hauser WA, Sacco RL: The incidence of deep and lobar intracerebral hemorrhage in whites, blacks, and Hispanics. Neurology 2005;65:518–522.

10 Howard G, Cushman M, Howard VJ, Kissela BM, Kleindorfer DO, Moy CS, Switzer J, Woo D: Risk factors for intracerebral hemorrhage: the reasons for geographic and racial differences in stroke (regards) study. [Erratum appears in Stroke 2013;44:E63]. Stroke 2013;44:1282–1287.
11 Irwin J, Wright P, Reeve P: Temporal trends and clinical characteristics of spontaneous intracerebral haemorrhage in the Waikato region of New Zealand: a hospital-based analysis. N Z Med J 2011;124:16–25.
12 Li X, Zhang JH, Qin X: Intracerebral hemorrhage and meteorological factors in chongqing, in the southwest of China. Acta Neurochir Suppl 2011;111: 321–325.
13 Palm F, Dos Santos M, Urbanek C, Greulich M, Zimmer K, Safer A, Grau AJ, Becher H: Stroke seasonality associations with subtype, etiology and laboratory results in the Ludwigshafen stroke study (lusst). Eur J Epidemiol 2013;28:373–381.
14 Appelros P, Stegmayr B, Terent A: Sex differences in stroke epidemiology: a systematic review. Stroke 2009;40:1082–1090.
15 Bushnell C, McCullough LD, Awad IA, Chireau MV, Fedder WN, Furie KL, Howard VJ, Lichtman JH, Lisabeth LD, Pina IL, Reeves MJ, Rexrode KM, Saposnik G, Singh V, Towfighi A, Vaccarino V, Walters MR: Guidelines for the prevention of stroke in women: a statement for healthcare professionals from the American Heart Association/American Stroke Association. Stroke 2014;45: 1545–1588.
16 Samarasekera N, Fonville A, Lerpiniere C, Farrall AJ, Wardlaw JM, White PM, Smith C, Al-Shahi Salman R: Influence of intracerebral hemorrhage location on incidence, characteristics, and outcome: population-based study. Stroke 2015;46:361–368.
17 Flaherty ML, Woo D, Haverbusch M, Sekar P, Khoury J, Sauerbeck L, Moomaw CJ, Schneider A, Kissela B, Kleindorfer D, Broderick JP: Racial variations in location and risk of intracerebral hemorrhage. Stroke 2005;36:934–937.
18 Al-Shahi R, Bhattacharya JJ, Currie DG, Papanastassiou V, Ritchie V, Roberts RC, Sellar RJ, Warlow CP: Prospective, population-based detection of intracranial vascular malformations in adults: the Scottish Intracranial Vascular Malformation Study (SIVMS). Stroke 2003;34:1163–1169.
19 van Beijnum J, Lovelock CE, Cordonnier C, Rothwell PM, Klijn CJ, Al-Shahi Salman R: Outcome after spontaneous and arteriovenous malformation-related intracerebral haemorrhage: population-based studies. Brain 2009;132:537–543.
20 Cordonnier C, Al-Shahi Salman R, Bhattacharya JJ, Counsell CE, Papanastassiou V, Ritchie V, Roberts RC, Sellar RJ, Warlow C: Differences between intracranial vascular malformation types in the characteristics of their presenting haemorrhages: prospective, population-based study. J Neurol Neurosurg Psychiatry 2008;79:47–51.
21 Ariesen MJ, Claus SP, Rinkel GJE, Algra A: Risk factors for intracerebral hemorrhage in the general population: a systematic review. Stroke 2003;34:2060–2065.
22 Sturgeon JD, Folsom AR, Longstreth WT Jr, Shahar E, Rosamond WD, Cushman M: Risk factors for intracerebral hemorrhage in a pooled prospective study. Stroke 2007;38:2718–2725.
23 O'Donnell MJ, Xavier D, Liu L, Zhang H, Chin SL, Rao-Melacini P, Rangarajan S, Islam S, Pais P, McQueen MJ, Mondo C, Damasceno A, Lopez-Jaramillo P, Hankey GJ, Dans AL, Yusoff K, Truelsen T, Diener H-C, Sacco RL, Ryglewicz D, Czlonkowska A, Weimar C, Wang X, Yusuf S, INTERSTROKE Investigators: Risk factors for ischaemic and intracerebral haemorrhagic stroke in 22 countries (the interstroke study): a case-control study. Lancet 2010;376:112–123.
24 Martini SR, Flaherty ML, Brown WM, Haverbusch M, Comeau ME, Sauerbeck LR, Kissela BM, Deka R, Kleindorfer DO, Moomaw CJ, Broderick JP, Langefeld CD, Woo D: Risk factors for intracerebral hemorrhage differ according to hemorrhage location. Neurology 2012;79:2275–2282.
25 Patra J, Taylor B, Irving H, Roerecke M, Baliunas D, Mohapatra S, Rehm J: Alcohol consumption and the risk of morbidity and mortality for different stroke types – a systematic review and meta-analysis. BMC Public Health 2010;10:258.
26 Casolla B, Dequatre-Ponchelle N, Rossi C, Henon H, Leys D, Cordonnier C: Heavy alcohol intake and intracerebral hemorrhage: characteristics and effect on outcome. Neurology 2012;79:1109–1115.
27 Jackson CA, Sudlow CLM: Is hypertension a more frequent risk factor for deep than for lobar supratentorial intracerebral haemorrhage? J Neurol Neurosurg Psychiatry 2006;77:1244–1252.
28 Samarasekera N, Smith C, Al-Shahi Salman R: The association between cerebral amyloid angiopathy and intracerebral haemorrhage: systematic review and meta-analysis. J Neurol Neurosurg Psychiatry 2012;83:275–281.

29 Devan WJ, Falcone GJ, Anderson CD, Jagiella JM, Schmidt H, Hansen BM, Jimenez-Conde J, Giralt-Steinhauer E, Cuadrado-Godia E, Soriano C, Ayres AM, Schwab K, Kassis SB, Valant V, Pera J, Urbanik A, Viswanathan A, Rost NS, Goldstein JN, Freudenberger P, Stogerer E-M, Norrving B, Tirschwell DL, Selim M, Brown DL, Silliman SL, Worrall BB, Meschia JF, Kidwell CS, Montaner J, Fernandez-Cadenas I, Delgado P, Greenberg SM, Roquer J, Lindgren A, Slowik A, Schmidt R, Woo D, Rosand J, Biffi A, International Stroke Genetics Consortium: Heritability estimates identify a substantial genetic contribution to risk and outcome of intracerebral hemorrhage. Stroke 2013;44:1578–1583.

30 Zhang R, Wang X, Tang Z, Liu J, Yang S, Zhang Y, Wei Y, Luo W, Wang J, Li J, Chen B, Zhang K: Apolipoprotein e gene polymorphism and the risk of intracerebral hemorrhage: a meta-analysis of epidemiologic studies. Lipids Health Dis 2014;13:47.

31 Biffi A, Sonni A, Anderson CD, Kissela B, Jagiella JM, Schmidt H, Jimenez-Conde J, Hansen BM, Fernandez-Cadenas I, Cortellini L, Ayres A, Schwab K, Juchniewicz K, Urbanik A, Rost NS, Viswanathan A, Seifert-Held T, Stoegerer E-M, Tomas M, Rabionet R, Estivill X, Brown DL, Silliman SL, Selim M, Worrall BB, Meschia JF, Montaner J, Lindgren A, Roquer J, Schmidt R, Greenberg SM, Slowik A, Broderick JP, Woo D, Rosand J, International Stroke Genetics Consortium: Variants at APOE influence risk of deep and lobar intracerebral hemorrhage. Ann Neurol 2010;68:934–943.

32 Biffi A, Cortellini L, Nearnberg CM, Ayres AM, Schwab K, Gilson AJ, Rost NS, Goldstein JN, Viswanathan A, Greenberg SM, Rosand J: Body mass index and etiology of intracerebral hemorrhage. Stroke 2011;42:2526–2530.

33 Sarwar N, Gao P, Seshasai SR, Gobin R, Kaptoge S, Di Angelantonio E, Ingelsson E, Lawlor DA, Selvin E, Stampfer M, Stehouwer CD, Lewington S, Pennells L, Thompson A, Sattar N, White IR, Ray KK, Danesh J: Diabetes mellitus, fasting blood glucose concentration, and risk of vascular disease: a collaborative meta-analysis of 102 prospective studies. Lancet 2010;375:2215–2222.

34 Wieberdink RG, Koudstaal PJ, Hofman A, Witteman JCM, Breteler MMB, Ikram MA: Insulin resistance and the risk of stroke and stroke subtypes in the nondiabetic elderly. Am J Epidemiol 2012;176:699–707.

35 Woo D, Deka R, Falcone GJ, Flaherty ML, Haverbusch M, Martini SR, Greenberg SM, Ayres AM, Sauerbeck L, Kissela BM, Kleindorfer DO, Moomaw CJ, Anderson CD, Broderick JP, Rosand J, Langefeld CD, Woo JG: Apolipoprotein e, statins, and risk of intracerebral hemorrhage. Stroke 2013;44:3013–3017.

36 Wu J, Uchino M, Sastry SM, Schaumberg DA: Age-related macular degeneration and the incidence of cardiovascular disease: a systematic review and meta-analysis. PLoS ONE 2014;9:e89600.

37 Klein BE, Howard KP, Gangnon RE, Dreyer JO, Lee KE, Klein R: Long-term use of aspirin and age-related macular degeneration. JAMA 2012;308:2469–2478.

38 Wieberdink RG, Ikram MK, Koudstaal PJ, Hofman A, Vingerling JR, Breteler MMB: Retinal vascular calibers and the risk of intracerebral hemorrhage and cerebral infarction: the Rotterdam study. Stroke 2010;41:2757–2761.

39 Baker ML, Hand PJ, Liew G, Wong TY, Rochtchina E, Mitchell P, Lindley RI, Hankey GJ, Wang JJ: Retinal microvascular signs may provide clues to the underlying vasculopathy in patients with deep intracerebral hemorrhage. Stroke 2010;41:618–623.

40 Hackam DG, Mrkobrada M: Selective serotonin reuptake inhibitors and brain hemorrhage: a meta-analysis. Neurology 2012;79:1862–1865.

41 Hu D, Huang J, Wang Y, Zhang D, Qu Y: Fruits and vegetables consumption and risk of stroke: a meta-analysis of prospective cohort studies. Stroke 2014;45:1613–1619.

42 Al-Shahi Salman R, Labovitz DL, Staph C: Spontaneous intracerebral haemorrhage. BMJ 2009;339:b2586.

Prof. Rustam Al-Shahi Salman
Centre for Clinical Brain Sciences (CCBS), University of Edinburgh, Edinburgh
First Floor, Chancellor's Building, 49 Little France Crescent
Edinburgh EH16 4SB (UK)
E-Mail Rustam.Al-Shahi@ed.ac.uk

Toyoda K, Anderson CS, Mayer SA (eds): New Insights in Intracerebral Hemorrhage.
Front Neurol Neurosci. Basel, Karger, 2016, vol 37, pp 13–26 (DOI: 10.1159/000437110)

Emergency Imaging of Intracerebral Haemorrhage

Farah Alobeidi · Richard I. Aviv

Department of Medical Imaging, Sunnybrook Health Sciences Centre, Toronto, Ont., Canada

Abstract

Spontaneous intracerebral haemorrhage (ICH) is a devastating condition with high mortality and morbidity despite advances in neurocritical care. Early deterioration is common in the first few hours after ICH onset, secondary to rapid haematoma expansion and growth. Rapid diagnosis and aggressive early management of these patients are therefore crucial. Imaging plays a key role in establishing the diagnosis and the underlying aetiology of ICH, identifying complications and predicting patients who are at high risk for haematoma expansion. In this chapter, we present an evidence-based imaging framework for the management of spontaneous ICH in the acute setting. Non-enhanced computed tomography is long established as the gold standard for ICH diagnosis but has limitations in demonstrating the underlying aetiology in cases of secondary ICH. There is now growing evidence for the ability of non-invasive angiography to establish the underlying aetiology and to predict further haematoma expansion. The presence of small enhancing foci within the haematoma on computed tomography angiography (CTA), the CTA Spot Sign, has been prospectively validated as a predictor of haematoma expansion. Early identification of patients at risk of haematoma expansion allows for the appropriate escalation of care to a neurosurgical team, admission to a neurocritical care unit, appropriate supportive therapy and targeted novel medical and surgical interventions. Catheter angiography, which remains the gold standard for identifying underlying secondary vascular lesions, should be used in selected cases. However, non-invasive vascular imaging should be considered as an important step in the diagnosis and early management of secondary ICH patients. Previous concerns related to the radiation dose, contrast-induced nephropathy and cost are addressed in this chapter. Recently, animal models have enabled the qualitative assessment of haematoma expansion, and our increased understanding of ICH may inform future trials of targeted medical and surgical therapies.

© 2016 S. Karger AG, Basel

Spontaneous intracerebral haemorrhage (ICH) is defined as ICH in the absence of trauma. It constitutes 10–15% of all stroke cases. ICH is a devastating condition with a 30–50% mortality rate in the first month and is a major cause of disability despite advances in neurocritical care. Moreover, early deterioration is common in the first few hours after ICH onset secondary to rapid haematoma expansion and growth [1]. ICH can be divided into primary ICH (PICH) and secondary ICH (SICH). PICH usually occurs in older patients and is often associated with hypertension or cerebral amyloid angiopathy. Secondary causes account for 28–40% of all ICH cases and include anticoagulation, vascular malformations, aneurysms and haemorrhage secondary to neoplasms or infarction [2–4]. It is important to rapidly establish the underlying cause of ICH to direct appropriate management.

Establishing the Diagnosis of Intracerebral Haemorrhage

ICH presents with non-specific clinical features such as abrupt neurological deficits, headache, vomiting, decreased levels of consciousness or coma. Although certain features such as rapid deterioration or elevated blood pressure are more suggestive of ICH than ischaemic stroke, it is not possible to differentiate between these two conditions based on clinical features alone. Non-enhanced computed tomography (NECT) is widely available and is the recommended gold standard for ICH diagnosis due to its sensitivity in detecting acute haemorrhage. Gradient echo or T2* susceptibility-weighted MRI are as sensitive as NECT in detecting acute haemorrhage and are more sensitive in detecting previous haemorrhage, but their use is limited in the acute setting due to cost and availability.

Establishing the Underlying Cause of Intracerebral Haemorrhage

Catheter angiography (CA) is considered as the gold standard for identifying underlying vascular lesions such as arteriovenous malformations (AVMs), dural arteriovenous fistulae or aneurysms due to its high spatial and temporal resolution. However, the main disadvantages of CA are its relative invasiveness, discomfort, restricted availability, high technical skill requirements, costs and complications; these drawbacks make CA unsuitable as a screening test. The overall reported neurological complication rate is 1.3%, with a 0.5% risk of permanent neurological disability [5]. Computed tomography (CT) angiography (CTA), on the other hand, is non-invasive, fast, relatively cheap and easily accessible. Retrospective and prospective studies have shown excellent sensitivity, specificity and accuracy (89–100%) of CTA for determining the aetiology of SICH [6, 7]. A further prospective study comparing CTA with CA in young (<45 years) and non-hypertensive patients demonstrated negative and positive predictive values of CTA and venography of 97.3 and 100%, respectively [4].

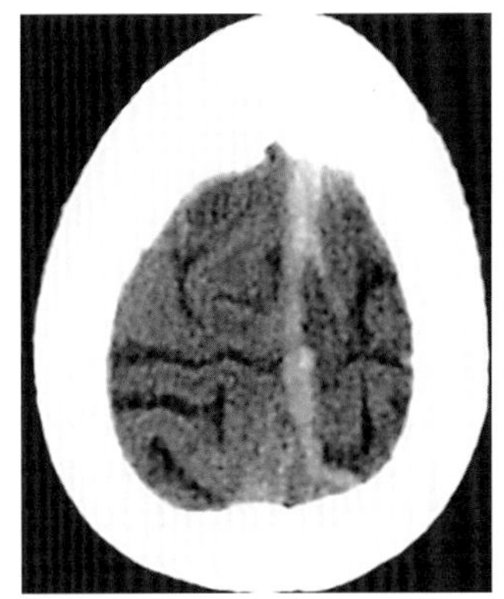

Fig. 1. High suspicion non-enhanced computed tomography (NECT) scan appearances demonstrating linear hyperdensity present at the vertex in the distribution of the superior sagittal sinus; this finding is consistent with the cord sign and is indicative of venous sinus thrombosis.

The American Heart Association (AHA)/American Stroke Association guidelines for ICH management have been modified to suggest CTA, CT venography, contrast-enhanced CT, contrast-enhanced MRI (CEMRI), magnetic resonance angiography and magnetic resonance venography for the evaluation of underlying structural lesions, including vascular malformations and tumours, when there is clinical or radiological suspicion of SICH [8]. However, the clinical features suggestive of SICH are very non-specific and include headache, neurological or constitutional symptoms. Radiological features on NECT suggestive of SICH are the presence of subarachnoid haemorrhage, unusual (non-circular) haematoma shape, the presence of oedema out of proportion to the time of ICH presentation, unusual haemorrhage location, the presence of a mass lesion and the cord sign in venous sinus thrombi (fig. 1). Imaging features are slightly more sensitive and specific than the clinical features; however, relying on imaging to select patients for CA results in unacceptable false negative rates considering the potential morbidity and mortality associated with missed SICH diagnoses. Halpin et al. prospectively evaluated patients with spontaneous ICH by CA based on their NECT findings. A group identified to exhibit features suspicious of an underlying vascular lesion on NECT underwent acute CA, which revealed positive results in 84% of patients. The second group, which was deemed to have no suspicious NECT features, underwent delayed CA within 3 months, and this test revealed positive results in 24% of cases [3]. In a different retrospective study, patients were stratified into low, intermediate and high probability of an underlying vascular lesion based on NECT. The positive and negative predictive values for the presence of underlying vascular aetiology were 84.2 and 97.8%, respectively, in the high and low probability groups. However, 72/421 (17.1%) patients in the intermediate probability group exhibited an underlying lesion on CTA [7]. Assuming that all intermediate and high risk patients require further vascular imaging and accepting a false negative rate of 2% in the low risk group, 71% of the patient cohort would require additional imaging. Hence, considering the NECT findings alone would require that up to 71% of the population undergo further vascular imaging, and the

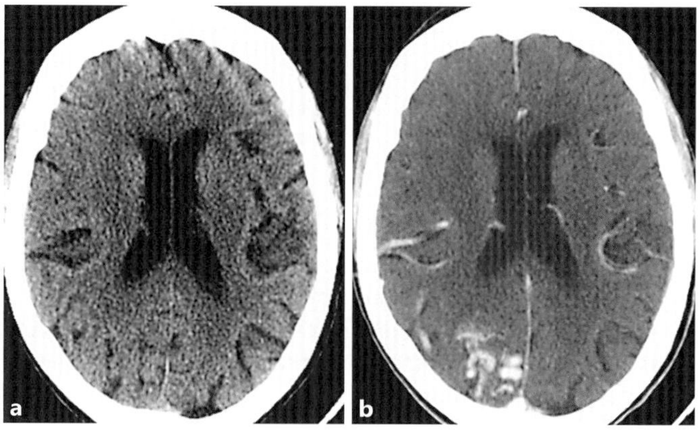

Fig. 2. Low suspicion NECT scan (**a**) demonstrating no abnormality. Following contrast administration (**b**), a 2 cm arteriovenous malformation is detected.

NECT findings may not reliably detect secondary causes of ICH (fig. 2) we advocate that every patient presenting with non traumatic SAH should undergo non-invasive vascular imaging such as CTA. Lastly, the reliance on a suspicious imaging finding to direct further vascular imaging leads to verification bias whereby only those patients under suspicion are selected for vascular imaging (fig. 3).

Moreover, there is a widespread false assumption that haemorrhage in the basal ganglia or the posterior fossa is almost exclusively due to hypertension and that these patients should not be further investigated with vascular imaging. A prospective study by Zhu et al. [2] found that younger patients (≤45) without pre-existing hypertension had a higher probability of an underlying vascular lesion. The authors concluded that CA should be considered for all spontaneous ICH patients except those over 45 years old with pre-existing hypertension experiencing haemorrhage in the thalamus, the putamen or the posterior fossa. This conclusion, which is appropriate for CA, should not be extrapolated to CTA studies, which are widely available and are associated with minimal risk. Many studies have demonstrated an underlying vascular cause based on CA or CTA in hypertensive patients and in those with haemorrhage in 'non-structural' locations of the basal ganglia and the posterior fossa [2, 3, 7]. In the same study, Zhu et al. demonstrated that underlying vascular lesions were seen overall in 58/206 patients (28%), including 9% of hypertensive patients. Among patients over >45 years old, 3.4% of hypertensive patients with ICH in a 'non-structural' location had an underlying cause, compared with 7% of normotensive patients with haemorrhage in a similar location. Halpin et al. [3] described 26 lesions occurring in the basal ganglia with a secondary cause in 31% of all patients and in 11% of hypertensive patients. Similar results were obtained by Almandoz et al. [9], who observed that 9.5% of cases with underlying lesions were hypertensive patients >46 years old, including 2.6% of cases in the basal ganglia or the thalamus. Therefore, the risk of an underlying cause in hypertensive patients with SICH in the basal ganglia or the thalamus is 2–3% and is ~10% in all locations [2, 3, 7]. These findings mirror those of an autopsy review of 144 patients who had died from massive ICH; in this study, 36% of hypertensive pa-

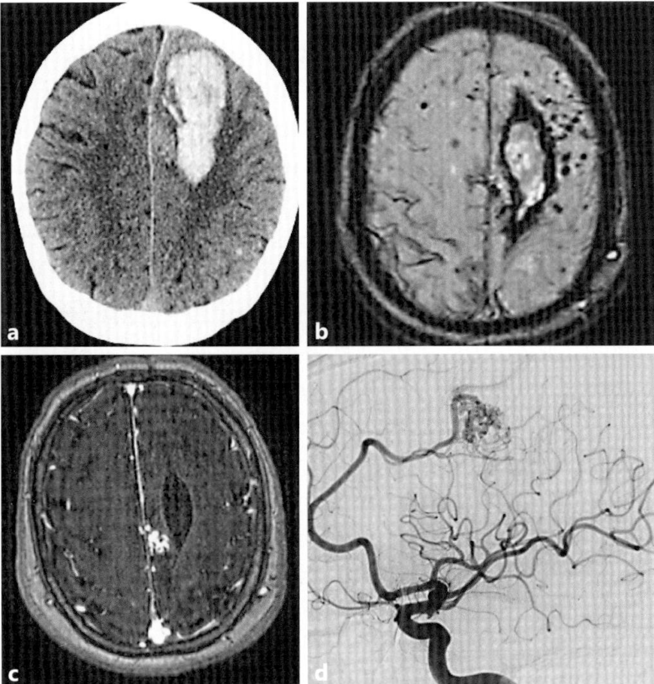

Fig. 3. Verification bias. A 65-year-old male patient presenting with lobar haemorrhage on NECT (**a**). The Lobar intracerebral haemorrhage (ICH) location is frequently seen in association with amyloid angiopathy, as confirmed on gradient echo MRI (**b**), on which multiple susceptibility foci are present throughout the bilateral frontal lobe and, to a lesser extent, the parietal lobe. Haemosiderin staining surrounds the lobar haematoma. Without proceeding to a vascular study, this patient was diagnosed with an amyloid-related ICH. However, contrast-enhanced magnetic resonance angiography (**c**) demonstrated an unexpected arteriovenous malformation along the medial edge of the haematoma, and this malformation was confirmed as the cause of ICH based on catheter angiography (**d**).

tients were found to have a secondary cause of ICH, with one-third harbouring an AVM or an aneurysm; 19 normotensive (13%) and 5 hypertensive (3%) SICH patients experienced haemorrhage in the basal ganglia [10]. These results support the screening of all patients with spontaneous ICH for secondary causes.

Screening Patients for Secondary Intracerebral Haemorrhage

The current AHA recommendations requiring NECT as a screening tool prior to further vascular assessment for SICH determination are based on the historical need for CA, which had intrinsic safety limitations that precluded it from being applied as a routine screening tool. Further, we have established that NECT has limited performance as a screening tool, necessitating alternative options to be sought. The SICH score was proposed as a potential screening method for selecting patients for CA and was established to predict the patient's risk of harbouring an underlying vascular aetiology based on clinical (age, sex, hypertension and impaired coagulation) and NECT characteristics [11]. However, external validation of the SICH score outside the United States showed that this measure had only modest calibration (agreement between the predicted and observed outcome) and discrimination (separation of those with and without an underlying vascular lesion) [12]. In another validation study of the SICH score compared with CA or intraoperative findings, the false negative rate for a low SICH score (and, therefore, the risk of SICH) was 5.8% [9].

CTA is a low-risk, non-invasive diagnostic test that demonstrates high sensitivity and specificity for SICH. We have previously argued that these test characteristics merit its use in all patients presenting with ICH. CTA is widely accessible and is relatively inexpensive compared to digital subtraction angiography and MRI. Cost utility analysis has demonstrated a clear role for CTA in ICH evaluation, with a dominant cost-effective imaging strategy of NECT and CTA prevailing when the risk of SICH is below 15% [13]. CTA is already established in the management of acute ischaemic stroke and subarachnoid haemorrhage, yet its use as part of a standard ICH protocol has lagged despite the greater incidence, morbidity and mortality of ICH than of subarachnoid haemorrhage [14]. One reason contributing to this slower uptake includes concern related to the radiation dose, which is interesting, as the probability of SICH in low risk ICH patients undergoing NECT is similar to that of an occult cervical spine fracture in acute trauma, and in this setting, CT of the cervical spine is widely accepted as the protocol of choice in high energy trauma patients [15] despite radiation concerns. Although the radiation dose for CTA is higher than that for axial NECT, the overall lifetime expected incidence of radiation effects remains very small, especially in an older ICH population. To minimise the radiation dose, we recommend intracranial CTA from the skull base to the vertex in the absence of subarachnoid haemorrhage. The rationale for this approach is that neck vessel imaging is less important in the acute stage of an unexpected treatable vascular lesion such as AVM or dural arteriovenous fistulae, as these patients are expected to undergo non-emergent CA or magnetic resonance angiography for planning purposes prior to therapeutic intervention.

An additional concern attenuating CTA uptake is the potential for worsening renal function following contrast administration. Contrast-induced nephropathy (CIN) is defined as a ≥25% relative or ≥0.5 mg/dl absolute increase in baseline the serum creatinine level 48–72 hours after exposure to a contrast agent [16]. Several studies have suggested that the role of contrast material in nephropathy induction may be overestimated by the failure to correct for baseline renal dysfunction in sick patients not receiving contrast [17, 18]. In a large retrospective study, Newhouse et al. [17] demonstrated that more than half of hospitalised patients not exposed to a contrast agent showed a change of at least 25% in their serum creatinine level over 3 days. In a retrospective cohort of acute stroke patients, the incidence of acute nephropathy was lower in patients who had received contrast than in those who had not, even after adjusting for risk factors [19]. Other studies have similarly found that intravenous contrast does not increase the risk of acute nephropathy compared to controls who did not receive contrast [18, 20, 21]. Although baseline renal dysfunction is an important risk factor for the subsequent development of CIN, it is not reliable enough to predict its development [16]. For at risk patients, the concern for the development of CIN is a relative, but not absolute, contraindication to the administration of iodinated contrast medium [22] and should be weighed against the potential benefits of performing the test. Patients without risk factors such as pre-existing renal dysfunction, proteinuria and hypertension are not at increased risk of developing CIN [22, 23], and there is no need to screen these patients to determine their baseline creatinine levels prior to imaging [23]. Further, baseline creatinine measurements can be waived in an emergency setting for at risk patients [24]. In one acute stroke study, an average of 73.3 ± 51 min elapsed before the serum creatinine levels were available [25], potentially producing unnecessary delays in treatment administration. Intravenous contrast agents are therefore safe in patients independent of the estimated baseline glomerular filtration rate when standard prophylactic measures, such as the use of low-osmolar contrast agents and adequate intravenous hydration, are taken [22, 24, 26].

The 'Spot Sign' and Haematoma Expansion

Haematoma expansion is a strong predictor of neurological deterioration [27] and an independent predictor of mortality and functional outcomes [1]. The CTA Spot Sign is the presence of focal areas of contrast enhancement within an acute haematoma [28] (fig. 4). A consensus definition and classification criteria for the CTA Spot Sign are shown in table 1 [29]. Contrast enhancement may appear as single or multiple focal or serpiginous foci within the margin of the parenchymal haematoma without connection to an outside vessel. The enhancing foci should be approximately double the background haematoma density, and their density usually approximates 120 Hounsfield Units. The Spot Sign is found in cases of PICH and by definition is not present in cases of SICH, which may mimic the Spot Sign (fig. 5) [30]. Vessels entering the haematoma from the periphery and communicating with the region of contrast extravasation should not be confused with the Spot Sign and are indicative of an underlying vascular lesion [30]. Careful review of axial CTA source images and non-enhanced images should be performed to exclude vascular and calcified non-vascular mimics, respectively. The recommended window width and level for Spot Sign identification are 200 and 100, respectively [31]. The CTA Spot Sign is also associated with increased risk of peri- and post-operative haemorrhage, triggering discussions over the optimal surgical strategy.

The CTA Spot Sign has been validated in single and multicentre studies as an independent predictor of haematoma expansion [28, 32–34], functional outcome [35] and mortality [25]. Single centre study data suggest that the CTA Spot Sign is present

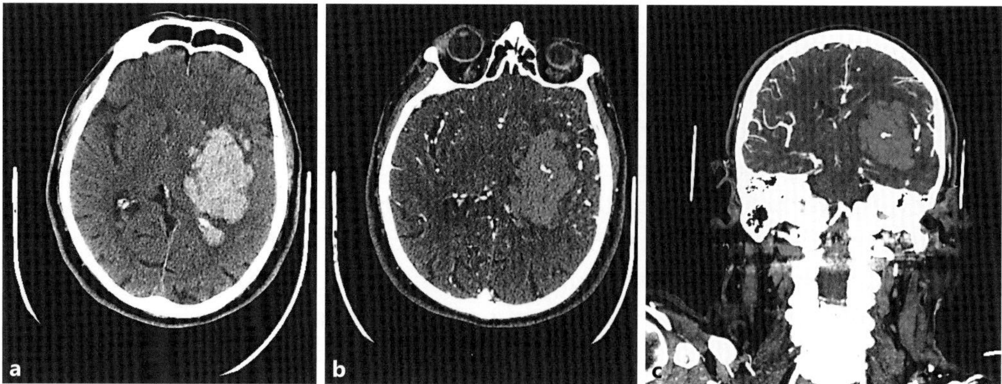

Fig. 4. A 66-year-old woman with acute onset right-sided weakness and a reduced level of consciousness. NECT (**a**) demonstrates a left deep haematoma. Computed tomography angiography (CTA) in the axial (**b**) and coronal planes (**c**) confirms the presence of a CTA Spot Sign showing no communication beyond the haematoma margin.

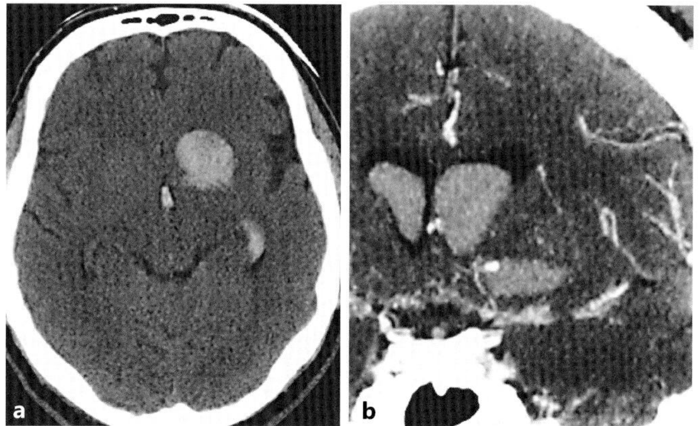

Fig. 5. A 72-year-old hypertensive male patient underwent NECT (**a**), which demonstrated a deep left haematoma. Without CTA, a common diagnosis would be hypertension-related haemorrhage. Coronal CTA (**b**) demonstrates a Spot Sign mimic. Contrast density not only within the haematoma margin but also communicating beyond the margin into a lenticulostriate vessel; this finding is consistent with the presence of a small lenticulostriate artery microaneurysm.

Table 1. Spot Sign classification [29]

Appearance	Serpiginous and/or spot-like appearance
Location	Within the margin of the parenchymal haematoma without connection to an outside vessel
Density	Approximately double the density (HU) compared to background haematoma
Lesion number	Single or multiple

HU = Hounsfield Units.

in ~30% of patients presenting within 6 hours of ictus [28, 32, 35, 36] using first-pass CTA. Lower prevalence relates to the heterogeneity in CTA timing and the rates of contrast extravasation, with only ~50% of CTA studies demonstrating arterial timing in one series. Spot Sign accuracy depends on the timing of CTA, with decreasing positive predictive value with increasing imaging delay from ictus, although its negative predictive value remains unchanged over time [34, 36]. Adding delayed imaging to CTA increases the prevalence of the CTA Spot Sign to up to 50% and improves its sensitivity and positive predictive value for haematoma expansion and poor clinical outcome [36, 37]. Other dynamic approaches, such as biphasic CT perfusion protocols, also improve Spot Sign detection and increase sensitivity above that of CTA or CECT for the prediction of haematoma expansion and poor outcome [38]. Optimal imaging strategies are not yet determined, but first-pass CTA is likely to miss ~10–20% of CTA Spot Signs.

Although haemostatic treatment and acute intensive blood pressure reduction reduce haematoma expansion, clinical outcomes remain poor in many patients [39]. This may be due to inadequate targeted patient selection for treatment. The Spot Sign score is a scoring system based on the number, dimensions and attenuation of Spot Signs and is used to predict significant haematoma expansion. This system had previously been suggested as a tool for patient selection for early haemostatic treatment [36]. However, in a prospective multicentre study, only the Spot Sign number independently predicted haematoma expansion, while other Spot Sign characteristics such as Spot Sign size, density and relative attenuation did not [40]. Therefore, a simple count of the number of Spot Signs may be all that is required to predict the risk of haematoma expansion. Spot Sign identification can be performed by non-radiologists in an emergency setting with high accuracy [41]. The inter-reader reliability was good to very good (kappa 0.77–0.94) [28, 32, 35, 36], reducing to moderate when a broad range of readers including neurology, emergency medicine and neuroradiology staff and fellows was included [41]. This reliability makes the Spot Sign a potential surrogate marker for considering haemostatic therapy. The 2010 update of the AHA/American Stroke Association guidelines was modified to recommend that the Spot Sign may stratify patients at higher risk for haematoma expansion [8]. The outcomes of 3 international studies assessing the utility of the CTA Spot Sign as a surrogate for patient selection for recombinant factor VIIa or tranexamic acid treatment are anticipated over the next few years.

Proposed Imaging Framework for Emergent Intracerebral Haemorrhage Management

There is a need to develop a standardised approach for the diagnostic work-up of acute ICH patients [42]. We have outlined the evidence for performing CTA as part of the standard protocol for all patients presenting with ICH. It is cost-effective to perform CTA at the same time as NECT. In PICH, a CTA may stratify patients for targeted haemostatic treatment based on the identification of the CTA Spot Sign. In SICH, CTA will limit the performance of unnecessary diagnostic CAs. In positive CTA cases undergoing endovascular treatment, CTA enables the interventional neuroradiologist to tailor the procedure by highlighting vessels of interest, thereby minimising the risk of stroke to other vascular territories. CTA also reduces the radiation time and the volume of contrast material used. A negative CTA result usually precludes any further diagnostic CA in older patients (>45–50 years old) with 'typical' hypertensive bleeds (older age, hypertension history, and basal ganglia haemorrhage). Younger and/or non-hypertensive patients with equivocal or negative CTA findings do undergo a CEMRI with a gradient echo or susceptibility-weighted sequence in many centres, usually within 2 days, to exclude other secondary causes such as tumour, cavernoma or microbleed-associated hypertensive or cerebral amyloid angiopathy-related haemorrhage. If the MRI result is negative, urgent diagnostic CA should be considered, particularly in the case of younger patients or those with isolated intraventricular or lobar ICH. Finally, a CEMRI should be performed in all patients with negative CA/CTA findings within 6–8 weeks to look for expected ICH evolution and thereby exclude an underlying lesion. This framework is outlined in figure 6 [43].

Future Directions

Understanding haematoma expansion in ICH allows for the better identification of patients harbouring SICH, thereby ensuring prompt and appropriate therapy. The CTA Spot Sign offers promise for future prognostication and risk stratification for targeted novel surgical and medical therapies. The results of treatment with haemostatic agents thus far have not demonstrated an improvement in clinical outcome [39] despite a reduction in haematoma growth [44]. Selective therapy for high-risk patients is more likely to yield improved outcomes. The results of the PRospective Evaluation of Diabetic Ischemic heart disease by Computed Tomography (PREDICT) study recommended the Spot Sign as an entry criterion for future trials for haemostatic therapy in ICH [34]. The Spot Sign for Predicting and Treating ICH Growth Study (STOP-IT), 'Spot Sign' Selection of Intracerebral Hemorrhage to Guide Hemostatic Therapy (SPOTLIGHT) and the Spot Sign and Tranexamic Acid On Preventing ICH Growth (STOP-AUST) trials are current randomised double-blinded multicentre trials in which the CTA Spot Sign is being used as a biomarker for high-risk patients who are being randomly allocated to treatment with haemostatic agents or placebo [45–47]. However, the CTA Spot Sign is limited due to its qualitative nature and differences in the rates of leakage [48]. In a single centre study, perfusion CT was more sensitive in assessing different rates of contrast leakage than CTA or post-contrast CT [48]. Quantitative analysis describing the rate and pattern of haematoma expansion in ICH patients may provide a better understanding of the underlying pathophysiology of haematoma expansion and may better inform future studies and

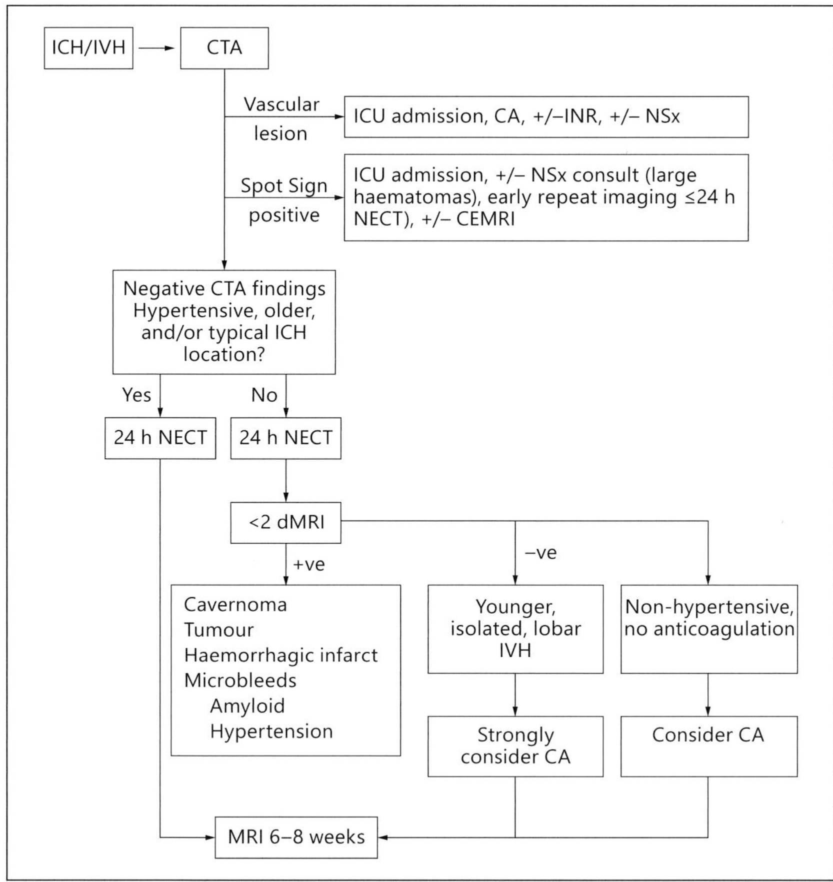

Fig. 6. Flow chart for the management of acute ICH [43]. ICH = Intracerebral haemorrhage; IVH = intraventricular haemorrhage; CTA = computed tomography angiography; ICU = intensive care unit; CA = catheter angiography; INR = interventional neuroradiology; NSx = neurosurgery; NECT = non-enhanced computed tomography; CEMRI = contrast-enhanced magnetic resonance imaging.

therapeutic strategies. Recently, an integrated real-time MRI animal model of contrast extravasation and haematoma expansion has been described [49]. Quantitative analysis of haematoma expansion using animal models has demonstrated in vivo patterns of haematoma growth for the first time [50]. Further studies on the effect of haemostatic agents on varying rates of contrast leakage are required.

Conclusion

Secondary causes of ICH are more common than previously thought, and this discrepancy is likely attributed to selection bias associated with the patients historically requiring CA. Hypertensive patients with haemorrhage in the basal ganglia were traditionally excluded from vascular imaging but demonstrate an underlying secondary vascular cause of ICH in approximately 3.4% of cases. NECT and clinical details cannot reliably assess SICH or haematoma expansion. CTA is a widely available, relatively low risk and low cost test with a high sensitivity and specificity for detecting an underlying lesion in SICH patients. Moreover, the CTA Spot Sign has been prospectively validated as a surrogate marker of haematoma expansion. An evidence-based framework for the imaging of ICH patients has been proposed. This framework includes CTA on all patients with ICH. This approach will reduce the overall number of invasive higher risk CA studies being performed for diagnostic purposes. Selecting high-risk patients for novel targeted medical and surgical therapies using the Spot Sign may improve outcomes and is currently being investigated. Future studies need to assess the impact of these therapies on various rates of contrast leakage.

References

1 Davis SM, Broderick J, Hennerici M, Brun NC, Diringer MN, Mayer SA, Begtrup K, Steiner T: Hematoma growth is a determinant of mortality and poor outcome after intracerebral hemorrhage. Neurology 2006;66:1175–1181.

2 Zhu XL, Chan MSY, Poon WS: Spontaneous intracranial hemorrhage: which patients need diagnostic cerebral angiography?: a prospective study of 206 cases and review of the literature. Stroke 1997;28: 1406–1409.

3 Halpin SF, Britton JA, Byrne JV, Clifton A, Hart G, Moore A: Prospective evaluation of cerebral angiography and computed tomography in cerebral haematoma. J Neurol Neurosurg Psychiatry 1994;57: 1180–1186.

4 Wong GKC, Siu DYW, Abrigo JM, Poon WS, Tsang FCP, Zhu XL, Yu SCH, Ahuja AT: Computed tomographic angiography and venography for young or nonhypertensive patients with acute spontaneous intracerebral hemorrhage. Stroke 2011;42:211–213.

5 Willinsky RA, Taylor SM, TerBrugge K, Farb RI, Tomlinson G, Montanera W: Neurologic complications of cerebral angiography: prospective analysis of 2,899 procedures and review of the literature. Radiology 2003;227:522–528.

6 Yeung R, Ahmad T, Aviv RI, De Tilly LN, Fox AJ, Symons SP: Comparison of CTA to DSA in determining the etiology of spontaneous ICH. Can J Neurol Sci 2009;36:176–180.

7 Delgado Almandoz JE, Schaefer PW, Forero NP, Falla JR, Gonzalez RG, Romero JM: Diagnostic accuracy and yield of multidetector CT angiography in the evaluation of spontaneous intraparenchymal cerebral hemorrhage. AJNR Am J Neuroradiol 2009;30: 1213–1221.

8 Morgenstern LB, Hemphill JC, Anderson C, Becker K, Broderick JP, Connolly ES, Greenberg SM, Huang JN, MacDonald RL, Messé SR, Mitchell PH, Selim M, Tamargo RJ: Guidelines for the management of spontaneous intracerebral hemorrhage: a guideline for healthcare professionals from the American Heart Association/American Stroke Association. Stroke 2010;41:2108–2129.

9 Delgado Almandoz JE, Jagadeesan BD, Moran CJ, Cross DT, Zipfel GJ, Lee J-M, Romero JM, Derdeyn CP: Independent validation of the secondary intracerebral hemorrhage score with catheter angiography and findings of emergent hematoma evacuation. Neurosurgery 2012;70:131–140.

10 McCormick WF, Rosenfield DB: Massive brain hemorrhage: a review of 144 cases and an examination of their causes. Stroke 1973;4:946–954.

11 Delgado Almandoz JE, Schaefer PW, Goldstein JN, Rosand J, Lev MH, González RG, Romero JM: Practical scoring system for the identification of patients with intracerebral hemorrhage at highest risk of harboring an underlying vascular etiology: the Secondary Intracerebral Hemorrhage Score. AJNR Am J Neuroradiol 2010;31:1653–1560.

12 van Asch CJJ, Velthuis BK, Greving JP, van Laar PJ, Rinkel GJE, Algra A, Klijn CJM: External validation of the secondary intracerebral hemorrhage score in The Netherlands. Stroke 2013;44:2904–2906.

13 Aviv RI, Kelly AG, Jahromi BS, Benesch CG, Young KC: The cost-utility of CT angiography and conventional angiography for people presenting with intracerebral hemorrhage. PLoS One 2014;9:e96496.

14 Broderick JP, Adams HP, Barsan W, Feinberg W, Feldmann E, Grotta J, Kase C, Krieger D, Mayberg M, Tilley B, Zabramski JM, Zuccarello M: Guidelines for the management of spontaneous intracerebral hemorrhage: a statement for healthcare professionals from a special writing group of the Stroke Council, American Heart Association. Stroke 1999;30: 905–915.
15 Blackmore CC, Mann FA, Wilson AJ: Helical CT in the primary trauma evaluation of the cervical spine: an evidence-based approach. Skeletal Radiol 2000; 29:632–639.
16 Mehran R, Nikolsky E: Contrast-induced nephropathy: definition, epidemiology, and patients at risk. Kidney Int Suppl 2006;69;S11–S15.
17 Newhouse JH, Kho D, Rao QA, Starren J: Frequency of serum creatinine changes in the absence of iodinated contrast material: implications for studies of contrast nephrotoxicity. AJR Am J Roentgenol 2008; 191:376–382.
18 Oleinik A, Romero JM, Schwab K, Lev MH, Jhawar N, Delgado Almandoz JE, Smith EE, Greenberg SM, Rosand J, Goldstein JN: CT angiography for intracerebral hemorrhage does not increase risk of acute nephropathy. Stroke 2009;40:2393–2397.
19 Lima FO, Lev MH, Levy RA, Silva GS, Ebril M, de Camargo EC, Pomerantz S, Singhal AB, Greer DM, Ay H, González RG, Koroshetz WJ, Smith WS, Furie KL: Functional contrast-enhanced CT for evaluation of acute ischemic stroke does not increase the risk of contrast-induced nephropathy. AJNR Am J Neuroradiol 2010;31:817–821.
20 McGillicuddy EA, Schuster KM, Kaplan LJ, Maung AA, Lui FY, Maerz LL, Johnson DC, Davis KA: Contrast-induced nephropathy in elderly trauma patients. J Trauma 2010;68:294–297.
21 Langner S, Stumpe S, Kirsch M, Petrik M, Hosten N: No increased risk for contrast-induced nephropathy after multiple CT perfusion studies of the brain with a nonionic, dimeric, iso-osmolal contrast medium. AJNR Am J Neuroradiol 2008;29:1525–1529.
22 ACR Committee on Drugs and Contrast Media: Manual on Contrast Media, version 9. Reston, VA, ACR Committee on Drugs and Contrast Media, 2013.
23 Tippins RB, Torres WE, Baumgartner BR, Baumgarten DA: Are screening serum creatinine levels necessary prior to outpatient CT examinations? Radiology 2000;216:481–484.
24 European Society of Urogenital Radiology: ESUR Guidelines on Contrast Media, version 8.1. http://www.esur.org/guidelines/, accessed 31 August 2015, European Society of Urogenital Radiology, 2012.
25 Kim J, Smith A, Hemphill JC, Smith WS, Lu Y, Dillon WP, Wintermark M: Contrast extravasation on CT predicts mortality in primary intracerebral hemorrhage. AJNR Am J Neuroradiol 2008;29:520–525.
26 Owen RJ, Hiremath S, Myers A, Fraser-Hill M, Barrett B: Consensus Guidelines for the Prevention of Contrast Induced Nephropathy. Ottawa, ON, Canadian Association of Radiologists, 2011, pp 1–16.
27 Leira R, Dávalos A, Silva Y, Gil-Peralta Y, Tejada J, Garcia M, Castillo J: Early neurologic deterioration in intracerebral hemorrhage: predictors and associated factors. Neurology 2004;63:461–467.
28 Wada R, Aviv RI, Fox AJ, Sahlas DJ, Gladstone DJ, Tomlinson G, Symons SP: CT angiography 'spot sign' predicts hematoma expansion in acute intracerebral hemorrhage. Stroke 2007;38:1257–1262.
29 Thompson AL, Kosior JC, Gladstone DJ, Hopyan JJ, Symons SP, Romero F, Dzialowski I, Roy J, Andrew M: Defining the CT angiography 'spot sign' in primary intracerebral hemorrhage. Can J Neurol Sci 2009;36:456–461.
30 Gazzola S: Vascular and non vascular mimics of the CT angiography 'spot sign' in patients with secondary intracerebral haemorrhge. Stroke 2008;39:1177–1183.
31 Huynh TJ, Symons SP, Aviv RI: Advances in CT for prediction of hematoma expansion in acute intracerebral hemorrhage. Imaging Med 2013;5:539–551.
32 Goldstein JN, Fazen LE, Snider R, Schwab K, Greenberg SM, Smith EE, Lev MH, Rosand J: Contrast extravasation on CT angiography predicts hematoma expansion in intracerebral hemorrhage. Neurology 2007;68:889–894.
33 Park SY, Kong MH, Kim JH, Kang DS, Song KY, Huh SK: Role of 'spot sign' on CT angiography to predict hematoma expansion in spontaneous intracerebral hemorrhage. J Korean Neurosurg Soc 2010; 48:399–405.
34 Demchuk AM, Dowlatshahi D, Rodriguez-Luna D, Molina CA, Blas YS, Dzialowski I, Kobayashi A, Boulanger JM, Lum C, Gubitz G, Padma V, Roy J, Kase CS, Kosior J, Bhatia R, Tymchuk S, Subramaniam S, Gladstone DJ, Hill MD, Aviv RI, PREDICT/Sunnybrook ICH CTA study group: Prediction of haematoma growth and outcome in patients with intracerebral haemorrhage using the CT-angiography spot sign (PREDICT): a prospective observational study. Lancet Neurol 2012;11:307–314.
35 Li N, Wang Y, Wang W, Ma L, Xue J, Weissenborn K, Dengler R, Worthmann H, Wang DZ, Gao P, Liu L, Wang Y, Zhao X: Contrast extravasation on computed tomography angiography predicts clinical outcome in primary intracerebral hemorrhage: a prospective study of 139 cases. Stroke 2011;42:3441–3446.

36 Delgado Almandoz JE, Yoo AJ, Stone MJ, Schaefer PW, Goldstein JN, Rosand J, Oleinik A, Lev MH, Gonzalez RG, Romero JM: Systematic characterization of the computed tomography angiography spot sign in primary intracerebral hemorrhage identifies patients at highest risk for hematoma expansion: the spot sign score. Stroke 2009;40:2994–3000.
37 Ederies A, Demchuk A, Chia T, Gladstone DJ, Dowlatshahi D, Bendavit G, Wong K, Symons SP, Aviv RI: Postcontrast CT extravasation is associated with hematoma expansion in CTA spot negative patients. Stroke 2009;40:1672–1676.
38 Koculym A, Huynh TJ, Jakubovic R, Zhang L, Aviv RI: CT perfusion spot sign improves sensitivity for prediction of outcome compared with CTA and postcontrast CT. AJNR Am J Neuroradiol 2013;34:965–970.S1.
39 Mayer SA, Brun NC, Begtrup K, Broderick J, Davis S, Diringer MN, Skolnick BE, Steiner T: Efficacy and safety of recombinant activated factor VII for acute intracerebral hemorrhage. N Engl J Med 2008;358:2127–2137.
40 Huynh TJ, Demchuk AM, Dowlatshahi D, Gladstone DJ, Krischek O, Kiss A, Hill MD, Molina CA, Rodriguez-Luna D, Dzialowski I, Silva Y, Czlonkowska A, Lum C, Boulanger J-M, Gubitz G, Bhatia R, Padma V, Roy J, Kase CS, Aviv RI: Spot sign number is the most important spot sign characteristic for predicting hematoma expansion using first-pass computed tomography angiography: analysis from the PREDICT study. Stroke 2013;44:972–977.
41 Huynh TJ, Flaherty TJ, Gladstone DJ, Broderick JP, Demchuk AM, Dowlatshahi D, Meretoja A, Davis SM, Mitchell PJ, Tomlinson GA, Chenkin J, Chia TL, Symons SP, Aviv RI: Multicenter accuracy and interobserver agreement of spot sign identification in acute intracerebral hemorrhage. Stroke 2014;45:107–112.
42 Cordonnier C, Klijn CJM, Van Beijnum J, Al-Shahi Salman R: Radiological investigation of spontaneous intracerebral hemorrhage: systematic review and trinational survey. Stroke 2010;41:685–690.
43 Khosravani H, Mayer SA, Demchuk A, Jahromi BS, Gladstone DJ, Flaherty M, Broderick J, Aviv RI: Emergency noninvasive angiography for acute intracerebral hemorrhage. AJNR Am J Neuroradiol 2013;34:1481–1487.
44 Mayer SA, Brun NC, Begtrup K, Broderick J, Davis S, Diringer MN, Skolnick BE, Steiner T: Recombinant activated factor VII for acute intracerebral hemorrhage. N Engl J Med 2005;352:777–785.
45 Clinicaltrials.gov: The spot sign for predicting and treating ICH growth study (STOP-IT). 2008 (updated 2014). http://clinicaltrials.gov/ct2/show/NCT00810888 (accessed December 14, 2014).
46 Clinicaltrials.gov: 'Spot sign' selection of intracerebral hemorrhage to guide hemostatic therapy (SPOTLIGHT). 2011 (updated 2014). https://clinicaltrials.gov/ct2/show/NCT01359202 (accessed December 14, 2014).
47 Clinicaltrials.gov: STOP-AUST:the spot sign and tranexamic acid on preventing ICH growth – AUStralasia trial. 2012 (updated 2014). https://clinicaltrials.gov/ct2/show/NCT01702636 (accessed December 14, 2014) .
48 d'Esterre CD, Chia TL, Jairath A, Lee TY, Symons SP, Aviv RI: Early rate of contrast extravasation in patients with intracerebral hemorrhage. AJNR Am J Neuroradiol 2011;32:1879–1884.
49 Aviv RI, Huynh T, Huang Y, Ramsay D, Van Slyke P, Dumont D, Asmah P, Alkins R, Liu R, Hynynen K: An in vivo, MRI-integrated real-time model of active contrast extravasation in acute intracerebral hemorrhage. AJNR Am J Neuroradiol 2014;35:1693–1699.
50 Liu R, Huynh TJ, Huang Y, Ramsay D, Hynynen K, Aviv RI: Modeling the pattern of contrast extravasation in acute intracerebral hemorrhage using dynamic contrast-enhanced MR. Neurocrit Care 2015;22:320–324.

Dr. Richard Aviv
Department of Medical Imaging, Sunnybrook Health Sciences Centre
2075 Bayview Avenue
Toronto, ON M4N 3M5 (Canada)
E-Mail richard.aviv@sunnybrook.ca

Toyoda K, Anderson CS, Mayer SA (eds): New Insights in Intracerebral Hemorrhage.
Front Neurol Neurosci. Basel, Karger, 2016, vol 37, pp 27–34 (DOI: 10.1159/000437111)

Evidence-Based Critical Care of Intracerebral Hemorrhage: An Overview

Lea Küppers-Tiedt[a] · Thorsten Steiner[a, b]

[a]Klinik für Neurologie, Klinikum Frankfurt Hoechst, Frankfurt a.M., and [b]Klinik für Neurologie, Universitätsklinikum Heidelberg, Heidelberg, Germany

Abstract

Outcome of intracerebral hemorrhage (ICH) is still poor and siginificantly influenced by complications during the acute phase, so optimized neurocritical care is crucial. Vital parameters, neurological status and laboratory values of ICH-patient should be monitored very closely with special attention on blood pressure and intracranial pressure. Systolic blood pressure should be kept <140 mm Hg and intracranial pressure <20 mm Hg. Administration of hemostatic agents in spontaneous ICH without intake of anticoagulants is actually not recommended out of clinical trials. Neurosurgical treatment of ICH is still an individual decision. Patients with a higher level of consciousness may profit from an early operation. © 2016 S. Karger AG, Basel

Introduction

Intracerebral hemorrhage (ICH) accounts for 9–27% of strokes worldwide [1] and is still characterized by poor outcomes. Mortality in patients with ICH is up to 50% within the first 6 months and up to 60% within 1 year. Predictors associated with death are increasing age, low Glasgow Coma Scale (GCS) score, increasing ICH volume, presence of intraventricular hemorrhage (IVH), and deep/infratentorial ICH [2]. The neurological outcome of ICH is also poor: of those who survive, only a small proportion reaches independent life after 1 year, with estimates varying between 12 and 39% [3].

So, optimal management of patients with ICH is crucial. A meta-analysis of 13 randomized controlled trials [4] shows that specialized neurocritical care in a stroke unit is beneficial to ICH patients.

In the following overview, we will illustrate the essentials of this neurocritical care of ICH.

Critical Care

Basic Procedures

The first important aspect of neurocritical care is monitoring vital parameters like blood pressure, oxygen saturation, body temperature and intracranial pressure, as well as blood test results like blood glucose and electrolyte levels. These parameters should be kept in a physiological range or, for patients with ICH, in an optimal range.

Blood Pressure

One of the most critical parameters for patients with ICH is blood pressure. Elevated blood pressure is very common in patients with ICH because hypertension is one of the major risk factors for ICH. ICH itself also leads to the activation of the sympathetic nervous system, causing hypertension and tachycardia. Qureshi et al. [5] observed systolic blood pressure (RRsyst) >140 mm Hg in 75% of patients with ICH.

Elevated blood pressure in the acute phase of ICH is associated with hematoma expansion and worsening of outcome [6]. On the other hand, rapid and intensive blood pressure reduction may critically reduce cerebral blood flow in the penumbra of the intracerebral hematoma. The first and second Intensive Blood Pressure Reduction in Acute Cerebral Haemorrhage Trials (INTERACT and INTERACT-2, respectively) [7, 8] and some smaller studies [9–13] showed that aggressive lowering of elevated blood pressure to a target of RRsyst <140 mm Hg is safe and does not affect the perihematoma blood flow in a critical manner. This treatment leads to a reduction in hematoma growth and may be associated with a better outcome than blood pressure reduction to a target of RRsyst <180 mm Hg.

Lowering blood pressure below 140 mm Hg within 6 h of an acute ICH is safe and, therefore, recommended. No specific antihypertensive drug can be recommended, but for better control, it should be given intravenously. The blood pressure should be monitored very closely, optimally continuously via invasive blood pressure measurement.

Body Temperature

Elevated body temperature (>37.5°C) is also very common (about 40%) in patients with ICH due to infections or damage to any structures of the central temperature homeostasis pathways [14]. It is an independent risk factor associated with poor outcome and death [15]. Insufficient data is available to establish whether treatment of fever leads to better functional outcome or reduced mortality in patients with ICH. However, according to data from ischemic stroke and experimental data, we consider normothermia as a basic principle of neuroprotection and recommend early treatment of elevated body temperature. Therefore, medication or any cooling devices can be used.

Blood Glucose/Electrolytes

It has been shown in many small trials that hyperglycemia (i.e. blood glucose levels >140–200 mg/dl or 7.8–11 mmol/l) is associated with hematoma expansion as well as higher mortality rates and worsening of neurological outcome in patients with ICH [16]. There are no specific recommendations for lowering the blood glucose levels to a certain level in acute ICH. However, according to the results from the treatment of acute ischemic stroke, we recommend treatment of hyperglycemia >200 mg/dl using i.v. or s.c. insulin. Maybe the threshold should be lowered to 140 mg/dl according to findings from other critical care conditions. Also, hypoglycemia (<40–50 mg/dl or 2.8–3.3 mmol/l) may lead to neurological deterioration in ICH patients. So, hypoglycemia should be corrected by oral or i.v. glucose [17].

Electrolyte disturbances, especially hyponatremia, are common under critical care conditions. Severe hyponatremia may lead to (aggravation of) brain edema and is therefore of particular interest in neurocritical care. Karamatsu et al. presented an observational study showing that 15.6% of ICH patients had hyponatremia <135 mmol/l. Hyponatremia was associated with increased early mortality [18]. It is unclear whether the correction of hyponatremia is beneficial to ICH patients, but based on the association of hyponatremia with an increased risk of brain edema, we advise paying attention to the sodium level.

Management of Elevated Intracranial Pressure

Increased intracranial pressure (ICP) is one of the leading causes of death among ICH patients. The sources of elevated ICP include large hematoma volumes, perifocal edema, hydrocephalus and secondary ischemia.

There is insufficient data available illustrating which patients will profit from ICP measurement or the threshold for ICP lowering.

For practical reasons and despite the lack of clear evidence, we suggest an approach according to ICP management applied in cases of severe traumatic brain injury [19].

According to many studies, mainly in traumatic brain injury, we consider an increased ICP >20 mm Hg as the treatment threshold [20].

The following interventions for ICP lowering are available:

- Upper body elevation 30°
- Analgesia, sedation, and intubation (GCS score <8)
- Osmotic therapy (e.g. mannitol, glycerol, or hypertonic saline) to raise serum osmolarity to 315–320 mOsm/l

- Barbiturates
- Hyperventilation (partial pressure of CO2 30–35 mm Hg)
- Hypothermia (32–34°C)
- Neurosurgical therapy like external ventricular drain (EVD) placement or decompressive hemicraniectomy
- No hypoosmolar solutions or glucocorticoids

Unfortunately, no clear evidence from randomized controlled trials is available for any of these methods for ICP lowering. Also, smaller studies show contradictory results [21].

Glycerol and mannitol were tested, with no benefits regarding case fatality and outcome parameters [22, 23]. Hypertonic 3% saline resulted in less perihematomal edema and a trend toward lower mortality in one nonrandomized study [24]. Also, mild hypothermia (35°C) prevented the increase in perihemorrhagic edema in patients with large ICH in a small study [25].

Several nonrandomized trials showed conflicting results for decompressive surgery in ICH patients [26, 27].

Despite the good efficacy of glucocorticoids in reducing edema in brain tumors, the use of dexamethasone has not shown any effect on case mortality or outcome in ICH patients in several studies and is therefore not recommended [28].

Prophylaxis of Deep Venous Thrombosis

Because of their immobility and their paretic limbs, patients with ICH are at high risk for deep venous thrombosis (DVT) and, consecutively, pulmonary embolism. Prophylaxis with low dose subcutaneous heparin showed no harm, especially no hematoma growth, in several studies [29]. Thigh-length graduated compression stockings did not prevent DVT based on the Clots in Legs Or sTockings after Stroke-1 (CLOTS-1) trial [30]. By contrast, the use of elastic stockings combined with intermittent pneumatic compression lowers the rate of DVT in patients with ischemic stroke and ICH and may lead to a better outcome [31, 32].

Antiepileptic Therapy

Epileptic seizures after ICH occur in 3–17% of patients, and the incidence of seizures increases up to 42% when subclinical seizures only seen on a continuous electroencephalogram are also considered [33]. Epileptic seizures should be treated with antiepileptic drugs because they might increase ICP.

Prophylactic treatment with antiepileptic drugs is controversial. There are many data available indicating that the use of phenytoin is associated with poor outcome. For other antiepileptic drugs (like valproic acid or levetiracetam), it is less clear whether their use reduces the incidence of early or late post-ICH seizures or leads to a better neurological outcome [34, 35]. In conclusion, there is not enough evidence to support the general use of prophylactic antiepileptic drugs in ICH.

Hemostatic Therapy

One of the biggest problems in ICH is the enlargement of the hemorrhage in the acute phase. So, it appears logically consistent to treat patients with ICH using hemostatic agents like recombinant activated factor VII or tranexamic acid.

In spontaneous ICH not related to antithrombotic drugs, recombinant activated factor VII lessens hematoma growth but exerts no benefit on the survival rate or outcome parameters and leads to increased thrombotic problems [36, 37]. In a pilot trial, tranexamic acid caused neither harm nor benefit in acute ICH [38]. So, actually, no specific hemostatic therapy can be recommended for ICH not associated with antithrombotic therapy. There are several studies ongoing.

The intake of anticoagulant drugs like vitamin K antagonists increases the risk of intracranial hemorrhage and worsens outcome [39]. There are no data from randomized controlled trials regarding the effect of normalizing coagulation on outcome or hematoma growth. However, from clinical observation and pharmacological considerations, it is standard to stop administering the anticoagulant drug in cases of ICH and to normalize coagulation using vitamin K (5–10 mg intravenously) and either fresh frozen plasma (e.g. 20 ml/kg) or prothrombin complex concentrate (e.g. 25–40 IU/kg) in patients receiving vitamin K antagonists. For patients on heparin, i.v. protamine sulfate should be used [21]. For novel oral anticoagulants (NOACs), there is no specific antidote available to date, but several candidates are currently tested in ongoing studies. Due to the shortness of experience with patients under NOACs, there is only a consensus of expert opinion available [40]. In accordance with the management of ICH associated with vitamin K antagonists, prothrombin complex concentrate should be given to patients with ICH associated with NOACs.

If ICH occurs under antiplatelet therapy, no specific therapy other than stopping the antiplatelet medication is recommended [21]. There is insufficient data available to establish whether platelet transfusion may lead to lesser hematoma growth or better outcome [41]. Actually, clinical trials on this topic are ongoing.

Neurosurgical Intervention

Neurosurgical options in acute ICH are the evacuation of the hematoma via open surgery (craniotomy) or minimally invasive approaches or stereotactic drainage of the blood clot. If a hydrocephalus occurs or in cases of IVH, an EVD can be inserted.

Hematoma evacuation in supratentorial ICH is still a contentious issue despite the many clinical studies that have been conducted. The International Surgical Trial in Intracerebral Haemorrhage (STICH)-1 trial [42], which compared hematoma evacuation within 24 h with best medical treatment, could not demonstrate the superiority of early surgery. In a post hoc analysis of the STICH-1-data, a nonsignificant advantage of early surgery was seen in a subgroup of patients with lobar hematomas without IVH. So, the STICH-2 trial investigated the effect of hematoma evacuation within 12 h in this subgroup of patients. Also in STICH-2, surgery was not superior to conservative treatment [43].

A meta-analysis of STICH-2 and 14 other trials of surgery for supratentorial ICH showed an advantage for early surgery, but the data are very heterogeneous and therefore should be interpreted with care. A meta-analysis of individual patient data published before STICH-2 arrived at the conclusion that patients with a higher level of consciousness (GCS score 9–12) might benefit from surgery within the first eight hours [44].

In conclusion, there is no evidence for routine hematoma evacuation of supratentorial ICH based on the data obtained so far. Patients with a GCS score of 9–12 may profit from early intervention. So, surgery for supratentorial ICH is still an individual decision. More clinical trials, especially studies examining minimally invasive methods partially in combination with thrombolytic agents, are ongoing.

Infratentorial ICHs, especially cerebellar hemorrhage, cause brainstem compression and hydrocephalus very frequently with rapid clinical deterioration and a lethal or worse outcome. There are no clinical trials available comparing hematoma evacuations with conservative management or drainage of cerebrospinal fluid. Nevertheless, an EVD should be inserted in cases of hydrocephalus, and hematoma evacuation should be considered if the fourth ventricle is obliterated regardless of hematoma volume or clinical condition [45] or if the hematoma diameter is >30–40 mm or the GCS score is <14 [46].

Up to 40% of ICH cases are associated with secondary IVH. The presence of IVH often causes hydrocephalus and is therefore associated with worsening of outcome. It seems reasonable to apply an EVD in cases of clinical and/or radiological evidence of hydrocephalus. A meta-analysis [47] concluded that the combination of EVD and intraventricular fibrinolysis has an additional positive effect on outcome in severe IVH. A randomized controlled trial on this topic (Clot Lysis Evaluation of Accelerated Resolution of Intraventricular Hemorrhage III, CLEAR III) is ongoing.

References

1 Feigin VL, Lawes CM, Bennett DA, et al: Worldwide stroke incidence and early case fatality reported in 56 population-based studies: a systematic review. Lancet Neurol 2009;8:355–369.

2 Poon MT, Fonville AF, Al-Shahi Salman R: Long-term prognosis after intracerebral haemorrhage: systematic review and meta-analysis. J Neurol Neurosurg Psychiatry 2014;85:660–667.

3 van Asch CJ, Luitse MJ, Rinkel GJ, et al: Incidence, case fatality, and functional outcome of intracerebral haemorrhage over time, according to age, sex, and ethnic origin: a systematic review and meta-analysis. Lancet Neurol 2010;9:167–176.

4 Langhorne P, Fearon P, Ronning OM, et al: Stroke unit care benefits patients with intracerebral hemorrhage: systematic review and meta-analysis. Stroke 2013;44:3044–3049.

5 Qureshi AI, Ezzeddine MA, Nasar A, et al: Prevalence of elevated blood pressure in 563,704 adult patients with stroke presenting to the ED in the United States. Am J Emerg Med 2007;25:32–38.

6 Ohwaki K, Yano E, Nagashima H, et al: Blood pressure management in acute intracerebral hemorrhage: relationship between elevated blood pressure and hematoma enlargement. Stroke 2004;35:1364–1367.

7 Anderson CS, Huang Y, Wang JG, et al: Intensive blood pressure reduction in acute cerebral haemorrhage trial (INTERACT): a randomised pilot trial. Lancet Neurol 2008;7:391–399.

8 Anderson CS, Heeley E, Huang Y, et al: Rapid blood-pressure lowering in patients with acute intracerebral hemorrhage. N Engl J Med 2013;368:2355–2365.

9 Qureshi AI, ATACH Investigators: Antihypertensive treatment of acute cerebral hemorrhage. Crit Care Med 2010;38:637–48.
10 Arima H, Anderson CS, Wang JG, et al: Lower treatment blood pressure is associated with greatest reduction in hematoma growth after acute intracerebral hemorrhage. Hypertension 2010;56:852–858.
11 Qureshi AI, Palesch YY, Martin R, et al: Effect of systolic blood pressure reduction on hematoma expansion, perihematomal edema and 3-month outcome among patients with intracerebral hemorrhage: results from the Antihypertensive Treatment of Acute Cerebral Hemorrhage Study. Arch Neurol 2010;67: 570–576.
12 Koch S, Romano JG, Forteza AM, et al: Rapid blood pressure reduction in acute intracerebral hemorrhage: feasibility and safety. Neurocrit Care 2008;8: 316–321.
13 Xu MY: Effect of blood pressure lowering strategy on the enlargement of hematoma and clinical outcome in patients with acute intracerebral haemorrhage. Chin J Cerebrovasc Dis 2011;8:23–27.
14 Honig A, Michael S, Eliahou R, et al: Central fever in patients with spontaneous intracerebral hemorrhage: predicting factors and impact on outcome. BMC Neurol 2015;15:6.
15 Greer DM, Funk SE, Reaven NL, et al: Impact of fever on outcome in patients with stroke and neurologic injury: a comprehensive meta-analysis. Stroke 2008;39:3029–3035.
16 Qureshi AI, Palesch YY, Martin R, et al: Association of serum glucose concentrations during acute hospitalization with hematoma expansion, perihematomal edema, and three month outcome among patients with intracerebral hemorrhage. Neurocrit Care 2011;15:428–435.
17 Adams HP Jr, del Zoppo G, Alberts MJ, et al: Guidelines for the early management of adults with ischemic stroke: a guideline from the American Heart Association/American Stroke Association Stroke Council, Clinical Cardiology Council, Cardiovascular Radiology and Intervention Council, and the Atherosclerotic Peripheral Vascular Disease and Quality of Care Outcomes in Research Interdisciplinary Working Groups: the American Academy of Neurology affirms the value of this guideline as an educational tool for neurologists. Stroke 2007;38: 1655–1711.
18 Kuramatsu JB, Bobinger T, Volbers B, et al: Hyponatremia is an independent predictor of in-hospital mortality in spontaneous intracerebral hemorrhage. Stroke 2014;45:1285–1291.
19 Chesnut RM, Temkin N, Carney N, et al: A trial of intracranial-pressure monitoring in traumatic brain injury. N Engl J Med 2012;367:2471–2481.
20 Brain Trauma Foundation, American Association of Neurological Surgeons, Joint Section on Neurotrauma and Critical Care: Guidelines for the management of severe head injury. J Neurotrauma 1996;13: 641–734.
21 Steiner T, Al-Shahi Salman R, Beer R, et al: European Stroke Organisation (ESO) guidelines for the management of spontaneous intracerebral hemorrhage. Int J Stroke 2014;9:840–855.
22 Yu YL, Kumana CR, Lauder IJ, et al: Treatment of acute cerebral hemorrhage with intravenous glycerol. A double-blind, placebo controlled, randomized trial. Stroke 1992;23:967–971.
23 Misra UK, Kalita J, Ranjan P, et al: Mannitol in intracerebral hemorrhage: a randomized controlled study. J Neurol Sci 2005;234:41–45.
24 Wagner I, Hauer EM, Staykov D, et al: Effects of continuous hypertonic saline infusion on perihemorrhagic edema evolution. Stroke 2011;42:1540–1545.
25 Kollmar R, Staykov D, Dorfler A, et al: Hypothermia reduces perihemorrhagic edema after intracerebral hemorrhage. Stroke 2010;41:1684–1689.
26 Shimamura N, Munakata A, Naraoka M, et al: Decompressive hemi-craniectomy is not necessary to rescue supratentorial hypertensive intracerebral hemorrhage patients: consecutive single-center experience. Acta Neurochir Suppl 2011;111:415–419.
27 Ma L, Liu WG, Sheng HS, et al: Decompressive craniectomy in addition to hematoma evacuation improves mortality of patients with spontaneous basal ganglia hemorrhage. J Stroke Cerebrovasc Dis 2010; 19:294–298.
28 Feigin VL, Anderson NE, Rinkel GJE, et al: Corticosteroids for aneurysmal subarachnoid hemorrhage and primary intracerebral hemorrhage. Cochrane Database Syst Rev 2005;(3):CD004583.
29 Orken DN, Kenangil G, Ozkurt H, et al: Prevention of deep venous thrombosis and pulmonary embolism in patients with acute intracerebral hemorrhage. Neurologist 2009;15:329–331.
30 Dennis M, Sandercock PA, Reid J, et al: Effectiveness of thigh-length graduated compression stockings to reduce the risk of deep vein thrombosis after stroke (CLOTS trial 1): a multicentre, randomised controlled trial. Lancet 2009;373:1958–1965.
31 Dennis M, Sandercock P, Reid J, et al: Effectiveness of intermittent pneumatic compression in reduction of risk of deep vein thrombosis in patients who have had a stroke (CLOTS 3): a multicentre randomised controlled trial. Lancet 2013;382:516–524.
32 CLOTS (Clots in Legs Or sTockings after Stroke) Trials Collaboration: Effect of intermittent pneumatic compression on disability, living circumstances, quality of life, and hospital costs after stroke: secondary analyses from CLOTS 3, a randomised trial. Lancet Neurol 2014;13:1186–1192.

33 Garrett MC, Komotar RJ, Starke RM, et al: Predictors of seizure onset after intracerebral hemorrhage and the role of long-term antiepileptic therapy. J Crit Care 2009;24:335–339.

34 Gilad R, Boaz M, Dabby R, et al: Are post intracerebral hemorrhage seizures prevented by anti-epileptic treatment? Epilepsy Res 2011;95:227–231.

35 Messé SR, Sansing LH, Cucchiara BL, et al: Prophylactic antiepileptic drug use is associated with poor outcome following ICH. Neurocrit Care 2009;11:38–44.

36 Al-Shahi Salman R: Haemostatic drug therapies for acute spontaneous intracerebral haemorrhage. Cochrane Database Syst Rev 2009;(4):CD005951.

37 Diringer MN, Skolnick BE, Mayer SA, et al: Thromboembolic events with recombinant activated factor VII in spontaneous intracerebral hemorrhage: results from the Factor Seven for Acute Hemorrhagic Stroke (FAST) trial. Stroke 2010;41:48–53.

38 Sprigg N, Renton CJ, Dineen RA, et al: Tranexamic acid for spontaneous intracerebral hemorrhage: a randomized controlled pilot trial. J Stroke Cerebrovasc Dis 2014;23:1312–1318.

39 Flibotte JJ, Hagan N, O'Donnell J, et al: Warfarin, hematoma expansion, and outcome of intracerebral hemorrhage. Neurology 2004;63:1059–1064.

40 Steiner T, Böhm M, Dichgans M, et al: Recommendations for the emergency management of complications associated with new direct oral anticoagulants (DOAC) Apixaban, dabigatran, and Rivaroxaban. Clin Res Cardiol 2013;102:399–412.

41 Campbell PG, Sen A, Yadla S, et al: Emergency reversal of antiplatelet agents in patients presenting with an intracranial hemorrhage: a clinical review. World Neurosurg 2010;74:279–285.

42 Mendelow AD, Gregson BA, Fernandes HM, et al: Early surgery versus initial conservative treatment in patients with spontaneous supratentorial intracerebral haematomas in the International Surgical Trial in Intracerebral Haemorrhage (STICH): a randomised trial. Lancet 2005;365:387–397.

43 Mendelow AD, Gregson BA, Rowan EN, et al: Early surgery versus initial conservative treatment in patients with spontaneous supratentorial lobar intracerebral haematomas (STICH II): a randomised trial. Lancet 2013;382:397–408.

44 Gregson BA, Broderick JP, Auer LM, et al: Individual patient data subgroup meta-analysis of surgery for spontaneous supratentorial intracerebral hemorrhage. Stroke 2012;43:1496–1504.

45 Kirollos RW, Tyagi AK, Ross SA, et al: Management of spontaneous cerebellar hematomas: a prospective treatment protocol. Neurosurgery 2001;49:1378–1386.

46 Kobayashi S, Sato A, Kageyama Y, et al: Treatment of hypertensive cerebellar hemorrhage – surgical or conservative management? Neurosurgery 1994;34:246–250.

47 Gaberel T, Magheru C, Parienti JJ, et al: Intraventricular fibrinolysis versus external ventricular drainage alone in intraventricular hemorrhage: a meta-analysis. Stroke 2011;42:2776–2781.

Dr. med. Lea Küppers-Tiedt, Prof. Dr. med. Thorsten Steiner
Klinik für Neurologie, Klinikum Frankfurt Hoechst
Gotenstrasse 6–8
DE–65929 Frankfurt a.M. (Germany)
E-Mail Lea.Kueppers-Tiedt@KlinikumFrankfurt.de, thorsten.steiner@KlinikumFrankfurt.de

Toyoda K, Anderson CS, Mayer SA (eds): New Insights in Intracerebral Hemorrhage.
Front Neurol Neurosci. Basel, Karger, 2016, vol 37, pp 35–50 (DOI: 10.1159/000437112)

New Insights into Blood Pressure Control for Intracerebral Haemorrhage

Lisa S. Manning · Thompson G. Robinson

Department of Cardiovascular Sciences and NIHR Biomedical Research Unit in Cardiovascular Disease, University of Leicester, Leicester, UK

Abstract

Although blood pressure (BP) levels may rise in the weeks preceding intracerebral haemorrhage (ICH), in contrast to findings in the ischaemic stroke population, the initial post-ICH BP is often much higher than the last pre-morbid level. Elevated BP is therefore common in acute ICH, often with markedly elevated levels, and is associated with poor outcomes, though the exact pathophysiological mechanisms remain unclear. The Antihypertensive Treatment of Acute Cerebral Haemorrhage (ATACH) trial and the INTEnsive blood pressure Reduction in Acute Cerebral haemorrhage Trial (INTERACT) demonstrated that early and intensive lowering of elevated BP in the acute ICH period is feasible and safe. Importantly, recent CT perfusion studies have shown that early, intense BP reduction does not reduce cerebral blood flow or promote cerebral ischaemia. The recent, large INTERACT2 trial confirmed the safety of early BP lowering in ICH and suggested that intensive target-driven BP reduction may improve outcomes, with a non-significant trend towards reduced death and major disability and a significant favourable shift of scores on the modified Rankin scale compared with guideline-based treatment. BP lowering in acute ICH may reduce haematoma growth, particularly when target levels are achieved early and are sustained, though the evidence is partly conflicting. Other aspects of BP may also be important following acute ICH, with maximum systolic BP and systolic BP variability being independent predictors of poor outcomes in a recent study. This chapter gives an overview of the current evidence regarding BP in ICH and covers the following topics: the incidence of elevated BP in acute ICH and the patterns of BP observed before and after the event; the effect of elevated BP on outcomes in ICH and the potential underlying pathophysiological mechanisms; the safety and feasibility of BP lowering; the effects of BP lowering on clinical and radiological outcomes; other important aspects of BP in ICH; and the choice of antihypertensive agent.

© 2016 S. Karger AG, Basel

Incidence and Pathophysiology of Elevated Blood Pressure in Intracerebral Haemorrhage

Elevated blood pressure (BP) is a frequent occurrence in acute stroke, with 75% of patients having a BP >140/90 mm Hg and with 50% and 15% having a systolic BP (SBP) >160 and >184 mm Hg, respectively [1]. In acute intracerebral haemorrhage (ICH), BP is often raised to markedly elevated levels on hospital admission [1, 2]. Though chronic hypertension is a major risk factor for incident and recurrent ICH, acute ICH can also occur during hypertensive crises and short-term increases in BP [3].

A recent population-based study comparing acute stroke BP levels and pre-morbid BP levels in patients with ischaemic stroke versus those with ICH has improved our understanding of BP trends in these two stroke subtypes. Rothwell et al. [4] found significantly higher acute stroke BPs in ICH compared with ischaemic stroke (mean first post-event BP of 189.8 vs. 158.5 mm Hg) and reported that, in contrast to findings in acute ischaemic stroke, the first acute stroke BP was much higher than pre-morbid levels in ICH (mean increase of 40.7 mm Hg) and that BP fell substantially in the first 24 h (mean decrease of 41.1 mm Hg). Furthermore, steep increases in BP were seen in the days and weeks prior to ICH, though the first post-stroke BP remained higher than the last pre-morbid BP, even in those with a pre-event rise. These findings suggest that whilst a recent pre-morbid BP increase may contribute to elevated BP in acute ICH, post-stroke factors are also involved. Contributory factors for this abrupt rise include damage to brain regions that regulate the autonomic nervous system [5]; activation of the neuroendocrine system (including the sympathetic nervous system, renin-angiotensin system, and glucocorticoid system) [6]; headache; infection; and increased BP related to psychological distress [7].

Whilst the temporal trend is for BP to spontaneously decline over the several days following ICH (with the steepest decline seen in the first 24 h) [1], elevated BP in the acute period is of important prognostic significance, as discussed below.

Prognostic Significance of Elevated Blood Pressure in Acute Intracerebral Haemorrhage

Evidence from earlier observational studies regarding the effect of BP in acute ICH is partly conflicting: though most reported significant associations between higher overall BP or mean arterial BP (MAP) parameters and higher mortality or reduced survival [8, 9], others did not [10]. However, recent evidence from larger cohorts is more compelling, showing a significant and nearly linear association between higher BP and the risk of poor outcomes. A systematic review [11] and a large multicentre Chinese study [2] reported that admission SBP and diastolic BP were significantly associated with increased odds of death or disability; an SBP greater than 140–150 mm Hg within the first 12 h of onset was associated with a doubling in the risk of death or disability (fig. 1). Unlike the U-shaped relationship between SBP and outcome in acute ischaemic stroke, in ICH, only one study has shown poor outcomes at very low levels of SBP [12].

Pathophysiological Effects of Blood Pressure in Intracerebral Haemorrhage

The exact pathological mechanisms underlying the association between elevated BP and outcome following ICH remain unclear. An underlying hypothesis relates to the effects of stroke on cerebral autoregulation. Cerebral autoregulation is impaired in acute stroke [13, 14], and thus, cerebral perfusion becomes increasingly pressure dependent. Elevated BP or steep increases in BP may promote ongoing bleeding and haematoma expansion and may enhance the formation of cerebral oedema through oncotic or hydrostatic pressure gradients in the perihaematomal region [15, 16]. Furthermore, mass effects related to ICH and cerebral oedema may lead to elevations in intracranial pressure, which may compromise cerebral perfusion further in the presence of elevated MAP.

Data from clinical studies that support the above proposed hypotheses are limited. Whilst some studies have reported an association between BP and haematoma growth, others have not. A number of earlier case series reported that individuals with elevated SBP were pre-disposed to haematoma expansion [17, 18]; one observational study found a significant association between SBP >200 mm Hg and haematoma growth in 186 patients [15]. However, two further studies, each enrolling 60 participants, found no such associations [19, 20]. Overall, the interpretation of these data is hampered by heterogeneity among the studies, particularly in regard to the definition of ICH growth and the timing of measures.

Evidence regarding a potential relation between BP and the formation of perihaematoma or cerebral oedema is also conflicting. One observational study reported that elevated 24 h SBP profiles were related to the presence of brain oedema on repeat imaging at 5 days in a cohort of 240 patients with either ICH or ischaemic stroke [21]. However, a recent post-hoc analysis of the ICH Acutely Decreasing Arterial Pressure Trial (ICH-ADAPT), which enrolled 67 patients with acute ICH and performed CT perfusion at 2 h and repeat CT at 24 h, found no association between high or low SBP load (percentage of time with SBP >180 or <150 mm Hg in the first 24 h) and the growth of perihaematomal oedema [22]. Others have hypothesised that abrupt elevations in BP following ICH are associated with worse outcome due to effects outside of the brain; for example, those with chronic hypertension are more likely to have cardiac disease and diastolic dysfunction and may decompensate secondary to the increased afterload caused by abrupt BP elevations following ICH.

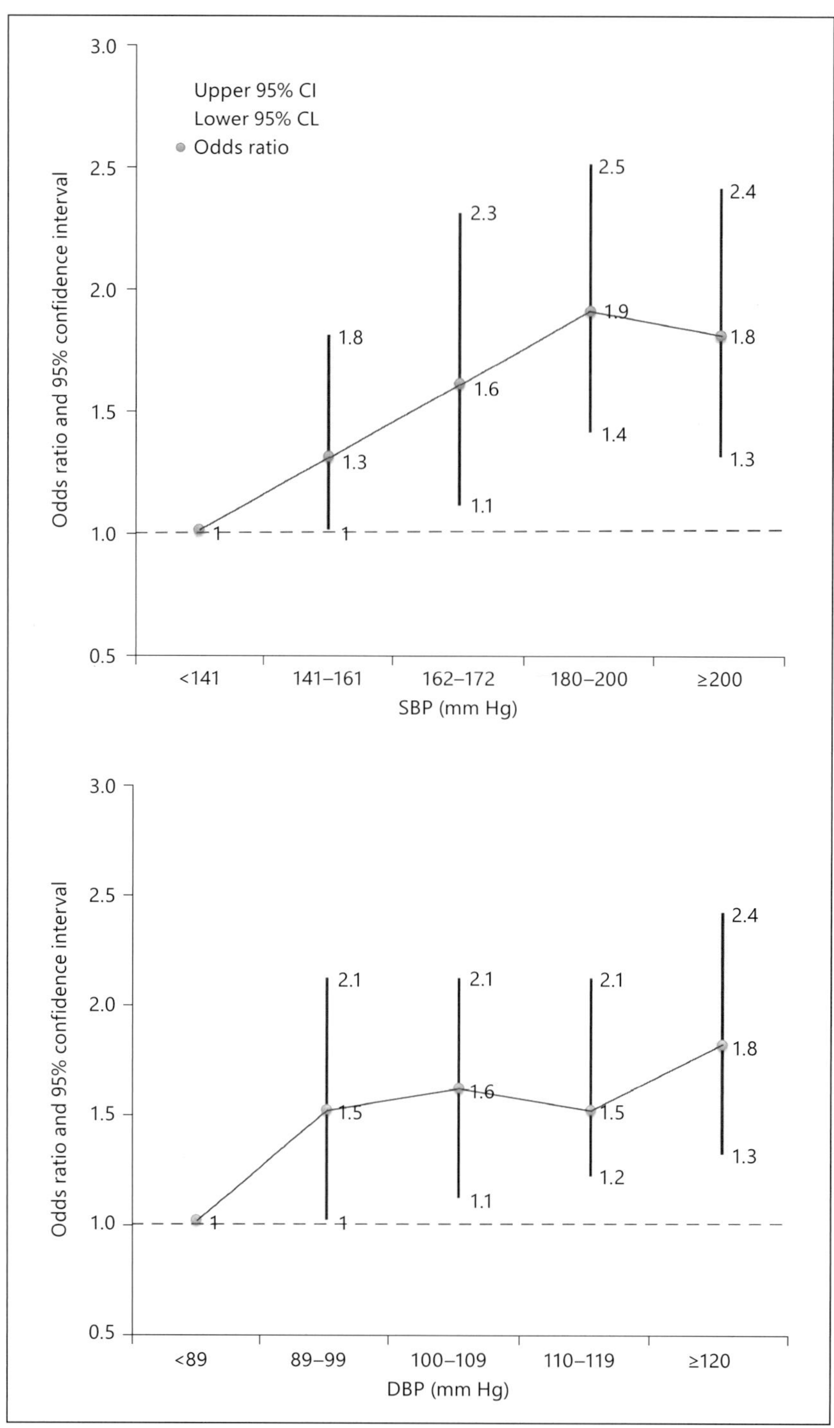

Fig. 1. The multiple adjusted odds ratios and 95% confidence intervals of death/disability according to quintiles of admission systolic blood pressure (SBP) and diastolic BP (p value for trend in both <0.005) from a multicentre Chinese study (n = 1,760). Reproduced with permission from [2].

Table 1. Summary of recommendations for BP management in acute ICH from international guidelines

Guidelines	Recommendations		
	BP level, mm Hg	Recommended action	Monitoring
American Heart Association/American Stroke Association (2007 and 2010) [24, 25]	SBP >200 or MAP >150	Consider aggressive BP reduction with IV agents	Monitor BP every 5 min
	SBP >180 or MAP >150 and suspicion of elevated ICP	Consider monitoring ICP and reducing BP with IV medication	Maintain a cerebral perfusion pressure of >60–80 mm Hg
	SBP >180 or MAP >130 with no suspicion of elevated ICP	Consider a modest reduction of BP, e.g., a target BP of 160/90 mm Hg	Monitor BP every 15 min
European Stroke Organisation (2014) [23]	Within 6 h of ICH onset, intense BP reduction to a target of <140 mm Hg systolic within 1 h is safe and may be superior to a target of <180 mm Hg. No specific agent can be recommended. The strength of this recommendation is weak and is based on evidence of moderate* quality.		

BP = Blood pressure; SBP = systolic blood pressure; MAP = mean arterial blood pressure; ICP = intracranial pressure; ICH = intracerebral haemorrhage; IV = intravenous.
* Moderate-quality evidence described as evidence for which 'further research is likely to have an important impact on our confidence in the estimate of effect and may change the estimate'.

Current Guidelines for Blood Pressure Control in Intracerebral Haemorrhage

Current guidelines for BP control in acute ICH are outlined in table 1 [23–25]. With the exception of the European Stroke Organisation guideline, which recommends a less cautious approach to BP management [23], all were published prior to the completion of two recent important studies. The recommendations were therefore based mainly on observational data that suggested the following: a reduction in MAP by >15% is associated with reduced cerebral blood flow [13]; a reduction in SBP to <160 mm Hg within 6 h is associated with a trend towards improved outcomes [26]; higher baseline BP may be associated with haematoma growth [27]; and rapid lowering of BP may be hazardous. Whether the monitoring of cerebral perfusion pressure improves outcomes when there is suspicion of raised intracranial pressure is unknown, but monitoring is often used to ensure that BP is not lowered disproportionately to maintain the cerebral perfusion pressure [24]. Future guidelines are likely to change in view of emerging evidence on the safety, feasibility and potential benefit of BP lowering from the ADAPT, Antihypertensive Treatment of Acute Cerebral Haemorrhage (ATACH) trial, and INTEnsive blood pressure Reduction in Acute Cerebral haemorrhage Trial (INTERACT)2, as discussed below.

Safety and Feasibility of Blood Pressure Lowering in Acute Intracerebral Haemorrhage

The cautious approach to BP lowering in acute ICH advised in previous guidelines is partly a consequence of extrapolating, from the penumbra of ischaemic stroke, a risk of inducing cerebral ischaemia in the perihaematomal region with rapid BP lowering, particularly in the presence of impaired autoregulation. However, recent careful studies with advanced cerebral imaging have reassured against such a hazard [28]: in ICH-ADAPT, 75 patients with ICH (<24 h from onset) and SBP >150 mm Hg were randomised to one of two intravenous (IV) BP-lowering protocols targeting an SBP of <150 or <180 mm Hg. CT perfusion was performed at 2 h post-randomisation to measure perihaematomal cerebral blood flow. The authors reported significantly lower SBP in the <150 mm Hg target group at 2 h (140 ± 19 vs. 162 ± 12 mm Hg, p = 0.001), with no significant difference in relative perihaematomal cerebral blood flow between the two groups, concluding that early BP lowering does not reduce perihaematomal cerebral blood flow. Furthermore, there was no consistent relation between the magnitude of BP change and perihaematomal cerebral blood flow. These findings are discordant with the hypothesis that rapid BP reduction may precipitate ischaemia in acute ICH and provide supportive data for the safety of early BP reduction.

A post-hoc analysis of data from the same group went on to show no association between BP treatment and perihaematomal oedema expansion and no relation between BP lowering and cerebral blood flow within 1 cm of the haematoma or in visibly oedematous tissues [22]. These findings add further support to the safety of BP lowering but suggest that BP reduction has no significant effect on the worsening of cerebral oedema.

The ATACH trial [29] and INTERACT [30] showed safety and efficacy with early target-driven BP reduction. The ATACH trial enrolled 60 patients with ICH (within <6 h of symptom onset) and SBP >170 mm Hg and reported on the safety of a nicardipine-based BP-lowering regimen with the aim of achieving and maintaining (for 18–24 h) one of three BP target levels (170–200/140–170/110–140 mm Hg). The pilot-phase INTERACT [30], undertaken in 404 patients with acute ICH (within <6 h of onset) and elevated SBP (150–220 mm Hg), randomised patients to either early intensive BP reduction (target SBP of 140 mm Hg within 1 h) or guideline-based BP management (target SBP of 180 mm Hg). Intensive BP lowering was safe and well tolerated, with no significant difference in the rates of serious adverse events or in neurological deterioration between groups. BP lowering was also feasible, with a mean SBP difference between randomised groups of 13.3 mm Hg at 1 h (p < 0.0001). Furthermore, there was a trend towards attenuation of haematoma growth (on 24 h CT) with intensive BP reduction, with a 33% lower relative risk of haematoma growth (95% CI 0–59%, p = 0.05), and an absolute risk reduction of 8% (95% CI 1–17%, p = 0.05). Table 2 shows a summary of findings from recent trials for lowering BP in ICH.

Table 2. Important recent BP-lowering trials for acute ICH

Name, year	Number of particpants	Time to randomisation*, h	Average baseline SBP, mm Hg	BP target(s)	Treatment	Key findings
INTERACT [30] (2008)	404	All <6 Median 3.39 (2.24–4.52)	Intensive group 182±19 Guideline group 180±18	140 mm Hg in intensive group 180 mm Hg in guideline group	Stepped IV protocol according to locally available agents	Early intensive BP lowering was safe, feasible, and seemed to reduce haematoma growth
ATACH [29] (2010)	60	All <6 Median ~1.75	209 (1st tier) 212 (2nd tier) 201 (3rd tier)	According to 3 tiers: 1st 170–220; 2nd 140–170; 3rd 110–140	IV nicardipine	It was possible to achieve groups with discernibly different SBPs to test the effect of various intensities of SBP reduction with IV nicardipine. The overall rate of SAEs and neurological deterioration was below the specified safety threshold
ICH-ADAPT [28] (2013)	75	All <24 h Median ~8.2	Intensive group 182±20 Guideline group 184±25	Intensive group <150 mm Hg Guideline group 180 mm Hg	1st line = IV labetalol; 2nd line = IV hydralazine or IV enalapril if target is not reached/labetalol is contraindicated	Rapid BP lowering did not reduce peri-haematomal cerebral blood flow, indicating that BP reduction in ICH does not induce cerebral ischaemia
INTERACT2 [31] (2013)	2,839	All <6	179±17	Intensive group <140 mm Hg Guideline group <180 mm Hg	IV and oral agents were to be initiated according to pre-specified treatment protocols that were based on the local availability of agents	Intensive lowering of blood pressure was safe but did not result in a significant reduction in the rate of the primary outcome of death or severe disability. An ordinal analysis of mRS scores indicated improved functional outcomes with intensive BP lowering

INTERACT = INTEnsive blood pressure Reduction in Acute Cerebral haemorrhage Trial; ATACH = Antihypertensive Treatment of Acute Cerebral Haemorrhage trial; ICH-ADAPT = ICH Acutely Decreasing Arterial Pressure Trial; * Time from symptom onset to randomisation, in hours; ICH = intracerebral haemorrhage; SBP = systolic blood pressure; BP = blood pressure; IV = intravenous; SAE = significant adverse event; mRS = modified Rankin scale.

Effect of Blood Pressure Lowering on Clinical Outcomes

The definitive main-phase INTERACT2 randomly assigned 2,839 patients (from 144 hospitals across 21 countries) with spontaneous ICH (within <6 h of onset) and elevated SBP (≤150–220 mm Hg) to a strategy of early intensive (SBP target <140 mm Hg within 1 h and maintained for 7 days) or guideline-recommended BP

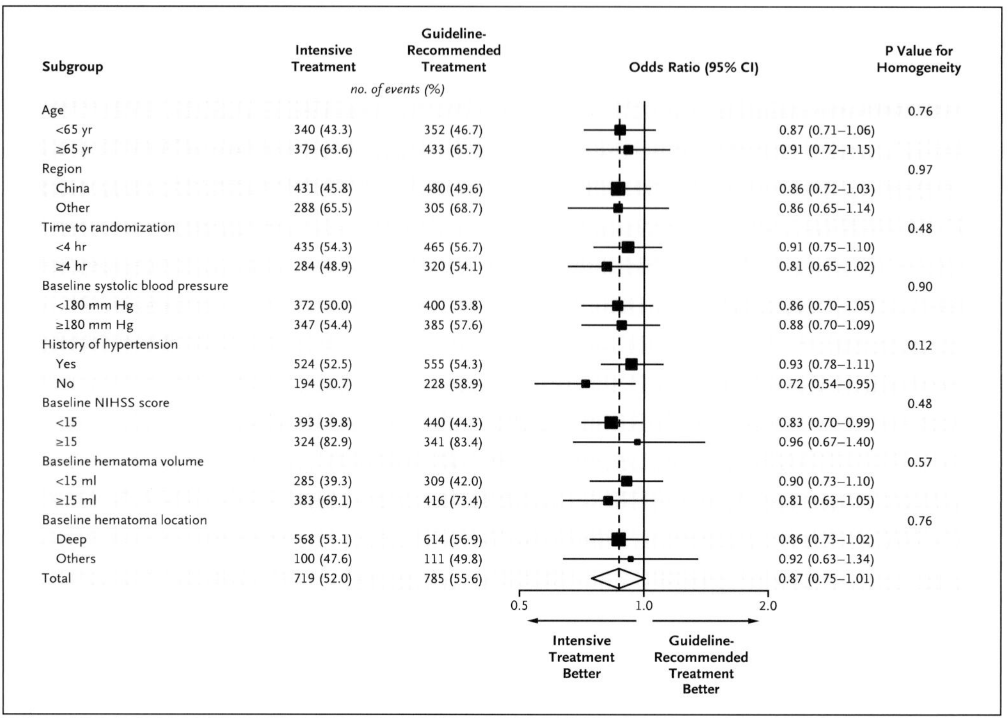

Subgroup	Intensive Treatment	Guideline-Recommended Treatment	Odds Ratio (95% CI)	P Value for Homogeneity
	no. of events (%)			
Age				0.76
<65 yr	340 (43.3)	352 (46.7)	0.87 (0.71–1.06)	
≥65 yr	379 (63.6)	433 (65.7)	0.91 (0.72–1.15)	
Region				0.97
China	431 (45.8)	480 (49.6)	0.86 (0.72–1.03)	
Other	288 (65.5)	305 (68.7)	0.86 (0.65–1.14)	
Time to randomization				0.48
<4 hr	435 (54.3)	465 (56.7)	0.91 (0.75–1.10)	
≥4 hr	284 (48.9)	320 (54.1)	0.81 (0.65–1.02)	
Baseline systolic blood pressure				0.90
<180 mm Hg	372 (50.0)	400 (53.8)	0.86 (0.70–1.05)	
≥180 mm Hg	347 (54.4)	385 (57.6)	0.88 (0.70–1.09)	
History of hypertension				0.12
Yes	524 (52.5)	555 (54.3)	0.93 (0.78–1.11)	
No	194 (50.7)	228 (58.9)	0.72 (0.54–0.95)	
Baseline NIHSS score				0.48
<15	393 (39.8)	440 (44.3)	0.83 (0.70–0.99)	
≥15	324 (82.9)	341 (83.4)	0.96 (0.67–1.40)	
Baseline hematoma volume				0.57
<15 ml	285 (39.3)	309 (42.0)	0.90 (0.73–1.10)	
≥15 ml	383 (69.1)	416 (73.4)	0.81 (0.63–1.05)	
Baseline hematoma location				0.76
Deep	568 (53.1)	614 (56.9)	0.86 (0.73–1.02)	
Others	100 (47.6)	111 (49.8)	0.92 (0.63–1.34)	
Total	719 (52.0)	785 (55.6)	0.87 (0.75–1.01)	

Fig. 2. The effect of early BP lowering on the odds ratio of death or major disability at 90 days by predefined subgroups in INTERACT2. Reproduced with permission from [31].

treatment (SBP <180 mm Hg) [31]. In those assigned to intensive treatment, oral or IV agents were given according to pre-specified protocols based on local availability. The primary outcome was death or major disability (modified Rankin Scale (mRS) score ≥3) at 90 days, and the key secondary outcome was physical function (at 90 days) across all seven levels of the mRS, as determined by the use of an ordinal shift analysis of scores. The mean SBP levels were significantly lower from 15 min to day 7 in the intensive versus guideline treatment groups; at 1 h, the mean SBP in the intensive group was 150, compared with 164 mm Hg in the guideline group ($p < 0.001$). The results showed a borderline significant reduction in the primary outcome in the intensive treatment group (OR 0.87, CI 0.75–1.01, $p = 0.06$), with a significant favourable shift of the mRS scores (pooled OR for shift 0.87, CI 0.77–1.00, $p = 0.04$). Moreover, early target-driven BP reduction was safe, with no increase in adverse events in the intensive treatment arm and with significantly better quality-of-life scores. There was no evidence of heterogeneity of the effect in any pre-specified subgroup (fig. 2). The absence of a difference in effect between those randomised before and within 4 h after onset is of particular note, given the rapid evolution of bleeding in the first few hours following ICH, at which point one may expect BP lowering to have the greatest effect.

Recent acute stroke BP-lowering trials enrolling those with both ICH and ischaemic stroke and commencing treatment later have mostly yielded neutral results. It is, of course, important to interpret these results in context, as they are not truly specific to ICH, and in most cases, ICH patients made up a relatively small proportion (10–15%) of the total cohort. The large Efficacy of Nitric Oxide in Stroke (ENOS) trial recruited 4,011 patients with acute stroke, with a median time to enrolment of 26 h from onset [32]. Patients were randomised to either a transdermal glyceryl trinitrate (GTN) patch or placebo. BP was significantly lower in the GTN group at day 1 (SBP difference of –7 mm Hg; $p < 0.001$), but there was no difference between the groups in terms of functional outcome (assessed using the mRS) at 90 days. Subgroup analysis showed a benefit in those treated within 6 h, suggesting that very early treatment may be beneficial. There was no heterogeneity of the effect on outcomes in the subgroup analysis by stroke type (ischaemic/ICH/unknown).

Interestingly, an earlier feasibility study, namely, the Rapid Intervention with GTN in Hypertensive Stroke Trial (RIGHT) [33], showed safety, efficacy, and a trend towards improved functional outcome with paramedic-administered transdermal GTN, given much earlier following acute stroke onset (median of 55 min), in 41 patients. This adds support to the hypothesis that earlier treatment may be beneficial but, of course, must be interpreted with care, given that the small cohort included those with ischaemic stroke and ICH and that GTN has other potential neuroprotective mechanisms of action in addition to BP lowering.

The Scandinavian Candesartan Acute Stroke Trial (SCAST) reported no benefit, but rather potential harm (risk of poor functional outcome: OR 1.17, CI 1.00–1.38, $p = 0.048$), for candesartan given within 30 h of acute stroke (ICH and ischaemic stroke) [34]. Interestingly, as in the ENOS subgroup analysis, for those treated within 6 h, there was a non-significant benefit of candesartan for reduced vascular events (p for interaction 0.08). In a post-hoc analysis including only patients with ICH ($n = 247$), candesartan was associated with a non-significant increase in the risk of vascular events and a significant worsening in functional outcome [35]. Although SBP was significantly lower at 7 days in the treatment group in the SCAST, the mean difference was relatively small (5 mm Hg), and the median time to randomisation was over 17 h.

The totality of evidence to date is that early BP reduction in acute ICH is safe and feasible. Moreover, it does not affect perihaematomal blood flow, and compared with a target SBP of 180 mm Hg, as recommended in previous guidelines, a strategy to reduce SBP to 140 mm Hg within 6 h of symptom onset may improve functional outcomes. The ongoing ATACH II trial [36], which is aiming to recruit 1,280 subjects within 4.5 h of ICH onset, should provide further evidence as to the effect of intensive BP reduction on outcomes early in the course of acute ICH. Although recent trials enrolling both those with ICH and ischaemic stroke have yielded neutral results, subgroup analyses have shown a trend towards treatment benefit in those treated early (<6 h). The pilot-phase Field Administration of Stroke Therapy-BP Lowering (FAST-BP) trial, using GTN patches administered by paramedics within 2 h of stroke onset, may provide additional reassurance of the feasibility, safety and efficacy of BP lowering in the field and may lead to the subsequent development of future trials to address the effects of very early BP lowering in acute stroke, including ICH.

Effects of Blood Pressure Lowering on Haematoma Growth

As previously discussed, the evidence for the effect of elevated BP in acute ICH on haematoma growth is partly conflicting. Nonetheless, haematoma growth is a strong predictor of death and dependency in ICH, and treatment approaches to reduce this growth may improve prognosis. As described above, the pilot-phase INTERACT showed attenuation of haematoma growth (on repeat CT at 24 h) with intensive BP reduction [30]. Based on the knowledge that greater haematoma growth is observed in those who present earlier to the hospital with ICH [15], many have hypothesised that earlier BP-lowering treatment will provide better protection against haematoma growth and poor outcomes. To determine the effect on haematoma growth based on the time to BP-lowering treatment, Arima et al. [37] undertook a secondary analysis of data from 296 participants in the INTERACT cohort who had available CT scans at baseline and at 24 and 72 h. Reductions in proportional haematoma growth progressively decreased with delays in the initiation of study treatment, suggesting that earlier initiation of treatment is likely to offer greater protection against haematoma growth.

It is perhaps surprising that in the main-phase INTERACT2, of 964 participants enrolled in the CT substudy (with repeat CT at 24 h), there was no significant relation between intensive treatment and a reduction in haematoma growth: relative difference between the intensive and the guideline treatment groups, 4.5% (95% CI –3.1 to 12.7, $p = 0.27$), and absolute difference, 1.4 ml (95% CI –0.6 to 3.4, $p = 0.18$), after adjustment for prognostic variables [31]. However, in an observational analysis of the INTERACT2 data, the time and intensity of BP-lowering treatment and consistency in BP lowering were found to be important [38]: greater reductions in SBP (<10, 10–20, 20–40, and >40 mm Hg) were significantly associated with lower degrees of haematoma growth (10.7, 3.1, 2.7, and 2.2 ml volumes, respectively; p for trend <0.01). For participants in the intensive treatment group, the lowest haematoma growth was observed in those who achieved the target SBP (<140 mm Hg), with the least haematoma growth seen in those who achieved target BP consistently. A further analysis of pooled data from INTERACT and INTERACT2 showed significantly less growth of perihaematomal oedema with intensive BP lowering [39]. The effects on oedema growth were reduced when haematoma expansion or volume was included in the analysis, suggesting that the observed effects were in part a result of reduced haematoma growth.

Thus, whilst the evidence for the effect of the initial BP level on haematoma growth is partly conflicting and the results from recent definitive trials are not statistically significant, evidence from secondary analyses suggests that early BP lowering provides maximal protection against haematoma growth when the reduction in SBP is greater and when the target BP is achieved earlier and is sustained. The ongoing ATACH2 trial may provide more evidence, though future pre-hospital trials to assess the radiological and functional effects of very early BP lowering are warranted.

Other Emerging Concepts

An alternative hypothesis that may help to explain some of the ongoing uncertainty as to the effect of BP lowering on outcomes in ICH relates to BP variability (BPV). Indeed, in INTERACT2, the finding of no difference in the effect on outcomes between those treated at <4 and at 4–6 h of onset suggests that other aspects of BP control may be important. Moreover, the different efficacies of different BP-lowering drugs in reducing stroke risk cannot be explained by the effects of mean BP alone [40], and, as described in a recent systematic review, different antihypertensive drugs have differential effects on BPV [41]. BPV can be defined as the variation in BP over a period of time. It is most commonly (and simply) measured as the standard deviation or the coefficient of variation, though more complex calculated parameters are also described. Until recently, evidence regarding the effect of BPV in acute ICH was scarce, with just one single-centre observational study reporting that systolic BPV within 24 h of ICH was an independent predictor of death or neurological deterioration in 117 patients [42].

A recent post-hoc analysis of the INTERACT2 dataset has concurred with these findings, suggesting that systolic BPV is an important prognostic factor in ICH [43]. Manning et al. assessed the association of systolic BPV in the first 24 h (hyperacute phase) and at days 2–7 (acute phase) (derived from five and 12 standardised BP measures, respectively) following ICH with outcomes at 90 days. The authors reported that systolic BPV in both phases was an independent predictor of death or major disability at 90 days. Furthermore, the greater the variability in SBP was, the stronger the association with poor outcome was, whether defined as death or disability or as a shift in mRS scores (fig. 3). The maximum SBP was an additional independent predictor of poor outcome, whilst few associations were found between diastolic BP or MAP parameters. Though this was a post-hoc analysis of randomised controlled trial data and thus has limitations, it also has potential implications for clinical practice and future research. Episodic hypertension, isolated high SBP readings and large fluctuations in SBP in the first 24 h and over the few days following ICH are associated with poor outcomes, independent of mean BP; therefore, efforts should be taken to ensure stability and consistency in BP lowering, not only in the first 24 h but also in the several days following ICH. Taken together with reports by Rothwell et al. [44] on the potential differential effects of different antihypertensive classes on BPV, the therapeutic effects of modulating BPV in acute ICH should be considered in future trials.

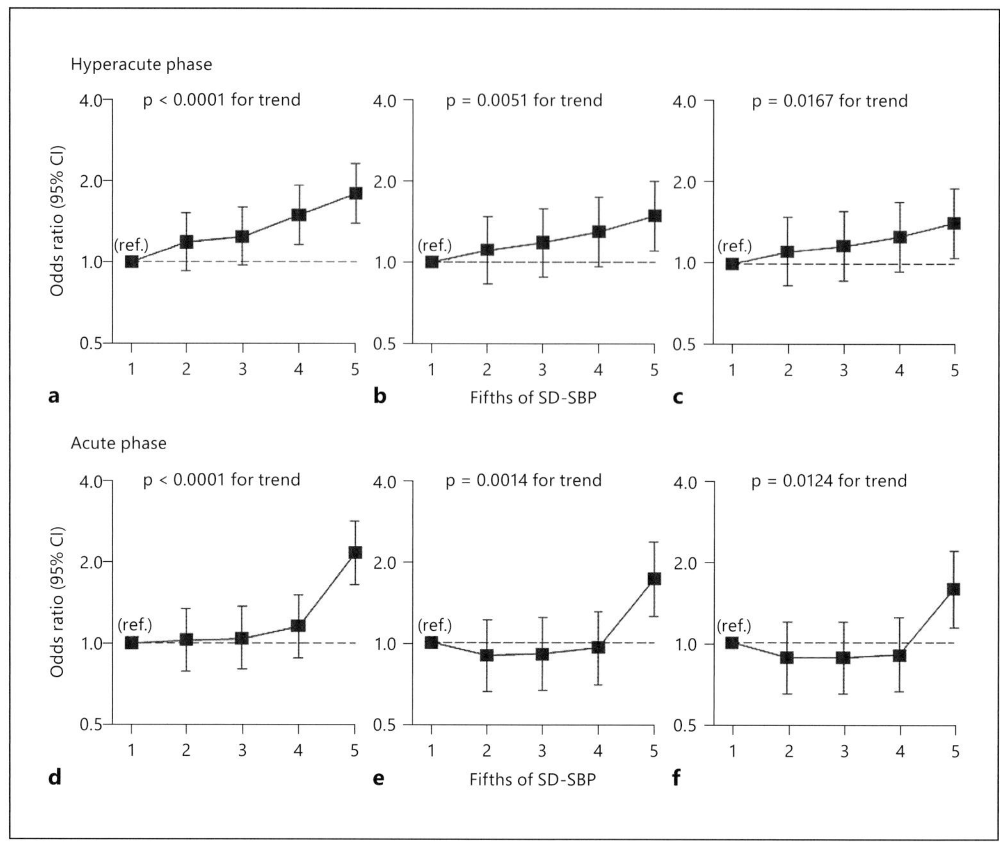

Fig. 3. The association between quintiles of SBP variability (standard deviation of SBP) in the hyperacute phase (first 24 h) and at days 2–7 after ICH and the odds ratios for death or dependency at 90 days in a post-hoc analysis of the INTEnsive blood pressure Reduction in Acute Cerebral haemorrhage Trial (INTERACT)2. Reproduced with permission from [43]. **a**, and **d** Analyses adjusted for age, sex and randomised treatment group. **b** and **e** Adjusted for all covariates above plus the baseline stroke severity (National Institutes of Health Stroke Scale), region (China/elsewhere), and haematoma volume. **c** and **f** Adjusted for all covariates above plus the mean SBP.

Specific Antihypertensive Agents

A wide range of agents are available for BP control, though a lack of comparative effectiveness studies means that there is no one ideal recommended drug in the context of acute ICH. Current guidelines cite labetalol and nicardipine as agents to consider as first-line treatment [23, 25], though other rapid-acting, readily titratable, parenteral agents such as clevidipine and urapidil are reasonable alternatives. A brief description of individual drugs and recent evidence related to them are given below.

Labetalol, a combined selective alpha 1 adrenergic and non-selective beta adrenergic receptor blocker, has a rapid onset (2–5 min) after IV administration, and its effects last from 2 to 4 h. It can be given as a bolus or infusion, without the need for invasive BP monitoring, and is one of several antihypertensive drugs used in INTERACT2. A recent systematic review of nicardipine versus labetalol in hypertensive crises, including ischaemic stroke, ICH, and subarachnoid haemorrhage, included 10 comparative studies (four specific to stroke) [45]. The authors reported comparable efficacy and safety, though nicardipine appeared to provide more predictable and consistent BP control. In the stroke population (ICH and ischaemic stroke), labetalol is safe and effectively reduces BP [46]. Although no specific trial data are available for esmolol (a rapidly acting cardio-selective beta blocker that may be given intravenously), it may be useful in certain settings, as it is not dependent on renal or hepatic function and therefore may be used in those with renal or hepatic impairment.

The second-generation dihydropyridine calcium channel blocker nicardipine has an onset of action of 5–10 min and has cerebral and vasodilatory properties that may improve cerebral perfusion. In a retrospective study comparing the drug with labetalol in a cohort of patients with ICH, subarachnoid haemorrhage, or ischaemic stroke, those receiving nicardipine were more likely to achieve the target BP within an hour and were less likely to need dose adjustments with additional agents [47].

The new third-generation dihydropyridine calcium channel blocker clevidipine may have a role in BP control in ICH. It has a rapid onset (<1 min) and is easily titratable. Several studies have confirmed its efficacy and safety in BP reduction in hypertensive crises in cardiac surgery and emergency department settings [48]. Most recently, the Evaluation of Patients with Acute Hypertension and Intracerebral Hemorrhage with Intravenous Clevidipine Treatment (ACCELERATE) trial [49], which included 35 hypertensive acute ICH patients, showed that clevidipine monotherapy quickly and safely achieved control of BP.

Nitroglycerine is a venodilator with an immediate onset of action that can be given intravenously or as a transdermal patch. As described previously, the recent RIGHT and large ENOS trials in acute stroke [32, 33] showed the safety and efficacy of transdermal GTN early after stroke but no overall effect on death or dependency versus placebo.

Sodium nitroprusside, an arterial and venous vasodilator, is cited as an agent to consider in European guidelines. However, it decreases cerebral perfusion pressure with increasing intracranial pressure and therefore should be used with caution in certain cases.

Finally, urapidil, a vasodilator that acts on peripheral vessels by alpha 1 adrenoreceptor blockade and on the central nervous system by alpha adrenoreceptor blockade, has a rapid onset of action, though wide individual dose variations are seen. A systematic review of hypertensive crises found it to be safe and effective for BP control [50]. Though not explicitly cited in current guidelines, given the large proportion of Chinese patients in INTERACT2, urapidil was the most commonly used agent.

Conclusions

In summary, elevated BP is common in acute ICH and is associated with poor outcomes, though the exact pathophysiological mechanisms remain unclear. In contrast to patterns of BP in acute ischaemic stroke, the initial post-ICH BP is often much higher than the last pre-morbid level. Early and intensive lowering of elevated BP in the acute ICH period is safe, may improve functional outcomes, and does not reduce cerebral blood flow or promote cerebral ischaemia. BP lowering may reduce haematoma growth, particularly when target levels are achieved early and are sustained. Other aspects of BP may be important in the acute stroke period, with maximum SBP and systolic BPV being independent predictors of poor outcomes in a recent study.

References

1 Qureshi AI, Ezzeddine MA, Nasar A, et al: Prevalence of elevated blood pressure in 563,704 adult patients with stroke presenting to the ED in the United States. Am J Emerg Med 2007;25:32–38.

2 Zhang Y, Reilly K, Tong W, et al: Blood pressure and clinical outcome among patients with acute stroke in Inner Mongolia, China. J Hypertens 2008;26:1446–1452.

3 Papadopoulos D, Iordanis M, Thomopoulos C, et al: Hypertension crisis. Blood Press 2010;19:328–336.

4 Fischer U, Cooney MT, Bull LM, et al: Acute post-stroke blood pressure relative to premorbid levels in intracerebral haemorrhage versus major ischaemic stroke: a population-based study. Lancet Neurol 2014;13:374–384.

5 Qureshi AI: Acute hypertensive response in patients with stroke: pathophysiology and management. Circulation 2008;118:176–187.

6 Olsson T, Marklund N, Gustafson Y, et al: Abnormalities at different levels of the hypothalamic-pituitary-adrenocortical axis early after stroke. Stroke 1992;23:1573–1576.

7 Carlberg B, Asplund K, Hägg E: Factors influencing admission blood pressure levels in patients with acute stroke. Stroke 1991;22:527–530.

8 Fogelholm R, Avikainen S, Murros K: Prognostic value and determinants of first-day mean arterial pressure in spontaneous supratentorial intracerebral hemorrhage. Stroke 1997;28:1396–1400.

9 Terayama Y, Tanahashi N, Fukuuchi Y, et al: Prognostic value of admission blood pressure in patients with intracerebral hemorrhage: Keio cooperative stroke study. Stroke 1997;28:1185–1188.

10 Lisk DR, Pasteur W, Rhoades H, et al: Early presentation of hemispheric intracerebral hemorrhage: prediction of outcome and guidelines for treatment allocation. Neurology 1994;44:133–139.

11 Willmot M, Leonardi-Bee J, Bath PMW: High blood pressure in acute stroke and subsequent outcome: a systematic review. Hypertension 2004;43:18–24.

12 Vemmos KN, Tsivgoulis G, Spengos K, et al: U-shaped relationship between mortality and admission blood pressure in patients with acute stroke. J Intern Med 2004;255:257–265.

13 Powers WJ, Zazulia AR, Videen TO, et al: Autoregulation of cerebral blood flow surrounding acute (6–22 h) intracerebral hemorrhage. Neurology 2001;57:18–24.

14 Oeinck M, Neunhoeffer F, Buttler K, et al: Dynamic cerebral autoregulation in acute intracerebral hemorrhage. Stroke 2013;44:2722–2728.

15 Kazui S, Minematsu S, Yamamoto H, et al: Predisposing factors to enlargement of intracerebral hematoma. Stroke 1997;28:2370–2375.

16 Sykora MM, Diedler JM, Rupp AP, et al: Impaired baroreceptor sensitivity predicts outcome in acute intracerebral haemorrhage. Crit Care Med 2008;36:3074–3079.

17 Broderick J, Brott T, Tomsick T: Ultra-early evaluation of intracerebral haemorrhage. J Neurosurg 1990;72:195–199.

18 Chen ST, Chen SD, Hsu CY, et al: Progression of hypertensive intracerebral hemorrhage. Neurology 1989;39:1509–1514.

19 Jauch EC, Lindsell CJ, Adeoye O, et al: Lack of evidence for an association between hemodynamic variables and hematoma growth in spontaneous intracerebral hemorrhage. Stroke 2006;37:2061.

20 Marti-Fabregas J, Martinez-Ramirez S, Martinez-Corral M, et al: Blood pressure is not associated with haematoma enlargement in acute intracerebral haemorrhage. Eur J Neurol 2008;15:1085–1090.
21 Vemmos KN, Tsivgoulis G, Spengos K, et al: Association between 24-h blood pressure monitoring variables and brain oedema in patients with hyperacute stroke. J Hypertens 2003;21:2167–2173.
22 McCourt R, Gould B, Gioia L, et al: Cerebral perfusion and blood pressure do not affect perihematoma edema growth in acute intracerebral hemorrhage. Stroke 2014;45:1292–1298.
23 Steiner T, Al-Shahi Salman R, Beer R, et al: European Stroke Organisation (ESO) guidelines for the management of spontaneous intracerebral hemorrhage. Int J Stroke 2014;9:840–855.
24 Morgenstern LB, Hemphill JC, Anderson C, et al: Guidelines for the management of spontaneous intracerebral hemorrhage: a guideline for healthcare professionals from the American Heart Association/American Stroke Association. Stroke 2010;41:2108–2129.
25 Broderick J, Connolly S, Feldmann E, et al: Guidelines for the management of spontaneous intracerebral hemorrhage in adults: 2007 update: a guideline from the American Heart Association/American Stroke Association Stroke Council, High Blood Pressure Research Council, and the Quality of Care and Outcomes in Research Interdisciplinary Working Group: the American Academy of Neurology affirms the value of this guideline as an educational tool for neurologists. Stroke 2007;38:2001–2023.
26 Qureshi AI, Mohammad YM, Yahia AM, et al: A prospective multicenterstudy to evaluate the feasibility and safety of aggressive antihypertensive treatment in patients with acute intracerebral hemorrhage. J Intensive Care Med 2005;20:44–52.
27 Ohwaki K, Yano E, Nagashima H, et al: Blood pressure management in acute intracerebral hemorrhage: relationship between elevated blood pressure and hematoma enlargement. Stroke 2004;35:1364–1367.
28 Butcher KS, Jeerakathil T, Hill M, et al: The intracerebral haemorrhage acutely decreasing arterial pressure trial (ICH ADAPT): final results. International Stroke Conference Oral Abstracts, 2013.
29 Antihypertensive Treatment of Acute Cerebral Hemorrhage (ATACH) Investigators: Antihypertensive treatment of acute cerebral hemorrhage. Crit Care Med 2010;38:637–648.
30 Anderson CS, Huang Y, Wang JG, et al: Intensive blood pressure reduction in acute cerebral haemorrhage trial (INTERACT): a randomised pilot trial. Lancet Neurol 2008;7:391–399.
31 Anderson CS, Heeley E, Huang Y, et al: Rapid blood-pressure lowering in patients with acute intracerebral hemorrhage. N Engl J Med 2013;368:2355–2365.
32 ENOS Trial Investigators, Bath PM, Woodhouse L, et al: Efficacy of nitric oxide, with or without continuing antihypertensive treatment, for management of high blood pressure in acute stroke (ENOS): a partial-factorial randomised controlled trial. Lancet 2015;385:617–628.
33 Ankolekar S, Fuller M, Cross I, et al: Feasibility of an ambulance-based stroke trial, and safety of glyceryl trinitrate in ultra-acute stroke: the rapid intervention with glyceryl trinitrate in hypertensive stroke trial (RIGHT, ISRCTN66434824). Stroke 2013;44:3120–3128.
34 Sandset EC, Bath PM, Boysen G, et al: The angiotensin-receptor blocker candesartan for treatment of acute stroke (SCAST): a randomised, placebo-controlled, double-blind trial. Lancet 2011;377:741–750.
35 Berge E, Jusufovic M, Sandset EC, et al: Blood pressure lowering treatment with candesartan in patients with acute haemorrhagic stroke. Cerebrovasc Dis 2014;37(suppl 1):1–709.
36 Qureshi AI, Palesch Y: Antihypertensive treatment of acute cerebral hemorrhage (ATACH) II: design, methods, and rationale. Neurocrit Care 2011;15:559–576.
37 Arima H, Huang Y, Wang JG, et al: Earlier blood pressure-lowering and greater attenuation of hematoma growth in acute intracerebral hemorrhage: INTERACT pilot phase. Stroke 2012;43:2236–2238.
38 Stapf C, Heeley E, Delcourt C, et al: Abstract 180: the relation of timing and degree of blood pressure control with hematoma growth – secondary analysis of the Interact2 trial. Stroke 2014;45:A180.
39 Anderson CS, Wu G, Arima H, et al: Early intensive BP lowering treatment reduces perihaematomal oedema in intracerebral haemorrhage: pooled analysis of INTERACT studies. Cerebrovasc Dis 2014;37(suppl 1):1–709.
40 Rothwell PM: Limitations of the usual blood-pressure hypothesis and importance of variability, instability, and episodic hypertension. Lancet 2010;375:938–948.
41 Webb AJ, Fischer U, Mehta Z, et al: Effects of antihypertensive-drug class on interindividual variation in blood pressure and risk of stroke: a systematic review and meta-analysis. Lancet 2010;375:906–915.
42 Rodriguez-Luna D, Piñeiro S, Rubiera M, et al: Impact of blood pressure changes and course on hematoma growth in acute intracerebral hemorrhage. Eur J Neurol 2013;20:1277–1283.

43 Manning L, Hirakawa Y, Arima H, et al: Blood pressure variability and outcome after acute intracerebral haemorrhage: a post-hoc analysis of INTERACT2, a randomised controlled trial. Lancet Neurol 2014;13:364–373.
44 Webb A, Fischer U, Rothwell P: Effects of beta blocker selectivity on blood pressure variability and stroke: a systematic review. Neurology 2011;77:713–737.
45 Peacock WF 4th, Hilleman DE, Levy PD, et al: A systematic review of nicardipine vs labetalol for the management of hypertensive crises. Am J Emerg Med 2012;30:981–993.
46 Potter JF, Robinson TG, Ford GA, et al: Controlling hypertension and hypotension immediately post-stroke (CHHIPS): a randomised, placebo-controlled, double-blind pilot trial. Lancet Neurol 2009; 8:48–56.
47 Lui-DeRyke X, Janisse J, Coplin W, et al: A comparison of nicardipine and labetalol for acute hypertension management following acute stroke. Neurocrit Care 2008;9:167–176.
48 Pollack C, Varon J, Garrison NA, et al: Clevidipine is safe and effective for treatment of patients with acute severe hypertension. Ann Emerg Med 2009;53:329–338.
49 Graffagnino C, Bergese S, Love J, et al: Clevidipine rapidly and safely reduces blood pressure in acute intracerebral haemorrhage: The ACCELERATE trial. Cerebrovasc Dis 2013;36:180.
50 Cherney D, Straus S: Management of patients with hypertensive urgencies and emergencies. A systematic review of the literature. J Gen Intern Med 2002; 17:937–945.

Prof. Thompson G. Robinson
Department of Cardiovascular Sciences and NIHR Biomedical Research Unit in Cardiovascular Disease, University of Leicester
Leicester Royal Infirmary, Infirmary Square
Leicester LE2 7LX (UK)
E-Mail tgr2@leicester.ac.uk

Toyoda K, Anderson CS, Mayer SA (eds): New Insights in Intracerebral Hemorrhage.
Front Neurol Neurosci. Basel, Karger, 2016, vol 37, pp 51–61 (DOI: 10.1159/000437113)

Emergency Reversal Strategies for Anticoagulation and Platelet Disorders

Marcel Levi

Department of Vascular Medicine and Department of Medicine, Academic Medical Center, University of Amsterdam, Amsterdam, The Netherlands

Abstract

Bleeding is the most important adverse effect of antithrombotic treatment and may be a major cause of morbidity, longstanding debilitation, and even mortality. In the case of severe hemorrhage in a patient who uses anticoagulant agents, it may be crucial to reverse anticoagulant treatment. Conventional anticoagulants such as vitamin K antagonists can be neutralized by the administration of vitamin K or prothrombin complex concentrates, whereas heparin and heparin derivatives can be counteracted by protamine sulfate. The antihemostatic effect of aspirin and other antiplatelet strategies can be corrected by the administration of platelet concentrate and/or desmopressin. Recently, a new generation of anticoagulants with a greater specificity toward activated coagulation factors as well as new antiplatelet agents have been introduced, and these drugs show efficacy and safety profiles that are at least as good as those of conventional agents in clinical studies. A limitation of these new agents may be the lack of a specific strategy to reverse their effects if a bleeding event occurs, although experimental studies show encouraging results for some of these agents.

© 2016 S. Karger AG, Basel

Introduction

Anticoagulant agents are frequently used for the prevention and treatment of a wide range of cardiovascular diseases. The most often used anticoagulants are heparin and its derivatives; vitamin K antagonists (VKAs) (such as warfarin or coumadin); and antiplatelet agents, including aspirin and thienopyridine derivatives such as clopidogrel or prasugrel. A myriad of clinical studies have demonstrated that these agents (alone or in combination) can prevent or treat acute or chronic thromboembolic complications [1]. The most important complication of treatment with

Table 1. Currently available reversal strategies for anticoagulant and antiplatelet agents

	Time until restoration of hemostasis after cessation of therapeutic dose	Reversing agent	Remark
VKAs	Warfarin: 60–80 h Acenocoumarol: 18–24 h Phenprocoumon: 8–10 days	Vitamin K i.v.: reversal in 12–16 h Vitamin K oral: reversal in 24 h PCCs: immediate reversal	Dose of vitamin K or PCCs depends on INR and body weight
Heparin	3–4 h	Protamine sulfate 25–30 mg; immediate reversal	1 mg of protamine per 100 anti-Xa units given in the last 2–3 h
LMW heparin	12–24 h	Protamine sulfate 25–50 mg; immediate (partial) reversal	1 mg of protamine per 100 anti-Xa units given in the last 8 h
Oral factor Xa inhibitors	Dependent on compound, usually within 12 h	PCCs (1,500–3,000 U)*	Based on laboratory end-points, no systematic experience in bleeding patients
Oral thrombin inhibitors	Dependent on compound, usually within 12 h	Possibly PCCs (1,500–3,000 U)*	Based on laboratory end-points, no systematic experience in bleeding patients
Aspirin	5–10 days (time to produce unaffected platelets)	DDAVP (0.3–0.4 μg/kg) and/or platelet concentrate; reversal in 15–30 min	Cessation not always required, also dependent on clinical situation and indication
Clopidogrel Prasugrel Cangrelor	1–2 days	Platelet concentrate, possibly in combination with DDAVP (0.3–0.4 μg/kg); reversal in 15–30 min	Cessation not always desirable, also dependent on clinical situation and indication

* Experimental treatment. VKAs = Vitamin K antagonists; i.v. = intravenous; LMW heparin = low-molecular-weight heparin; PCC = prothrombin complex concentrate; INR = international normalized ratio; DDAVP = de-amino d-arginine vasopressin or desmopressin.

anticoagulants is hemorrhage, which may be serious, may cause long-term debilitating disease, and may even be life-threatening [2]. Nevertheless, in many situations, clinical studies have shown a favorable balance between efficacy and safety in favor of anticoagulant treatment. However, if severe bleeding occurs, such as in the case of intracerebral hemorrhage, reversal of the anticoagulant effect of the various agents may be required (table 1) [3]. Depending on the clinical situation, i.e. the severity of the bleeding, this reversal may take place in a few hours, but in some cases, immediate reversal is necessary [4, 5]. Generally, each (immediate) reversal of anticoagulant treatment must also take into consideration the indication for the antithrombotic agents. For example, the interruption of combined aspirin and clopidogrel treatment in a patient in whom an intracoronary stent has recently been inserted will markedly increase the risk of acute stent thrombosis, with consequent downstream cardiac ischemia or infarction. Likewise, in a patient with a prosthetic mitral valve and atrial fibrillation, the interruption of VKAs may increase the risk of valve thrombosis and cerebral or systemic embolism. Each of these specific clinical situations requires a careful and balanced assessment of the benefits and risks of reversing anticoagulants (and potential strategies to keep the period of reversal as short as possible).

Incidence and Risk Factors for Bleeding in Patients on Old and New Anticoagulants

Currently, VKAs (such as warfarin, coumadin, acenocoumarol and phenprocoumon) are the most frequently used anticoagulant agents for the long-term prevention and treatment of a wide range of cardiovascular diseases. In well-controlled patients in clinical trials, treatment with VKAs increased the risk of major bleeding by 0.5%/year and the risk of intracranial hemorrhage by about 0.2%/year [6]. However, in three real-life surveys, this incidence varied from 1.35 to 3.4%/year [7–9]. The incidence of intracranial hemorrhage was 0.2%/year in the clinical trials, compared with 0.4–0.6%/year in the unselected samples. Similarly, antiplatelet agents significantly increase the risk and the extent of intracranial hemorrhage [10–12]. One must realize that the relatively uncomplicated trial populations may poorly reflect the real-life setting in which anticoagulants are prescribed. For example, in 6 pivotal trials that demonstrated the superiority of warfarin to placebo in the prevention of thromboembolic complications in patients with atrial fibrillation, 28,787 patients were screened, but only 12.6% of these patients were included in the studies [13]. Recently, a new generation of oral anticoagulants with direct inhibitory properties toward thrombin or factor Xa has been developed, and these agents are currently being evaluated in clinical trials. Specific details regarding these agents will be discussed below; however, generally speaking, the most important side effect of these agents is still (major) hemorrhage.

The most important risk factor for hemorrhage in users of anticoagulants is the intensity of the anticoagulant effect [6]. Studies indicate that with a target international normalized ratio (INR) of >3.0, the incidence of major bleeding is twice as high as with a target INR of 2.0–3.0 [14]. In a meta-analysis of studies in patients with prosthetic heart valves, a lower INR target range resulted in a lower frequency of major bleeding and intracranial hemorrhage but similar antithrombotic efficacy [15]. A retrospective analysis of outpatients using warfarin who presented with intracranial hemorrhage demonstrated that the risk of this complication doubled for each 1-unit increase in the INR [16]. Additionally, for low-molecular-weight (LMW) heparin, the bleeding risk is related to its dose: low-dose prophylactic heparin doubles the risk of major hemorrhage, although the absolute incidence is very low [17]. Higher doses of LMW heparin are usually given for short time periods but are also associated with major bleeding. In a retrospective analysis from a study of patients with acute coronary syndromes, it was shown that with every 10 s prolongation of the activated partial thromboplastin time (aPTT), the incidence of major hemorrhage increased by 7% [18]. For new oral antithrombin or anti-factor Xa agents (such as dabigatran, apixaban, and rivaroxaban), a clear relationship between the dose and the incidence of bleeding complications has been demonstrated as well.

Patient characteristics constitute another important determinant of the bleeding risk [19]. Elderly patients have a 2-fold increased risk of bleeding [20], and the relative risk of intracranial hemorrhage (particularly at higher intensities of anticoagulation) is 2.5-fold higher (95% CI 2.3–9.4) in patients >85 years old compared with patients aged 70–74 years [21]. Co-morbidities, such as renal or hepatic insufficiency, may also significantly increase the risk of bleeding. A case-control study of 1,986 patients on VKAs showed that this comorbidity increased the risk of bleeding by about 2.5-fold [13]. Another very important determinant of the risk of bleeding is the combined use of medications that affect both the coagulation system and platelet function. Two meta-analyses, comprising 6 trials with a total of 3,874 patients and 10 trials with a total of 5,938 patients, found that the relative risk of major bleeding when antithrombotic agents were combined with aspirin was 2.4 (95% CI 1.2–4.8) and 2.5 (95% CI 1.7–3.7), respectively [22, 23].

Reversal of Conventional Anticoagulants

When interrupting the administration of VKAs, important differences in the half-lives of the various agents (9 h for acenocoumarol, 36–42 h for warfarin, and 90 h for phenprocoumon) need to be taken into account [24]. The most straightforward intervention to counteract the effect of VKAs is the administration of vitamin K [25]. A recent randomized controlled trial did not find any difference in bleeding or other complications in nonbleeding patients with INR values of 4.5–10 who were treated with vitamin K or placebo [26]. In patients with clinically significant bleeding, however, the administration of vitamin K is crucial to reverse the anticoagulant effect of VKAs. Vitamin K can be given orally and intravenously, whereas the parenteral route has the advantage of a more rapid onset of the treatment [27]. After the administration of intravenous (i.v.) vitamin K, the INR will start to drop within 2 h and will be completely normalized within 12–16 h [28], whereas after oral administration, it will take up to 24 h to normalize the INR [25]. An often-voiced concern with the use of parenteral vitamin K is the occurrence of anaphylactic reactions; however, with the more modern micelle preparations, the incidence of this complication is very low [29]. In the case of very serious or even life-threatening bleeding, immediate correction of the INR is mandatory and can be achieved by the administration of vitamin K-dependent coagulation factors. Prothrombin complex concentrates (PCCs), containing all vitamin K-dependent coagulation factors, are more useful. In a prospective study in patients using VKAs and presenting with bleeding, the administration of PCCs resulted in at least satisfactory and sustained hemostasis in 98% of patients [30].

In recent years, the safety of PCCs, particularly regarding the transmission of blood-borne infectious diseases, has markedly improved owing to several techniques, such as pasteurization, nanofiltration, and the addition of solvent detergent.

Heparin has a relatively short half-life of about 60–90 min; therefore, the anticoagulant effect of therapeutic doses of heparin will be mostly eliminated at 3–4 h after the termination of continuous i.v. administration [31]. The anticoagulant effect of high-dose subcutaneous heparin, however, will take a longer time to abolish. If more immediate neutralization of heparin is required, i.v. protamine sulfate is the antidote of choice. Protamine, derived from fish sperm, binds to heparin to form a stable biologically inactive complex. Each milligram of protamine will neutralize approximately 100 units of heparin. Hence, the protamine dose in a patient on a stable therapeutic heparin dose of 1,000–1,250 U/h should be about 25–30 mg (sufficient to block the amount of heparin given in the last 2–3 h). The reversal of LMW heparin is more complex, as protamine sulfate will only neutralize anti-factor IIa activity and has no or only a partial effect on the smaller heparin fragments causing the anti-factor Xa activity of the compound [32, 33]. A practical approach is to give 1 mg of protamine per 100 anti-factor Xa units of LMW heparin given in the last 8 h (whereas 1 mg of enoxaparin equals 100 anti-factor Xa units). If bleeding continues, a second dose of 0.5 mg per 100 anti-factor Xa units can be given. There are some other strategies to reverse (mostly unfractionated) heparin, such as platelet factor-4, heparanase, or extracorporeal heparin-removal devices, but none of these approaches has been properly evaluated, and they are not currently approved for clinical use [5].

Reversal of New Direct Factor Xa Inhibitors

In recent years, a large number of new antithrombotic agents have been developed and tested in clinical trials, and many of these new agents will become widely available for clinical practice in the very near future [34]. One of the main advantages of these new agents is their relatively stable pharmacokinetic and pharmacodynamic properties (at least in the populations studied so far), which obviates the need for repeated control of the intensity of anticoagulation and for dose adjustments.

Some of these new classes of anticoagulants are directed at factor Xa. The prototypes of these agents are rivaroxaban and apixaban, which have shown promising results in clinical studies [35–38]. Taken together, the results of these studies indicate that compared with LMW heparin, direct factor Xa inhibitors result in a lower bleeding risk at doses achieving equivalent efficacy and in a similar bleeding risk at doses achieving higher efficacy. This means that in some clinical situations, these drugs may represent an important improvement; however, the risk of (major) bleeding is still present. It should be noted that most trials thus far were conducted in a relatively young population with limited co-morbidities (e.g., renal insufficiency). It is not yet clear how the benefit-risk ratio of the new agents will work out in 'real-life' populations of anticoagulant agent users, who are likely to be older and affected by various other disorders that may affect the bleeding risk. Moreover, the combined use of the new anticoagulant agents and antiplatelet agents was discouraged in clinical trials, whereas this is increasingly common in clinical practice and may also have a serious impact on the risk of hemorrhage.

Depending on the severity of the clinical situation and in view of the half-lives of the direct Xa inhibitors, the cessation of medication may be sufficient to reverse the anticoagulant effect in the case of bleeding. However, if immediate reversal of anticoagulation is required, there is no solid evidence regarding the anticoagulant effect of any of the orally available factor Xa inhibitors thus far. It was shown that the administration of PCCs resulted in a correction of the prolonged prothrombin time and restored depressed thrombin generation after rivaroxaban treatment in a controlled trial in healthy human volunteers [39, 40]. In view of the relatively wide availability of PCCs, this would be an interesting option if the results can be confirmed in patients on oral factor Xa inhibitors who present with bleeding complications. Alternatively, activated PCCs have been studied and shown to have similar effects; however, these agents may be associated with more thromboembolic complications. Lastly, a specific antidote for anti-factor Xa agents (a truncated form of enzymatically inactive factor Xa that binds to and reverses the anticoagulant action of the factor Xa inhibitors) is currently being evaluated [41]. Monitoring of the reversal of the anticoagulant effect of factor Xa inhibitors is most simply done by measuring the prothrombin time, although there is some variability between reagents for measuring the prothrombin time, and for some agents, the anti-factor Xa assay is more reliable [42, 43].

Reversal of Direct Thrombin Inhibitors

Another important group of new anticoagulants consists of direct thrombin inhibitors. Thrombin is the central enzyme in the coagulation process, not only mediating the conversion of fibrinogen to fibrin but also acting as the most important physiological activator of platelets and various other coagulation factors. The prototype of these thrombin inhibitors is hirudin, originally derived from the saliva from leeches *(Hirudo medicinalis)* and currently produced by recombinant technology. Dabigatran is a direct thrombin inhibitor with good and relatively stable bioavailability after oral ingestion and does not have the adverse effect of causing bleeding. Dabigatran was shown to be effective in the prevention and treatment of both venous and arterial thromboembolism. However, the risk of major bleeding is still present and requires adequate management strategies. As mentioned for the anti-factor Xa agents, clinical trials in patients using antithrombin agents excluded many patients with common co-morbidities and discouraged the simultaneous use of agents affecting platelet function. Therefore, the risk of hemorrhage in these trials may represent an underestimation of the real-life bleeding risk.

For each of the direct thrombin inhibitors, no established reversing agent is available in the case of serious bleeding complicating the anticoagulant treatment. Fortunately, the half-lives of most of the agents are relatively short; hence, in the case of less serious bleeding, interruption of the treatment will be sufficient to reverse the anticoagulant effect. However, if immediate reversal is required, it is not clear which would be the best strategy. In a controlled clinical study in healthy subjects, melagatran-induced effects on the aPTT, thrombin generation and platelet activation were not affected by the administration of recombinant factor VIIa [44]. Based on these results, it seems that factor VIIa is not effective in reversing direct thrombin inhibition. Additionally, the administration of PCC did not cause any reversal of the anticoagulant effect of dabigatran in the above-mentioned controlled trial in healthy human subjects [39]. However, experimental animal studies in a model of intracerebral hemorrhage showed that dabigatran could be effectively reversed by PCCs [45]. Specific antidotes for the thrombin inhibitors are under development. Idarucizumab is a fragment of an antibody that is a specific antidote for the oral direct thrombin inhibitor dabigatran [41]. Monitoring of the anticoagulant effect of thrombin inhibitors in routine clinical practice is difficult. The aPTT is not very useful. The ecarin clotting time may be more accurate but is not readily available in most routine clinical settings. The most convenient and practically applicable measure for monitoring the anticoagulant effect may be the diluted thrombin time, which needs to be standardized for the specific agent that was used [46].

Reversal of Antiplatelet Agents

Aspirin is effective in the secondary prevention of atherothrombotic disease, and particularly coronary artery disease, cerebrovascular thromboembolism and peripheral arterial disease [47]. As a consequence, aspirin is the most widely used antithrombotic agent worldwide. Aspirin increases the risk of bleeding, and particularly gastrointestinal bleeding, and is associated with a small but consistent increase in intracerebral hemorrhage. In addition, it has been shown that the use of aspirin is associated with increased perioperative blood loss in major procedures, although this does not necessarily translate into clinically relevant end-points, such as the requirement for transfusion or re-operation [48]. Over the last few years, the approach to the patient who uses aspirin and who presents with bleeding or needs to undergo an invasive procedure has changed considerably. In fact, in current clinical practice, bleeding can almost always be managed with local hemostatic procedures or conservative strategies without interrupting aspirin use, and most invasive procedures also do not require the cessation of aspirin when adequate attention is given to local hemostasis. In contrast, interruption of aspirin has been associated with an increased risk of thromboembolic complications, potentially due to rebound hypercoagulability. Nevertheless, under special clinical circumstances, such as intracranial bleeding or the need to undergo a neurosurgical or ophthalmic procedure, the antihemostatic effect of aspirin needs to be reversed immediately. The most rigorous measure to achieve that is the administration of platelet concentrate after the cessation of aspirin. Another approach is the administration of de-amino d-arginine vasopressin (DDAVP, desmopressin) [49]. The combined effect of platelet concentrate and the subsequent administration of DDAVP has also been advocated to correct aspirin's effect on platelets. The standard dose of DDAVP is 0.3–0.4 μg/kg in 100 ml saline over 30 min, and its effect is immediate.

Thienopyridine derivatives (such as clopidogrel, prasugrel and cangrelor) act by blocking the adenosine diphosphate receptor on platelets. Importantly, the combination of aspirin and clopidogrel, prasugrel or cangrelor is vastly superior to aspirin alone in patients who have received intracoronary stents and in other patients with high-risk coronary artery disease. There is ample evidence that dual platelet inhibition by aspirin plus a thienopyridine derivative has significantly higher efficacy than aspirin alone in patients with acute coronary syndromes who have undergone coronary interventions for at least a year (and possibly longer) since the event. However, the increased efficacy of the combined use of these agents is also associated with a significantly higher bleeding risk [50]. Taken together, these results indicate that dual platelet inhibition, particularly with clopidogrel or, even more notably, with prasugrel or cangrelor, is highly effective in high-risk patients with coronary artery disease, but the bleeding risk with dual platelet inhibition is something to take into account, and strategies to reverse the antiplatelet effect may be warranted in the case of serious bleeding.

The decision of whether or not to interrupt or even reverse antithrombotic treatment with dual platelet inhibition in the case of serious bleeding will depend not only on the specific clinical situation but also on the indication for the antithrombotic treatment (see above). Especially in patients with recent implantation of an intracoronary stent (in the last 6–12 weeks), cardiologists will often not agree or only reluctantly agree with the cessation of treatment [51]. In this period, re-endothelialization of the stent has not yet occurred, and the patient is very vulnerable to acute thrombotic occlusion of the stent. In patients with drug-eluting stents, this period may be even longer. If, however, the decision is made to stop and even reverse the treatment with aspirin and clopidogrel, the administration of platelet concentrate is probably the best way to correct the hemostatic defect [52]. In addition, DDAVP was shown to correct the defect in platelet aggregation caused by clopidogrel and thus may be another option [53].

Conclusion

Conventional anticoagulant treatment can be reversed by specific interventions when the clinical situation requires the immediate correction of hemostasis. For the new generation of anticoagulants, no specific antidotes or reversing agents are available; although some interventions are promising, they need further evaluation. Antiplatelet therapy with aspirin, either alone or in combination with thienopyridine derivatives such as clopidogrel and prasugrel, can be reversed, but this is often not required and sometimes not desirable in view of the indication for this treatment.

References

1 Hirsh J, Guyatt G, Albers GW, Harrington R, Schunemann HJ: Antithrombotic and thrombolytic therapy: American College of Chest Physicians Evidence-Based Clinical Practice Guidelines, ed 8. Chest 2008; 133:110S–112S.

2 Mannucci PM, Levi M: Prevention and treatment of major blood loss. N Engl J Med 2007;356:2301–2311.

3 Levi M, Eerenberg E, Kamphuisen PW: Periprocedural reversal and bridging of anticoagulant treatment. Neth J Med 2011;69:268–273.

4 Levi M: Emergency reversal of antithrombotic treatment. Intern Emerg Med 2009;4:137–145.

5 Levi MM, Eerenberg E, Lowenberg E, Kamphuisen PW: Bleeding in patients using new anticoagulants or antiplatelet agents: risk factors and management. Neth J Med 2010;68:68–76.

6 Schulman S, Beyth RJ, Kearon C, Levine MN: Hemorrhagic complications of anticoagulant and thrombolytic treatment: American College of Chest Physicians Evidence-Based Clinical Practice Guidelines, ed 8. Chest 2008;133:257S–298S.

7 Palareti G, Leali N, Coccheri S, Poggi M, Manotti C, D'Angelo A, Pengo V, Erba N, Moia M, Ciavarella N, Devoto G, Berrettini M, Musolesi S: Bleeding complications of oral anticoagulant treatment: an inception-cohort, prospective collaborative study (ISCOAT). Italian Study on Complications of Oral Anticoagulant Therapy. Lancet 1996;348:423–428.

8 Abdelhafiz AH, Wheeldon NM: Results of an open-label, prospective study of anticoagulant therapy for atrial fibrillation in an outpatient anticoagulation clinic. Clin Ther 2004;26:1470–1478.

9 Jackson SL, Peterson GM, Vial JH, Daud R, Ang SY: Outcomes in the management of atrial fibrillation: clinical trial results can apply in practice. Intern Med J 2001;31:329–336.

10 Toyoda K, Okada Y, Minematsu K, Kamouchi M, Fujimoto S, Ibayashi S, Inoue T: Antiplatelet therapy contributes to acute deterioration of intracerebral hemorrhage. Neurology 2005;65:1000–1004.

11 Toyoda K, Yasaka M, Nagata K, Nagao T, Gotoh J, Sakamoto T, Uchiyama S, Minematsu K: Antithrombotic therapy influences location, enlargement, and mortality from intracerebral hemorrhage. The Bleeding with Antithrombotic Therapy (BAT) Retrospective Study. Cerebrovasc Dis 2009;27:151–159.

12 Thompson BB, Bejot Y, Caso V, Castillo J, Christensen H, Flaherty ML, Foerch C, Ghandehari K, Giroud M, Greenberg SM, Hallevi H, Hemphill JC III, Heuschmann P, Juvela S, Kimura K, Myint PK, Nagakane Y, Naritomi H, Passero S, Rodriguez-Yanez MR, Roquer J, Rosand J, Rost NS, Saloheimo P, Salomaa V, Sivenius J, Sorimachi T, Togha M, Toyoda K, Turaj W, Vemmos KN, Wolfe CD, Woo D, Smith EE: Prior antiplatelet therapy and outcome following intracerebral hemorrhage: a systematic review. Neurology 2010;75:1333–1342.

13 Levi M, Hovingh GK, Cannegieter SC, Vermeulen M, Buller HR, Rosendaal FR: Bleeding in patients receiving vitamin K antagonists who would have been excluded from trials on which the indication for anticoagulation was based. Blood 2008;111:4471–4476.

14 Saour JN, Sieck JO, Mamo LA, Gallus AS: Trial of different intensities of anticoagulation in patients with prosthetic heart valves. N Engl J Med 1990;322: 428–432.

15 Vink R, Kraaijenhagen RA, Hutten BA, van den Brink RB, de Mol BA, Buller HR, Levi M: The optimal intensity of vitamin K antagonists in patients with mechanical heart valves: a meta-analysis. J Am Coll Cardiol 2003;42:2042–2048.

16 Hylek EM, Singer DE: Risk factors for intracranial hemorrhage in outpatients taking warfarin. Ann Intern Med 1994;120:897–902.

17 Geerts WH, Bergqvist D, Pineo GF, Heit JA, Samama CM, Lassen MR, Colwell CW: Prevention of venous thromboembolism: American College of Chest Physicians Evidence-Based Clinical Practice Guidelines, ed 8. Chest 2008;133:381S–453S.

18 Anand SS, Bates S, Ginsberg JS, Levine M, Buller H, Prins M, Haley S, Kearon C, Hirsh J, Gent M: Recurrent venous thrombosis and heparin therapy: an evaluation of the importance of early activated partial thromboplastin times. Arch Intern Med 1999; 159:2029–2032.

19 Levi M, Eerenberg E, Kamphuisen PW: Bleeding risk and reversal strategies for old and new anticoagulants and antiplatelet agents. J Thromb Haemost 2011;9:1705–1712.

20 Hutten BA, Lensing AW, Kraaijenhagen RA, Prins MH: Safety of treatment with oral anticoagulants in the elderly. A systematic review. Drugs Aging 1999; 14:303–312.

21 Fang MC, Chang Y, Hylek EM, Rosand J, Greenberg SM, Go AS, Singer DE: Advanced age, anticoagulation intensity, and risk for intracranial hemorrhage among patients taking warfarin for atrial fibrillation. Ann Intern Med 2004;141:745–752.

22 Hart RG, Benavente O, Pearce LA: Increased risk of intracranial hemorrhage when aspirin is combined with warfarin: a meta-analysis and hypothesis. Cerebrovasc Dis 1999;9:215–217.

23 Rothberg MB, Celestin C, Fiore LD, Lawler E, Cook JR: Warfarin plus aspirin after myocardial infarction or the acute coronary syndrome: meta-analysis with estimates of risk and benefit. Ann Intern Med 2005; 143:241–250.

24 Ansell J, Hirsh J, Hylek E, Jacobson A, Crowther M, Palareti G: Pharmacology and management of the vitamin K antagonists: American College of Chest Physicians Evidence-Based Clinical Practice Guidelines, ed 8. Chest 2008;133:160S–198S.

25 Dentali F, Ageno W, Crowther M: Treatment of coumarin-associated coagulopathy: a systematic review and proposed treatment algorithms. J Thromb Haemost 2006;4:1853–1863.

26 Crowther MA, Ageno W, Garcia D, Wang L, Witt DM, Clark NP, Blostein MD, Kahn SR, Vesely S, Schulman S, Kovacs MJ, Rodger MA, Wells P, Anderson D, Ginsberg JS, Selby R, Siragusa S, Silingardi M, Dowd MB, Kearon C: Oral vitamin K versus placebo to correct excessive anticoagulation in patients receiving warfarin. Ann Intern Med 2009;150:293–300.

27 Crowther MA, Douketis JD, Schnurr T, Steidl L, Mera V, Ultori C, Venco A, Ageno W: Oral vitamin K lowers the international normalized ratio more rapidly than subcutaneous vitamin K in the treatment of warfarin-associated coagulopathy. A randomized, controlled trial. Ann Intern Med 2002;137: 251–254.

28 Lubetsky A, Yonath H, Olchovsky D, Loebstein R, Halkin H, Ezra D: Comparison of oral vs intravenous phytonadione (vitamin K1) in patients with excessive anticoagulation: a prospective randomized controlled study. Arch Intern Med 2003;163:2469–2473.

29 Dentali F, Ageno W: Management of coumarin-associated coagulopathy in the non-bleeding patient: a systematic review. Haematologica 2004;89:857–862.

30 Pabinger I, Brenner B, Kalina U, Knaub S, Nagy A, Ostermann H: Prothrombin complex concentrate (Beriplex P/N) for emergency anticoagulation reversal: a prospective multinational clinical trial. J Thromb Haemost 2008;6:622–631.

31 Hirsh J, Bauer KA, Donati MB, Gould M, Samama MM, Weitz JI: Parenteral anticoagulants: American College of Chest Physicians Evidence-Based Clinical Practice Guidelines, ed 8. Chest 2008;133:141S–159S.

32 Lindblad B, Borgstrom A, Wakefield TW, Whitehouse WM Jr, Stanley JC: Protamine reversal of anticoagulation achieved with a low molecular weight heparin. The effects on eicosanoids, clotting and complement factors. Thromb Res 1987;48:31–40.

33 Massonnet-Castel S, Pelissier E, Bara L, Terrier E, Abry B, Guibourt P, Swanson J, Jaulmes B, Carpentier A, Samama M: Partial reversal of low molecular weight heparin (PK 10169) anti-Xa activity by protamine sulfate: in vitro and in vivo study during cardiac surgery with extracorporeal circulation. Haemostasis 1986;16:139–146.

34 Garcia D, Libby E, Crowther MA: The new oral anticoagulants. Blood 2010;115:15–20.

35 Agnelli G, Gallus A, Goldhaber SZ, Haas S, Huisman MV, Hull RD, Kakkar AK, Misselwitz F, Schellong S: Treatment of proximal deep-vein thrombosis with the oral direct factor Xa inhibitor rivaroxaban (BAY 59–7939): the ODIXa-DVT (Oral Direct Factor Xa Inhibitor BAY 59–7939 in Patients With Acute Symptomatic Deep-Vein Thrombosis) study. Circulation 2007;116:180–187.

36 Shantsila E, Lip GY: Apixaban, an oral, direct inhibitor of activated Factor Xa. Curr Opin Investig Drugs 2008;9:1020–1033.

37 ROCKET AF Study Investigators: Rivaroxaban-once daily, oral, direct factor Xa inhibition compared with vitamin K antagonism for prevention of stroke and Embolism Trial in Atrial Fibrillation: rationale and design of the ROCKET AF study. Am Heart J 2010; 159:340–347.

38 Buller HR, Lensing AW, Prins MH, Agnelli G, Cohen A, Gallus AS, Misselwitz F, Raskob G, Schellong S, Segers A: A dose-ranging study evaluating once-daily oral administration of the factor Xa inhibitor rivaroxaban in the treatment of patients with acute symptomatic deep vein thrombosis: the Einstein-DVT Dose-Ranging Study. Blood 2008;112:2242–2247.

39 Eerenberg ES, Kamphuisen PW, Sijpkens MK, Meijers JC, Buller HR, Levi M: Reversal of rivaroxaban and dabigatran by prothrombin complex concentrate: a randomized, placebo-controlled, crossover study in healthy subjects. Circulation 2011;124: 1573–1579.

40 Levi M, Moore KT, Castillejos CF, Kubitza D, Berkowitz SD, Goldhaber SZ, Raghoebar M, Patel MR, Weitz JI, Levy JH: Comparison of three-factor and four-factor prothrombin complex concentrates regarding reversal of the anticoagulant effects of rivaroxaban in healthy volunteers. J Thromb Haemost 2014;12:1428–1436.
41 Gomez-Outes A, Suarez-Gea ML, Lecumberri R, Isabel A, Fernandez T, Vargas-Castrillon E: Specific antidotes in development for reversal of novel anticoagulants: a review. Recent Pat Cardiovasc Drug Discov 2014;9:2–10.
42 Barrett YC, Wang Z, Frost C, Shenker A: Clinical laboratory measurement of direct factor Xa inhibitors: anti-Xa assay is preferable to prothrombin time assay. Thromb Haemost 2010;104:1263–1271.
43 Hillarp A, Baghaei F, Fagerberg B, I, Gustafsson KM, Stigendal L, Sten-Linder M, Strandberg K, Lindahl TL: Effects of the oral, direct factor Xa inhibitor rivaroxaban on commonly used coagulation assays. J Thromb Haemost 2011;9:133–139.
44 Woltz M, Levi M, Sarich TC, Bostrom SL, Ericksson UG, Erikkson-Lepkowska M, Svensson M, Weitz JI, Elg M, Wahlander K: Effect of recombinant factor VIIa on melagatran-induced inhibition of thrombin generation and platelet activation in healthy volunteers. Thromb Haemost 2004;91:1090–1096.
45 Van RJ, Stangier J, Haertter S, Liesenfeld KH, Wienen W, Feuring M, Clemens A: Dabigatran etexilate – a novel, reversible, oral direct thrombin inhibitor: interpretation of coagulation assays and reversal of anticoagulant activity. Thromb Haemost 2010;103:1116–1127.
46 Lindahl TL, Baghaei F, Blixter IF, Gustafsson KM, Stigendal L, Sten-Linder M, Strandberg K, Hillarp A: Effects of the oral, direct thrombin inhibitor dabigatran on five common coagulation assays. Thromb Haemost 2011;105:371–378.
47 Patrono C, Baigent C, Hirsh J, Roth G: Antiplatelet drugs: American College of Chest Physicians Evidence-Based Clinical Practice Guidelines, ed 8. Chest 2008;133:199S–233S.
48 Merritt JC, Bhatt DL: The efficacy and safety of perioperative antiplatelet therapy. J Thromb Thrombolysis 2004;17:21–27.
49 Mannucci PM: Desmopressin (DDAVP) in the treatment of bleeding disorders: the first 20 years. Blood 1997;90:2515–2521.
50 Yusuf S, Zhao F, Mehta SR, Chrolavicius S, Tognoni G, Fox KK: Effects of clopidogrel in addition to aspirin in patients with acute coronary syndromes without ST-segment elevation. N Engl J Med 2001;345: 494–502.
51 Grines CL, Bonow RO, Casey DE Jr, Gardner TJ, Lockhart PB, Moliterno DJ, O'Gara P, Whitlow P: Prevention of premature discontinuation of dual antiplatelet therapy in patients with coronary artery stents: a science advisory from the American Heart Association, American College of Cardiology, Society for Cardiovascular Angiography and Interventions, American College of Surgeons, and American Dental Association, with representation from the American College of Physicians. Catheter Cardiovasc Interv 2007;69:334–340.
52 Vilahur G, Choi BG, Zafar MU, Viles-Gonzalez JF, Vorchheimer DA, Fuster V, Badimon JJ: Normalization of platelet reactivity in clopidogrel-treated subjects. J Thromb Haemost 2007;5:82–90.
53 Leithauser B, Zielske D, Seyfert UT, Jung F: Effects of desmopressin on platelet membrane glycoproteins and platelet aggregation in volunteers on clopidogrel. Clin Hemorheol Microcirc 2008;39:293–302.

Dr. Marcel Levi
Department of Vascular Medicine and Department of Medicine
Academic Medical Center, University of Amsterdam
Meibergdreef 9
NL–1105 AZ Amsterdam (The Netherlands)
E-Mail m.m.levi@amc.uva.nl

Toyoda K, Anderson CS, Mayer SA (eds): New Insights in Intracerebral Hemorrhage.
Front Neurol Neurosci. Basel, Karger, 2016, vol 37, pp 62–77 (DOI: 10.1159/000437114)

Reperfusion-Related Intracerebral Hemorrhage

Mikito Hayakawa

Department of Cerebrovascular Medicine, National Cerebral and Cardiovascular Center, Suita, Osaka, Japan

Abstract

The efficacy of intravenous thrombolysis (IVT) for acute ischemic stroke patients has been well established worldwide, with endovascular therapy performed in patients who have failed or are ineligible for IVT and who have major vessel occlusion. The most feared complication of acute stroke reperfusion therapy is intracerebral hemorrhage (ICH), as these patients have a poor clinical outcome and high mortality. The fundamental mechanisms responsible for reperfusion-related ICH include increased permeability and disruption of the blood-brain barrier. Recombinant tissue plasminogen activator may exacerbate the blood-brain barrier disruption through its pharmacological action during IVT. Furthermore, interactions between the device and the vessel walls and contrast intoxication may also be related to ICH, which includes the occurrence of subarachnoid hemorrhage after endovascular therapy. Numerous factors have been reported to be associated with or to be able to predict ICH, and several scoring systems have been developed for predicting symptomatic ICH (sICH) after IVT. However, a scoring system with enough power to detect an unacceptably high risk of sICH or to provide information on when to withdraw IVT has yet to be definitively established. In current clinical practice, acute stroke patients without contraindications for IVT who have been identified by conventional computed tomography scans normally undergo IVT, irrespective of any clinical predictors of ICH after IVT. Strategies that have been suggested for preventing reperfusion-related ICH in high-risk patients include intensive blood pressure control, tight glycemic control, and the avoidance of early aggressive antithrombotic therapy. If sICH, and especially massive parenchymal hematoma, does occur, hematoma expansion needs to be prevented through the use of tight blood pressure control and other methods. Although evidence of efficacy has yet to be established, surgical removal is performed not only for the purpose of saving lives but also for improving the functional outcome. In order to develop therapeutic strategies for reperfusion-related ICH that will lead to an improved stroke prognosis, further studies are warranted.
© 2016 S. Karger AG, Basel

The efficacy of intravenous thrombolysis (IVT) for acute ischemic stroke patients using the recombinant tissue plasminogen activator (rt-PA) alteplase has been well established worldwide [1]. In patients who have failed or are ineligible for IVT and who have major artery occlusion, endovascular therapy (EVT) is also performed. In 2014, the Multicenter Randomized Clinical Trial of Endovascular Treatment for Acute Ischemic Stroke in the Netherlands (MR CLEAN) reported that acute reperfusion strategies that also used EVT were more effective than those that did not [2].

Intracerebral hemorrhage (ICH) can occur during reperfusion therapy and has been shown to be associated with a poor clinical outcome and high mortality. Therefore, ICH is one of the most feared complications of acute stroke reperfusion therapy.

In this chapter, the pathophysiology, frequency, clinical impact, predictors and treatment of ICH associated with reperfusion therapy, including IVT and EVT, are reviewed.

Pathophysiology

The pathophysiology of the complex phenomenon, reperfusion-related ICH, has yet to be completely elucidated. However, the fundamental mechanisms that lead to the extravasation of blood elements into the brain parenchyma have been reported to be increased permeability and disruption of the blood-brain barrier (BBB) [3]. The BBB consists of both the endothelial cell tight junctions of capillaries and the surrounding basal lamina, consisting of extracellular matrix (ECM) proteins. The end-feet of astrocytes encompass the outside of the basal lamina [4].

When ischemia suddenly occurs, endothelial swelling induces opening of the tight junctions, thereby causing increases in the permeability of the BBB. Furthermore, degradation of the ECM of the basal lamina occurs. Matrix metalloproteinase (MMP)-2 and MMP-9, which are generated in the astrocyte end-feet, play important roles in the ECM degradation process. Although reperfusion is essential for brain tissue survival, it can cause additional brain injury by itself during a process referred to as 'reperfusion injury'. During reperfusion, and especially when there is a delay before reperfusion begins, there is induction of oxygen free radicals, inflammatory responses, cytokine production and reactive hyperemia due to loss of vascular autoregulation. All of these events contribute to BBB disruption and to subsequent hemorrhagic transformation (HT), ICH and vasogenic edematous changes in the infarcted brain tissues [3, 5].

Using nonenhanced computed tomography (CT), the European Cooperative Acute Stroke Study (ECASS) devised a classification scheme that radiographically classified HT into 4 categories: hemorrhagic infarction (HI) type 1 (small hyperdense petechiae along the margins of the infarcted area), HI type 2 (more confluent petechiae throughout the infarcted area, but without a mass effect), parenchymal hematoma (PH) type 1 (a hematoma occupying ≤30% of the infarcted area) and PH type 2

(PH-2; a hematoma occupying >30% of the infarcted area, with a significant mass effect) [6]. HI seems to result from multifocal red blood cell extravasation, which can occur without antegrade reperfusion, while PH may represent ICH arising from a single damaged vessel due to ischemia and reperfusion injury [7, 8]. Posthoc analysis of the ECASS I and II trials, which were randomized controlled trials (RCTs) of IVT within 6 h of stroke onset, found that out of the 4 categories, only PH-2 had an impact on early neurological deterioration and long-term disability and mortality in patients when compared with patients without HT [9, 10]. In addition, most (73.5%) of the symptomatic ICH (sICH) in the ECASS II trial corresponded to PH [11].

Definition and Frequency of Symptomatic Intracerebral Hemorrhage

Among the reported clinical trials, the definitions of sICH have varied widely. The National Institute of Neurological Disorders and Stroke (NINDS) trial was the first RCT that showed the clinical efficacy of IVT when performed within 3 h of stroke onset [12]. In this trial, any ICH that was not seen on the baseline CT scan of a patient with neurological deterioration was classified as sICH. In the ECASS II trial, the National Institutes of Health Stroke Scale (NIHSS) score was required to show a ≥4-point increase in order to define ICH as symptomatic [13]. The ECASS III trial examined IVT within a time window of 3–4.5 h, and defined sICH as any ICH with a suspected causal relationship and a ≥4-point increase in the NIHSS score [14]. In the Safe Implementation of Thrombolysis in Stroke-Monitoring Study (SITS-MOST), a large European postmarketing surveillance study, sICH was defined as PH-2 combined with a ≥4-point increase in the NIHSS score [15]. However, due to methodological differences between these analyses, a direct comparison of the sICH rates between these studies is difficult to perform.

Table 1 shows the sICH rates for the prospective acute reperfusion therapy trials. The rates of ICH after IVT were higher than those observed after nonthrombolytic treatments. In a pooled analysis of 24 IVT studies, the sICH rate varied according to the definition used, with rates of 7.61 ± 0.94% for the NINDS definition, 5.67 ± 1.15% for the ECASS II definition, and 3.25 ± 2.27% for the SITS-MOST definition [16]. A recent pooled analysis of 9 RCTs of IVT showed that there was a significantly improved clinical outcome, irrespective of age or stroke severity, for IVT using alteplase within a 4.5-h window, despite an increased risk of fatal PH-2 within 7 days (2.7% in the IVT arm versus 0.4% in the control arm) [1]. Rt-PA may exacerbate BBB disruption via mechanisms that seem to increase ICH, such as the plasmin-mediated degradation of ECM proteins of the basal lamina, the activation of MMPs (especially MMP-9), and binding to low-density lipoprotein receptor-related protein 1, among others [3, 17]. Furthermore, the rates seemed to be higher in the EVT studies versus the IVT studies. However, the data for the EVT candidates should be interpreted cautiously, as these patients generally had major artery occlusions and higher stroke severities

Table 1. Summary of intracerebral hemorrhage data in prospective acute stroke reperfusion trials

Trial (year)	Arm	N	sICH, %	p	PH-2, %	p	SAH, %	p
RCT comparing IVT with placebo or control								
NINDS (1995)	Placebo	312	0.6	<0.0011	NA		0	
	Treatment	312	6.4		NA		0	
ECASS III (2008)	Placebo	403	0.2	0.008	0.2	0.02	NA	
	Treatment	418	2.4		1.9		NA	
IST-3 (2012)	Control	1,520	1.1	<0.001	NA		NA	
	Treatment	1,515	6.9		NA		NA	
RCT comparing intraarterial thrombolysis with control								
PROACT II (1999)	Control	59	2	0.06	NA		NA	
	Treatment	121	10		NA		NA	
MELT (2007)	Control	57	2	0.206	NA		NA	
	Treatment	57	9		NA		NA	
Single-arm study of Merci thrombectomy								
MERCI (2005)		141	7.8		1.4		3.5	
Multi MERCI (2008)		164	9.8		2.4*		1.2*	
Single-arm study of Penumbra thromboaspiration								
Pivotal stroke trial (2009)		125	11.2		1.6		3.2	
RCT comparing stent retriever with Merci retriever								
SWIFT (2012)	Merci	55	11	0.057	9.1	0.11	16.4	0.03
	Solitaire	58	2		1.7		3.4	
TREVO2 (2012)	Merci	90	9	0.782	6	0.5642	23	0.0786
	Trevo	88	7		8		12	
Single-arm study of ADAPT using new-generation large-bore aspiration catheter								
ADAPT FAST (2014)		98	0		NA		NA	
RCT comparing EVT plus medical therapy (including preceding IVT) or EVT alone with medical therapy alone								
IMS III (2013)	IVT	222	5.9	0.83	6.3	0.90	5.8	0.02
	IVT + EVT	434	6.2		6.0		11.5	
SYNTHESIS Expansion (2013)	IVT	181	6	0.99	NA		NA	
	EVT	181	6		NA		NA	
MR CLEAN (2014)	Medical	267	6.4	NS	5.2*	NS	0*	NS
	EVT	233	7.7		6.0*		0.9*	

ADAPT FAST = A Direct Aspiration first Pass Technique For Acute Stroke Thrombectomy; ECASS = European Cooperative Acute Stroke Study; EVT = endovascular reperfusion therapy; IMS = Interventional Management of Stroke; IST = International Stroke Trial; IVT = intravenous thrombolysis; MELT = Middle Cerebral Artery Embolism Local Fibrinolytic Intervention Trial; MERCI = Mechanical Embolus Removal in Cerebral Ischemia; MR CLEAN = Multicenter Randomized Clinical Trial of Endovascular Treatment for Acute Ischemic Stroke in the Netherlands; NA = not assessed; NINDS = National Institute of Neurological Disorders and Stroke; NS = not significant; PH-2 = parenchymal hematoma type 2; PROACT = Prolyse in Acute Cerebral Thromboembolism; RCT = randomized controlled trial; SAH = subarachnoid hemorrhage; sICH = symptomatic intracerebral hemorrhage; SWIFT = Solitaire FR With the Intention For Thrombectomy; TREVO = Thrombectomy Revascularization of Large Vessel Occlusions in Acute Ischemic Stroke; * symptomatic cases only.

compared with the IVT candidates. In fact, sICH rates for the EVT arms were similar to those for the non-EVT arms in the Interventional Management of Stroke (IMS) III [18], the SYNTHESIS Expansion [19] and the MR CLEAN [2] trials.

A posthoc analysis of the NINDS trial demonstrated that while the sICH definition used for the ECASS II trial and the modified SITS-MOST (any PH with a ≥4-point increase in the NIHSS score) exhibited a significant relationship with the increase in the modified Rankin scale score and with death, the definition for the NINDS trial did not [20]. In a single-center study, Gumbinger et al. [21] showed that all of the definitions from the NINDS, ECASS II, and ECASS III studies and the SITS-MOST significantly predicted an unfavorable outcome, which was defined as a 3-month modified Rankin Scale score ≥3 and death. The best prediction for this unfavorable outcome was achieved by the NINDS definition (odds ratio [OR], 10.42; 95% confidence interval [95% CI], 2.49–93.06), followed by the SITS-MOST definition (OR, 8.87; 95% CI, 1.23–387.52). In addition, the SITS-MOST definition proved to be best for predicting the highest risk of death (OR, 14.35; 95% CI, 3.25–85.86).

Predictors of and Factors Related to Intravenous Thrombolysis-Related Intracerebral Hemorrhage

Clinical Factors

To date, numerous factors have been reported to be associated with or to be able to predict ICH. Whiteley et al. [22] performed a meta-analysis of 55 studies that included 65,264 acute ischemic stroke patients in order to identify the pre-IVT predictors for ICH after IVT. This analysis demonstrated that ICH after IVT was associated with older age (OR per 1-year increase, 1.03; 95% CI, 1.01–1.04), a higher stroke severity (OR per 1-point increase in the NIHSS score, 1.08; 95% CI, 1.06–1.11) and higher glucose levels (OR per 1-mmol/l increase, 1.10; 95% CI, 1.05–1.14). Furthermore, there was an approximate doubling of the ORs for ICH in the presence of atrial fibrillation, congestive heart failure, renal impairment, or premorbid antiplatelet use.

Elevated blood pressure (systolic >185 mm Hg or diastolic >110 mm Hg) is one of the designated exclusion criteria for IVT. Although pretreatment blood pressure protocol violations have been reported to be independently associated with sICH (OR, 2.59; 95% CI, 1.07–6.25) [23], the previously mentioned meta-analysis found that the pretreatment systolic blood pressure was not a significant predictor of ICH (OR per mm Hg, 1.01; 95% CI, 1.00–1.01, p = 0.13) [22]. In studies that did not find any blood pressure protocol violations, the early average systolic blood pressure or systolic blood pressure variability, rather than the baseline blood pressure, was found to be useful for predicting sICH [24–26]. Although it has yet to be definitively clarified whether intensive lower blood pressure control can prevent the occurrence of ICH after IVT, this hypothesis is now being investigated by the Enhanced Control of Hypertension and Thrombolysis Stroke Study (ENCHANTED, NCT01422616).

The meta-analysis by Whiteley et al. [22] reported a trend toward a higher risk of ICH when warfarin was used (OR, 2.46; 95% CI, 0.92–6.59, $p = 0.07$). The Get With The Guidelines-Stroke Registry, which examined over 20,000 IVT patients, found that there was no increased risk of sICH in patients taking oral anticoagulants, provided that their international normalized ratio (INR) was ≤1.7 (OR, 1.01; 95% CI, 0.82–1.25) [27]. In contrast, Ruecker et al. [28] reported that the patients with an INR ≤1.7 who took warfarin until the day of or the day before stroke onset had an approximately 4-fold higher risk of sICH.

Both the meta-analysis by Whiteley et al. [22] and a pooled analysis of 7 RCTs of IVT [29] showed that the time of thrombolysis was not independently associated with ICH after IVT. However, data from a real clinical setting analyzed for 58,353 patients in the Get With the Guidelines-Stroke program demonstrated that a faster onset-to-treatment time was associated with a reduced incidence of sICH (OR per 15-min decrease, 0.96; 95% CI, 0.95–0.98) [30].

Dosage of Recombinant Tissue Plasminogen Activator

Although the standard dosage of alteplase that is used throughout most of the world is 0.9 mg/kg, with the exception of the ongoing ENCHANTED study, the majority of the reports in the literature have not performed any direct comparison of dosages. The ECASS I trial examined the administration of 1.1 mg/kg alteplase during a 6-h extended time window after stroke onset and found that the PH-2 rate was as high as 11.1% [9]. Therefore, the dosage was decreased to 0.9 mg/kg in the ECASS II trial, which resulted in a PH-2 rate of 7.6% [13]. A Japanese trial investigated the dosage of duteplase, an rt-PA that is very similar to alteplase, and found that a lower dosage (20 million international units) was less likely to cause massive ICH compared with a higher dosage (30 million international units) [31]. Therefore, the rt-PA dosage appears to be the critical determinant for ICH after IVT.

Ethnicity is another important risk factor for ICH. Spontaneous ICH is more frequently observed in Asian people, and especially the Japanese, compared with other races [32]. The Japan Alteplase Clinical Trial (J-ACT) investigated the efficacy of IVT by administering 0.6 mg/kg alteplase, which corresponds to 20 million international units of duteplase, in patients weighing 60 kg [33]. Based on the results of this study, the low dosage was approved for use in Japan. Further data from the Japan Post-Marketing Alteplase Registration Study (J-MARS) indicated that sICH rates were comparable to those in the SITS-MOST and that the outcomes at 3 months were good [34]. Chao et al. [35] additionally showed that low-dose alteplase was both effective and safe, especially for elderly Chinese patients. In contrast, several other Asian studies reported that low-dose alteplase worsened the clinical outcome or increased the incidence of sICH compared with standard-dose alteplase [36, 37]. These findings were most likely due to a decrease in the rate of timely reperfusion or problems related to the delayed reperfusion. Thus, the efficacy of low-dose alteplase (especially for Asian patients) remains controversial at the present time.

Imaging Findings

When assessing acute stroke, a conventional noncontrast CT scan is an essential modality for ruling out the possibility of ICH. In the ECASS I trial, higher ICH rates were most likely seen because the study included patients who were observed to have a large hypodense area (>1/3 of the middle cerebral artery [MCA] territory) on baseline CT, concomitant with use of high-dose alteplase and an extended time window [9]. The NINDS trial analyzed the data for the subjects after excluding all of the patients with >1/3 MCA hypodensity. Since the results showed the efficacy of IVT for acute ischemic stroke patients, with acceptable rates of sICH after IVT [12], subsequent IVT and EVT studies now tend to exclude those patients with >1/3 MCA hypodensity. The Alberta Stroke Program Early CT Score (ASPECTS) has been widely used as a simple semiquantitative 10-point grading system of the infarct volume in the MCA territory. When using this grading system, the MCA territory is allotted 10 points, with 1 point subtracted for each area that displays early ischemic change [38]. A score of <7 is reported to correlate well with an infarcted area of >1/3 of the MCA territory [39]. The meta-analysis performed by Whitley et al. [22] demonstrated that the ASPECTS can be used as an independent predictor of ICH after IVT (OR of a lower ASPECTS, 3.46; 95% CI, 1.92–6.21).

The usefulness of nonenhanced magnetic resonance imaging (MRI) to predict ICH after IVT has also been reported. Diffusion-weighted imaging (DWI) MRI can more accurately demonstrate early ischemic changes compared with conventional CT scans and has additionally been reported to be a useful tool for detecting patients at high risk for ICH [40]. The Stroke Acute Management with Urgent Risk-factor Assessment and Improvement (SAMURAI) study examined the use of DWI-ASPECTS for predicting sICH after IVT when using low-dose alteplase and reported the cut-off point to be ≤5 (OR, 4.74; 95% CI, 1.54–13.64) [40].

Today, modern clinical settings are evaluating acute stroke by using gadolinium-enhanced MRI to obtain perfusion-weighted images (PWIs). The Diffusion and Perfusion Imaging Evaluation For Understanding Stroke Evolution (DEFUSE) trial tested the efficacy of IVT for acute stroke patients who were selected based on a PWI-DWI mismatch. This study demonstrated that a patient with a 'malignant profile', which was defined as the presence of a ≥100-ml lesion on DWI and/or a ≥100-ml lesion on PWI, with a time-to-maximum residue function delay of ≥8 s, had an increased risk of sICH when successfully reperfused [41]. Recently, a pooled analysis of the DEFUSE trial and the Echoplanar Imaging Thrombolysis Evolution Trial (EPITHET) more accurately defined the cut-off for the 'malignant profile' as a lesion of ≥85 ml on PWI, with a time-to-maximum residue function delay of ≥8 s [42]. Furthermore, in another pooled analysis of the DEFUSE trial and EPITHET, a very low cerebral blood volume, which was defined as a cerebral blood volume <2.5th percentile of brain tissue contralateral to the infarct, was shown to have a much higher accuracy for predicting PH during reperfusion than the 'malignant profile' model did [43].

Table 2. Scoring systems used to predict symptomatic intracerebral hemorrhage after intravenous thrombolysis

Score	Parameter	Definition of sICH
MSS	Age (>60 years), NIHSS score (>10), glucose (>150 mg/dl), platelet count (<150,000/mm^3)	NINDS
HAT	NIHSS score (<15, 15–20, ≥20), glucose (>200 mg/dl) or history of diabetes, hypodensity on CT (≥1/3 of MCA territory)	NINDS
GRASPS	Age (≤60, 61–70, 71–80, >80 years), NIHSS score (0–5, 6–10, 11–15, 16–20, >20), glucose (<100, 100–149, ≥150 mg/dl), systolic blood pressure (<120, 120–149, 150–179, ≥180 mm Hg), ethnicity (Asian), sex (male)	NINDS
SEDAN	Age (>75 years), NIHSS score (≥10), glucose (8.1–12.0, >12.0 mmol/l), early infarct signs, hyperdense artery signs	ECASS II
SITS	Age (≥72 years), NIHSS score (7–12, ≥13), glucose (≥180 mg/dl), systolic blood pressure (≥146 mm Hg), weight (≥95 kg), onset-to-treatment time (≥180 min), aspirin monotherapy, aspirin + clopidogrel therapy, history of hypertension	SITS-MOST

ECASS = European Cooperative Acute Stroke Study; GRASPS = Glucose Race Age Sex Pressure Stroke Severity; HAT = Hemorrhage After Thrombolysis; MSS = Multicenter Stroke Survey; NIHSS = National Institutes of Health Stroke Scale; NINDS = National Institute of Neurological Disorders and Stroke; sICH = symptomatic intracerebral hemorrhage; SEDAN = Sugar on admission, Early infarct signs and (hyper) Dense cerebral artery sign on admission CT head scan, Age, and the National Institutes of Health Stroke Scale; SITS-MOST = Safe Implementation of Thrombolysis in Stroke-Monitoring Study.

Scoring Systems to Predict Intracerebral Hemorrhage

As seen in table 2, several scoring systems for predicting the risk of sICH after IVT have been developed. Strbian et al. [44] evaluated 6 different scoring systems: the MSS (Multicenter Stroke Survey); HAT (Hemorrhage After Thrombolysis); SEDAN (Sugar on admission, Early infarct signs and [hyper] Dense cerebral artery sign on admission CT head scan, Age, and the NIHSS); GRASPS (Glucose Race Age Sex Pressure Stroke Severity); SITS (Safe Implementation of Thrombolysis in Stroke); and SPAN (Stroke Prognostication using Age and NIH stroke scale)-100 positive index. For each of the systems, the researchers examined the ability to estimate the risk of sICH according to the ECASS II definition and found the performances of all of these scores to be moderate or poor (the area under the curve of the receiver-operator characteristics of each score was 0.56–0.70). To date, there have yet to be any scoring systems developed that have enough power to detect an unacceptably high risk for sICH and to provide definitive information on the decision to withdraw IVT in patients.

As a consequence, if an acute stroke patient without any contraindications for IVT is identified on the basis of a conventional CT scan, current stroke clinical practice indicates that such a patient should undergo IVT, irrespective of any clinical predictors of ICH after IVT. However, multimodal MRI (or CT) might be of use for excluding patients who could clearly be harmed by IVT due to an excess risk of ICH, despite the lack of any clearcut contraindication for IVT.

Predictors of and Factors Related to Endovascular Therapy-Related Intracerebral Hemorrhage

Reperfusion-related ICH after EVT is roughly classified into 2 categories: ICH caused by reperfusion at the deep ischemic core and ICH following vessel or tissue injury directly caused by the EVT procedure and/or devices, such as subarachnoid hemorrhage (SAH). While the mechanism of the former type is common to both IVT and EVT, the latter mechanism is inherent in EVT.

Theoretically, EVT has a lower risk of ICH than IVT does in the absence of thrombolytic agent use. One of the exclusion criteria for IVT is abnormal hemostasis (INR >1.7, platelet count <100,000/mm^3, and/or an activated partial thrombin time >45 s). Even so, a pooled analysis of the Mechanical Embolus Removal in Cerebral Ischemia (MERCI) and the Multi MERCI trials, which were prospective studies that used a first-generation mechanical thrombectomy device known as the Merci retriever, showed that abnormal hemostasis was not related to major sICH risk [45]. However, contrast media may contribute to the BBB disruption that leads to ICH after EVT due to a neurotoxic effect associated with its hyperosmolality and inherent chemotoxicity. Yoon et al. [46] investigated the relationship between CT findings after intraarterial thrombolysis and subsequent ICH. Contrast enhancement was defined as a hyperdense lesion that disappeared on a 24-h follow-up CT scan (fig. 1a–d). Contrast extravasation was defined as a hyperdense lesion with a maximum number of Hounsfield units >90 that persisted on a follow-up CT scan (fig. 1e–g). Compared with the patients without any hyperdense lesions, the patients with contrast enhancement had a lower incidence of hemorrhagic transformation (14.3 vs. 43.9%, $p = 0.047$). However, patients with contrast extravasation exhibited a higher incidence of both PH-2 (100 vs. 43.9%, $p = 0.006$) and sICH (100 vs. 38.9%, $p < 0.001$). Similar results were reported from the posthoc analysis of the IMS I and II trials, which were prospective studies of EVT following IVT [47]. The analysis also showed that the number of microcatheter injections was an independent positive predictor of ICH. Contrast extravasation may reflect degradation of the basal lamina, leading to BBB disruption due to contrast toxicity, while contrast enhancement may be caused by leakage of contrast medium due to the increased permeability of the BBB. Furthermore, mechanical injury of the vessel walls caused by passage of the device or by injection-pressure transmission may contribute to contrast extravasation, thereby leading to PH and/or sICH.

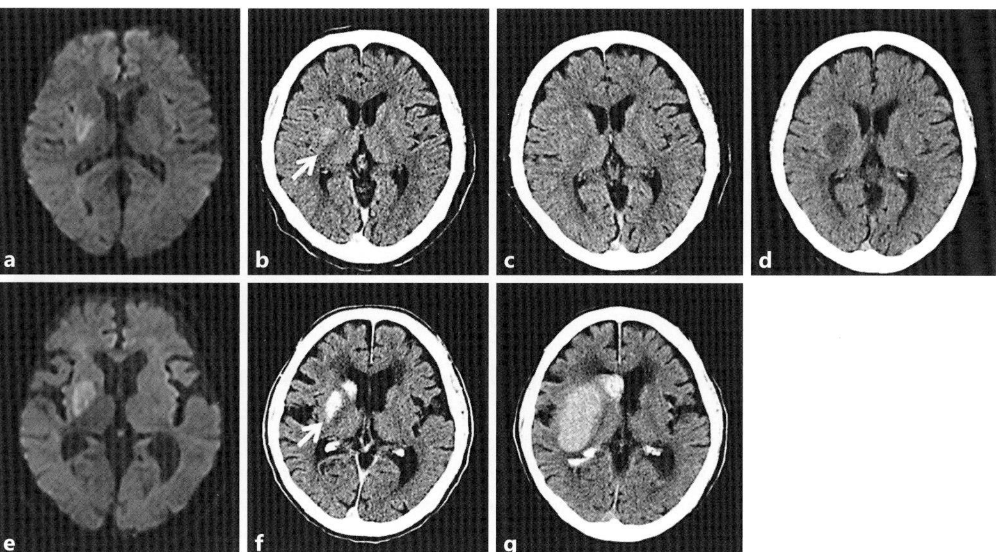

Fig. 1. Upper row: A 69-year-old woman with right middle cerebral artery occlusion who underwent intravenous thrombolysis using 0.6 mg/kg alteplase, followed by endovascular reperfusion therapy (EVT). **a** Diffusion-weighted magnetic resonance imaging on admission showing a hyperintense lesion at the right basal ganglia. **b** Noncontrast computed tomography (CT) immediately after EVT using the Solitaire FR and Penumbra 5MAX ACE for successful reperfusion, showing a subtle hyperdense lesion at the right basal ganglia (white arrow). **c** Follow-up CT at 3 h after the completion of EVT, showing disappearance of the hyperdense lesion. **d** Follow-up CT at 24 h after onset, showing an infarct of the right basal ganglia, without any hemorrhagic transformation. Lower row: An 80-year-old man with acute right intracranial internal carotid artery occlusion who underwent EVT 7 h after the last-known-well time (time of puncture). **e** Diffusion-weighted magnetic resonance imaging on admission showing a hyperintense lesion at the right basal ganglia. **f** Noncontrast CT immediately after EVT using the Solitaire FR for successful reperfusion, showing a clear hyperdense lesion at the right basal ganglia, with a maximum Hounsfield unit measurement of 92 (white arrow). **g** Follow-up CT at 4 h after the completion of EVT, showing a massive hematoma at the right basal ganglia.

Although SAH can occur in the patients undergoing EVT, it rarely occurs after IVT [12]. Smith [48] reported that the SAH incidence rates after Merci thrombectomy were 9.9% (symptomatic SAH; 2.7%) in the Multi MERCI trial (part 1) [48], while Shi et al. [49] reported a rate of 14.1% (symptomatic SAH; 1.6%) for a single-center experience. Shi et al. [49] also showed that patients with extensive SAH or coexisting PH tended to exhibit neurological deterioration and worse clinical/vital outcomes. The Multi MERCI trial reported that the concomitant use of abciximab and intraarterial rt-PA were risk factors for SAH [48]. The independent risk factors found for SAH after EVT (including Merci thrombectomy and intraarterial thrombolysis) were hypertension, distal M1 occlusion, rescue angioplasty after Merci failure and vessel perforation [49]. Along with apparent (intraprocedurally detectable) vessel perforation, the

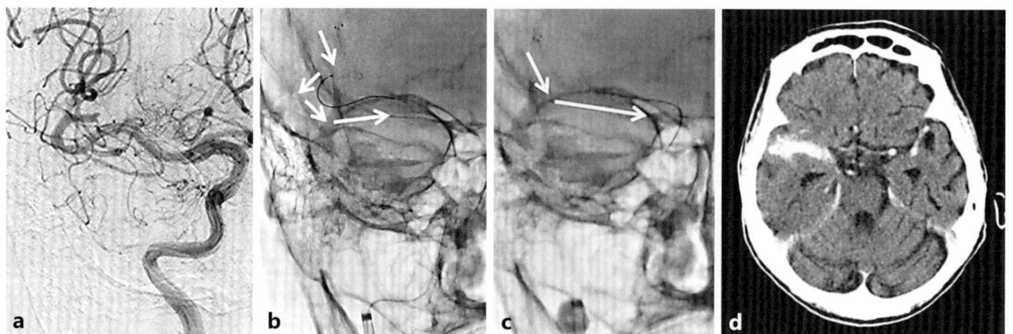

Fig. 2. An 80-year-old woman presenting with acute ischemic stroke. **a** Right internal carotid artery angiogram showing occlusion of the M2 portion of the right middle cerebral artery. **b** Solitaire FR retriever bent steeply in line with the vessel curvature (white arrows). **c** Upon use of the stent retriever, the curved vessel straightened (white arrows). Angiogram immediately after thrombectomy did not show any contrast extravasation, which suggested vessel rupture or perforation. **d** Noncontrast CT immediately after the completion of EVT, showing a clear hyperdense area at the right Sylvian fissure, which indicated subarachnoid hemorrhage.

mechanism of SAH after EVT (especially after thrombectomy) is considered to include angiographically undetectable minor trauma of perforating arteries or small branching cortical vessels due to the shear force that occurs during device traction [50] (fig. 2). Moreover, contrast injection stress and/or contrast neurotoxicity may influence the onset of SAH after EVT.

The Solitaire FR With the Intention For Thrombectomy (SWIFT) trial and the Thrombectomy Revascularization of Large Vessel Occlusions in Acute Ischemic Stroke (TREVO) 2 trial compared stent retrievers with the Merci retriever, with both trials showing not only the superiority of the recanalization performance of the stent retrievers but also the lower ICH/SAH rates in the stent retriever arms, indicating excellent safety of the stent retrievers [51, 52]. The results of these studies led to these stent retrievers becoming the mainstream thrombectomy devices in use today. Furthermore, the use of a direct aspiration first pass technique with a large-bore aspiration catheter such as the Penumbra 5MAX ACE has also been shown to be a rapid, effective and safe endovascular recanalization procedure [53]. The SAH incidence rates were 3.4% in the Solitaire arm and 16.4% in the Merci arm ($p = 0.03$) in the SWIFT trial and were 12% in the Trevo arm and 23% in the Merci arm ($p = 0.0786$) in the TREVO2 trial. Yoon et al. [50] reported that the rate of isolated SAH (unrelated to PH) after first-line Solitaire thrombectomy was 16.2%. Furthermore, SAH after the Solitaire procedure did not cause a deterioration in clinical outcomes compared with those of patients without SAH. Overall, the current results appear to suggest that the clinical significance of SAH after EVT may differ depending upon the thrombectomy devices used (SAH after Solitaire thrombectomy seemed to be benign). However, this issue has yet to be definitively clarified.

Management

Strategies to Prevent Reperfusion-Related Intracerebral Hemorrhage

Strategies that have been suggested for preventing ICH after IVT and/or EVT include intensive blood pressure control, tight glycemic control and the avoidance of early aggressive antithrombotic therapy for high-risk ICH patients [54].

As mentioned above, the ENCHANTED trial is currently investigating whether intensive blood pressure control can effectively prevent ICH after IVT. However, intensive blood pressure control could induce enlargement of the infarction and lead to a worse clinical outcome if there is insufficient reperfusion. Thus, after IVT, physicians must maintain the blood pressure at least within the target range that has been defined in the guidelines (<180/105 mm Hg).

Hyperglycemia has been demonstrated to be an enhancing factor of ICH after IVT, as it can damage the BBB through mechanisms such as direct injury of the neuronal membrane and increased production of oxygen free radicals [54]. Although there is no definitive evidence that documents the efficacy of a rapid, aggressive hyperglycemia correction in order to prevent ICH, the last edition of the American Heart Association/American Stroke Association guidelines for the early management of ischemic stroke, which was revised in 2013, has stated that treating hyperglycemia to achieve blood glucose levels in the range of 140–180 mg/dl, along with close monitoring of the patients in order to prevent hypoglycemia, is a reasonable course of action in acute ischemic stroke patients [55].

Neuroprotective agents might also be effective against ICH after IVT. The efficacy of the free-radical-trapping agent NXY-059 was tested in acute ischemic stroke patients in the Stroke-Acute Ischemic NXY Treatment (SAINT) 1 and 2 trials. Unfortunately, the use of NXY-059 proved to be futile for preventing ICH after IVT and improving clinical outcomes [56]. In Japan, the free-radical-scavenging agent edaravone has been approved as a neuroprotectant and is now being widely used throughout Japan for patients receiving IVT and/or EVT. It has been demonstrated in animal models that edaravone has a preventive effect against ICH after IVT. It has been proposed that the primary mechanism of action that makes it possible for edaravone to prevent ICH occurs via the ability of edaravone to inhibit the activation of MMP-9 [57].

Strategies When Symptomatic Intracerebral Hemorrhage Occurs

Once sICH, especially PH-2, occurs, the primary goal is to prevent hematoma expansion, which is closely related to further neurological deterioration. Moreover, if the hematoma is life-threatening, surgical hematoma removal may be required.

Previous editions of the American Heart Association guidelines for the management of spontaneous ICH that were published in 2007 recommended the infusion of platelets and cryoprecipitate for sICH after IVT, even though there was no demonstrated evidence for this action [58]. As of 2010, this recommendation has no longer been described in the revised editions of these guidelines [59].

Intensive blood pressure control is thought to be essential for preventing hematoma expansion. The Intensive Blood Pressure Reduction in Acute Cerebral Hemorrhage Trial-2 (INTERACT-2) showed intensive blood pressure reduction (systolic target <140 mm Hg in less than 1 h within 6 h of onset) tends to be beneficial in the 3-month functional outcome and has an acceptable safety compared with guideline-based management (systolic target <180 mm Hg) [60]. As a consequence, the revised edition of the European Stroke Organisation guidelines for the management of spontaneous ICH published in 2014 has also recommended the use of intensive blood pressure control [61]. Furthermore, the RCT methods for the current ongoing Antihypertensive Treatment of Acute Cerebral Hemorrhage (ATACH)-II trial (NCT 01176565) is following a much more strict methodology than that used for the INTERACT-2 trial. A study by Mokin et al. [62] also reported that systolic blood pressure reductions after the occurrence of PH had a strong negative correlation with hematoma expansion.

If PH-2 occurs after IVT and/or EVT and there is an impending herniation or a life-threatening event, early surgical hematoma removal not only is required but also may be helpful in improving the functional outcome [63]. Although the safety of surgical hematoma removal immediately after IVT or intraarterial thrombolysis remains unknown, since the half-life of rt-PA is under 5 min and approximately 80% of rt-PA is cleared within 10 min after discontinuation of the infusion, it is likely that this procedure would be relatively safe [64].

Conclusion

Reperfusion-related ICH secondary to IVT and/or EVT is one of the critical issues that can be encountered when treating acute ischemic stroke. Although this chapter has tried to describe the current knowledge available on the clinical aspects of reperfusion-related ICH, it should be noted that reliable preventive and treatment strategies for reperfusion-related ICH have yet to be definitively established, despite the positive results that have been reported for the use of new-generation thrombectomy devices and for the selection of patients when using multimodal MRI or CT, among other approaches. In order to establish therapeutic strategies for reperfusion-related ICH that will lead to improvements in stroke prognosis, further studies are warranted.

Acknowledgment

I would like to profoundly thank Dr. Kazunori Toyoda (National Cerebral and Cardiovascular Center) for his valuable advice.

References

1 Emberson J, Lees KR, Lyden P, et al: Effect of treatment delay, age, and stroke severity on the effects of intravenous thrombolysis with alteplase for acute ischaemic stroke: a meta-analysis of individual patient data from randomised trials. Lancet 2014;384: 1929–1935.

2 Berkhemer OA, Fransen PS, Beumer D, et al: A randomized trial of intraarterial treatment for acute ischemic stroke. N Engl J Med 2014;372:11–20.

3 Khatri P, McKinney AM, Swenson B, et al: Blood-brain barrier, reperfusion injury, and hemorrhagic transformation in acute ischemic stroke. Neurology 2012;79(suppl 1):S52–S57.

4 del Zoppo GJ: Stroke and neurovascular protection. N Engl J Med 2006;354:553–555.

5 Lakhan SE, Kirchgessner A, Tepper D, et al: Matrix metalloproteinases and blood-brain barrier disruption in acute ischemic stroke. Front Neurol 2013;4: 32.

6 Hacke W, Kaste M, Fieschi C, et al: Intravenous thrombolysis with recombinant tissue plasminogen activator for acute hemispheric stroke. The European Cooperative Acute Stroke Study (ECASS). JAMA 1995;274:1017–1025.

7 Cerebral Embolism Study Group: Immediate anticoagulation of embolic stroke: brain hemorrhage and management options. Stroke 1984;4:778–789.

8 Ogata J, Yutani C, Imakita M, et al: Hemorrhagic infarct of the brain without a reopening of the occluded arteries in cardioembolic stroke. Stroke 1989;20: 876–883.

9 Fiorelli M, Bastianello S, von Kummer R, et al: Hemorrhagic transformation within 36 hours of a cerebral infarct: relationships with early clinical deterioration and 3-month outcome in the European Cooperative Acute Stroke Study I (ECASS I) cohort. Stroke 1999;30:2280–2284.

10 Berger C, Fiorelli M, Steiner T, et al: Hemorrhagic transformation of ischemic brain tissue: asymptomatic or symptomatic? Stroke 2001;32:1330–1335.

11 Larrue V, von Kummer R, Muller A, et al: Risk factors for severe hemorrhagic transformation in ischemic stroke patients treated with recombinant tissue plasminogen activator: a secondary analysis of the European-Australasian Acute Stroke Study (ECASS II). Stroke 2001;32:438–441.

12 The National Institute of Neurological Disorders and Stroke rt-PA Study Group: Tissue plasminogen activator for acute ischemic stroke. N Engl J Med 1995;333:1581–1587.

13 Hacke W, Kaste M, Fieschi C, et al: Randomised double-blind placebo-controlled trial of thrombolytic therapy with intravenous alteplase in acute ischaemic stroke (ECASS II). Lancet 1998;352:1245–1251.

14 Hacke W, Kaste M, Bluhmki E, et al: Thrombolysis with alteplase 3 to 4.5 h after acute ischemic stroke. N Engl J Med 2008;359:1317–1329.

15 Wahlgren N, Ahmed N, Davalos A, et al: Thrombolysis with alteplase for acute ischaemic stroke in the Safe Implementation of Thrombolysis in Stroke-Monitoring Study (SITS-MOST): an observational study. Lancet 2007;369:275–282.

16 Seet RC, Rabinstein AA: Symptomatic intracranial hemorrhage following intravenous thrombolysis for acute ischemic stroke: a critical review of case definitions. Cerebrovasc Dis 2012;34:106–114.

17 Adibhalta RM, Hatcher JF: Tissue plasminogen activator (tPA) and matrix metalloproteinases in the pathogenesis of stroke: therapeutic strategies. CNS Neurol Disord Drug Targets 2008;7:243–253.

18 Broderick JP, Palesch YY, Demchuk AM, et al: Endovascular therapy after intravenous t-PA versus t-PA alone for stroke. N Engl J Med 2013;368:893–903.

19 Ciccone A, Valvassori L, Nichelatti M, et al: Endovascular treatment for acute ischemic stroke. N Engl J Med 2013;368:904–913.

20 Rao NM, Levine SR, Gornbein JA, et al: Defining clinically relevant cerebral hemorrhage after thrombolytic therapy for stroke. Analysis of the National Institute of Neurological Disorders and Stroke tissue-type plasminogen activator trials. Stroke 2014; 45:2728–2733.

21 Gumbinger C, Gruschka P, Böttinger M, et al: Improved prediction of poor outcome after thrombolysis using conservative definitions of symptomatic hemorrhage. Stroke 2012;43:240–242.

22 Whiteley WN, Slot KB, Fernandes P, et al: Risk factors for intracranial hemorrhage in acute ischemic stroke patients treated with recombinant tissue plasminogen activator. A systematic review and meta-analysis of 55 studies. Stroke 2012;43:2904–2909.

23 Tsivgoulis G, Frey JL, Flaster M, et al: Pre-tissue plasminogen activator blood pressure levels and risk of symptomatic intracerebral hemorrhage. Stroke 2009;40:3631–3634.

24 Butcher K, Christensen S, Parsons M, et al: Post-thrombolysis blood pressure elevation is associated with hemorrhagic transformation. Stroke 2010;41: 72–77.

25 Endo K, Kario K, Koga M, et al: Impact of early blood pressure variability on stroke outcomes after thrombolysis: the SAMURAI rt-PA Registry. Stroke 2013; 44:816–818.

26 Tomii Y, Toyoda K, Nakashima T, et al: Effects of hyperacute blood pressure and heart rate on stroke outcomes after intravenous tissue plasminogen activator. J Hypertens 2011;29:1980–1987.

27 Xian Y, Liang L, Smith EE, et al: Risks of intracranial hemorrhage among patients with acute ischemic stroke receiving warfarin and treated with intravenous tissue plasminogen activator. JAMA 2012;307:2600–2608.
28 Ruecker M, Matosevic B, Willeit P, et al: Subtherapeutic warfarin therapy entails an increased bleeding risk after stroke thrombolysis. Neurology 2012;79:31–38.
29 Lees KR, Bluhmki E, von Kummer R, et al: Time to treatment with intravenous alteplase and outcome in stroke: an updated pooled analysis of ECASS, ATLANTIS, NINDS, and EPITHET trials. Lancet 2010;375:1695–1703.
30 Saver JL, Fonarow GC, Smith EE, et al: Time to treatment with intravenous tissue plasminogen activator and outcome from acute ischemic stroke. JAMA 2013;309:2480–2488.
31 Yamaguchi T, Kikuchi H, Hayakawa T, et al: Clinical efficacy and safety of intravenous tissue plasminogen activator in acute embolic stroke: a randomized, double-blind, dose comparison study of duteplase; in Yamaguchi T, Mori E, Minematsu K, del Zoppo GJ (eds): Thrombolytic Therapy in Acute Ischemic Stroke III. Tokyo, Japan, Springer-Verlag, 1995, pp 223–229.
32 Toyoda K: Pharmacotherapy for the secondary prevention of stroke. Drugs 2009;69:633–647.
33 Yamaguchi T, Mori E, Minematsu K, et al: Alteplase at 0.6 mg/kg for acute ischemic stroke within 3 hours of onset: Japan Alteplase Clinical Trial (J-ACT). Stroke 2006;37:1810–1815.
34 Nakagawara J, Minematsu K, Okada Y, et al: Thrombolysis with 0.6 mg/kg intravenous alteplase for acute ischemic stroke in routine clinical practice. The Japan post-Marketing Alteplase Registration Study (J-MARS). Stroke 2010;41:1984–1989.
35 Chao AC, Liu CK, Chen CH, et al: Different doses of recombinant tissue-type plasminogen activator for acute stroke in Chinese patients. Stroke 2014;45:2359–2365.
36 Sharma VK, Tsivgoulis G, Tan JH, et al: Feasibility and safety of intravenous thrombolysis in multiethnic Asian stroke patients in Singapore. J Stroke Cerebrovasc Dis 2010;6:424–430.
37 Liao X, Wang Y, Pan Y, et al: Standard-dose intravenous tissue-type plasminogen activator for stroke is better than low doses. Stroke 2014;45:2354–2358.
38 Barber PA, Demchuk AM, Zhang J, et al: Validity and reliability of a quantitative computed tomography score in predicting outcome of hyperacute stroke before thrombolytic therapy ASPECTS Study Group. Alberta Stroke Programme Early CT Score. Lancet 2000;355:1670–1674.
39 Demaerschalk BM, Silver B, Wong E, et al: ASPECT scoring to estimate >1/3 middle cerebral artery territory infarction. Can J Neurol Sci 2006;33:200–204.
40 Nezu T, Koga M, Kimura K, et al: pretreatment ASPECTS on DWI predicts 3-month outcome following rt-PA. SAMURAI rt-PA Registry. Neurology 2010;75:555–561.
41 Albers GW, Thiji VN, Wechsler L, et al: Magnetic resonance imaging profiles predict clinical response to early reperfusion: the diffusion and perfusion imaging evaluation for understanding stroke evolution (DEFUSE) study. Ann Neurol 2006;60:508–517.
42 Mlynash M, Lansberg MG, De Silva DA, et al: Refining the definition of the malignant profile. Insights from the DEFUSE-EPITHET pooled data set. Stroke 2011;42:1270–1275.
43 Campbell BC, Christensen S, Parsons MW, et al: Advanced imaging improves prediction of hemorrhage after stroke thrombolysis. Ann Neurol 2013;73:510–519.
44 Strbian D, Michel P, Seiffge DJ, et al: Symptomatic intracranial hemorrhage after stroke thrombolysis. Comparison of prediction scores. Stroke 2014;45:752–758.
45 Nogueira RG, Smith WS; MERCI and Multi MERCI Writing Committee: Safety and efficacy of endovascular thrombectomy in patients with abnormal hemostasis: pooled analysis of MERCI and multi MERCI trials. Stroke 2009;40:516–522.
46 Yoon W, Seo JJ, Kim JK, et al: Contrast enhancement and contrast extravasation on computed tomography after intra-arterial thrombolysis in patients with acute ischemic stroke. Stroke 2004;35:876–881.
47 Khatri P, Broderick JP, Khoury JC, et al: Microcatheter contrast injections during intra-arterial thrombolysis may increase intracranial hemorrhage risk. Stroke 2008;39:3283–3287.
48 Smith WS: Safety of mechanical thrombectomy and intravenous tissue plasminogen activator in acute ischemic stroke. Results of the multi Mechanical Embolus Removal in Cerebral Ischemia (MERCI) trial, part I. AJNR Am J Neuroradiol 2006;27:1177–1182.
49 Shi ZS, Liebeskind DS, Loh Y, et al: Predictors of subarachnoid hemorrhage in acute ischemic stroke with endovascular therapy. Stroke 2010;41:2775–2781.
50 Yoon W, Jung MY, Jung SH, et al: Subarachnoid hemorrhage in a multimodal approach heavily weighted toward mechanical thrombectomy with Solitaire stent in acute stroke. Stroke 2013;44:414–419.
51 Saver JL, Jaha R, Levy EI, et al: Solitaire flow restoration device versus the Merci Retriever in patients with acute ischaemic stroke (SWIFT): a randomised, parallel-group, non-inferiority trial. Lancet 2012;380:1241–1249.
52 Nogueira RG, Lutsep HL, Gupta R, et al: Trevo versus Merci retrievers for thrombectomy revascularisation of large vessel occlusions in acute ischaemic stroke (TREVO 2): a randomised trial. Lancet 2012;380:1231–1240.

53 Turk AS, Frei D, Fiorella D, et al: ADAPT FAST study: a direct aspiration first pass technique for acute stroke thrombectomy. J Neurointerv Surg 2014;6:260–264.
54 Mokin M, Kan P, Kass-Hout T, et al: Intracerebral hemorrhage secondary to intravenous and endovascular intraarterial revascularization therapies in acute ischemic stroke: an update on risk factors, predictors, and management. Neurosurg Focus 2012; 32:E2.
55 Jauch EC, Saver JL, Adams HP Jr, et al: Guidelines for the early management of patients with acute ischemic stroke: a guideline for healthcare professionals from the American Heart Association/American Stroke Association. Stroke 2013;44:870–947.
56 Diener HC, Lees KR, Lyden P, et al: NXY-059 for the treatment of acute stroke: pooled analysis of the SAINT I and II Trials. Stroke 2008;39:1751–1758.
57 Yagi K, Kitazato KT, Uno M, et al: Edaravone, a free radical scavenger, inhibits MMP-9-related brain hemorrhage in rats treated with tissue plasminogen activator. Stroke 2009;40:626–631.
58 Broderick J, Connolly S, Feldmann E, et al: Guidelines for the management of spontaneous intracerebral hemorrhage in adults: 2007 update: a guideline from the American Heart Association/American Stroke Association Stroke Council, High Blood Pressure Research Council, and the Quality of Care and Outcomes in Research Interdisciplinary Working Group. Stroke 2007;38:2001–2023.
59 Morgenstern LB, Hemphill JC 3rd, Anderson C, et al: Guidelines for the management of spontaneous intracerebral hemorrhage: a guideline for healthcare professionals from the American Heart Association/American Stroke Association. Stroke 2010;41:2108–2129.
60 Anderson CS, Heeley E, Huang Y, et al: Rapid blood-pressure lowering in patients with acute intracerebral hemorrhage. N Engl J Med 2013;368:2355–2365.
61 Steiner T, Al-Shahi Salman R, Beer R, et al: European Stroke Organisation (ESO) guidelines for the management of spontaneous intracerebral hemorrhage. Int J Stroke 2014;9:840–855.
62 Mokin M, Kass-Hout T, Kass-Hout O, et al: Blood pressure management and evolution of thrombolysis-associated intracerebral hemorrhage in acute ischemic stroke. J Stroke Cerebrovasc Dis 2012;21: 852–859.
63 Fargen KM, Hoh BL, Fautheree GL, et al: Aggressive intervention to treat a young woman with intracranial hemorrhage following unsuccessful intravenous thrombolysis for left middle cerebral artery occlusion. Case report. J Neurosurg 2011;115:359–363.
64 Tanswell P, Seifried E, Su PCA, et al: Pharmacokinetics and systemic effects of tissue-type plasminogen activator in normal subjects. Clin Pharmacol Ther 1989;46:155–162.

Dr. Mikito Hayakawa
Department of Cerebrovascular Medicine, National Cerebral and Cardiovascular Center
5-7-1 Fujishirodai, Suita
Osaka 565-8565 (Japan)
E-Mail mikito-h@jc4.so-net.ne.jp

Toyoda K, Anderson CS, Mayer SA (eds): New Insights in Intracerebral Hemorrhage.
Front Neurol Neurosci. Basel, Karger, 2016, vol 37, pp 78–92 (DOI: 10.1159/000437115)

Cerebral Microbleeds: Detection, Associations and Clinical Implications

Yusuke Yakushiji

Division of Neurology, Department of Internal Medicine, Saga University Faculty of Medicine, Saga, Japan

Abstract

Vigorous investigations for cerebral microbleeds (CMBs) have been made since the late 1990s. CMBs on paramagnetic-sensitive magnetic resonance sequences correspond pathologically to clusters of hemosiderin-laden macrophages and have emerged as an important new imaging marker of cerebral small vessel disease, including intracerebral hemorrhage (ICH). The prevalence of CMBs varies according to the specific disease settings (stroke subtypes and dementing disorders) and is highest (60%) in ICH patients. The associations of CMBs with aging, hypertension and apolipoprotein E genotype are consistent with the two major underlying pathogeneses of CMBs: hypertensive arteriopathy and cerebral amyloid angiopathy (CAA). The distributional patterns of CMBs might help us to understand the predominant small vessel disease pathogenesis in the brain; the strictly lobar type of CMBs often reflects the presence of advanced CAA, while the other types of CMBs, such as 'deep or infratentorial CMBs', including the mixed type, are strongly associated with hypertension. CMBs might be associated with cognitive function (especially executive function), gait performance, and cerebrovascular events (spontaneous, antithrombotic drug-related or post-thrombolysis ICH). In the field of CAA, an understanding of CAA-related CMBs might help to guide decision making with regard to new therapeutic approaches, including the use of monoclonal antibodies against vascular amyloid. These concepts of CMBs might allow us to advance research on ICH as well as for dementia.

© 2016 S. Karger AG, Basel

Introduction

Advances in magnetic resonance (MR) imaging (MRI) techniques have allowed detection of the residual bleeding effects of cerebral small vessel disease (SVD), which can be visualized as small foci of chronic blood products in brain tissue, commonly referred to as 'microbleeds'. The term 'microbleeds' first appeared in 1996 [1], but subsequently, many different terms have been applied (e.g., asymptomatic microbleeds, brain microbleeds, cerebral microbleeds [CMBs], petechial hemorrhage) to describe such lesions. However, recent neuroimaging consensus recommends the designation of 'CMBs' [2], which is the most frequently used term. CMBs are defined as small, rounded, homogeneous, hypointense lesions that are visible on paramagnetic-sensitive MR sequences, such as T2*-weighted gradient-recalled echo (GRE) or susceptibility-weighted sequences [2, 3]. CMBs correspond pathologically to clusters of hemosiderin-laden macrophages [4]. Thus, CMBs are an aspect of cerebral SVD. Patient- and population-based MRI analyses suggest that CMBs have adverse implications and are associated with cerebrovascular diseases and dementia. Therefore, this chapter will discuss CMBs, their associated conditions, and their clinical relevance.

Pathological Features (1): Blood-Breakdown Products

Pathological studies suggest that CMBs on paramagnetic-sensitive MR sequences generally correlate with small collections of blood-breakdown products that have presumably leaked from damaged small vessels into the brain parenchyma [4, 5]. These CMBs are detected based on hemosiderin phagocytosis by macrophages adjacent to small blood vessels [4]. CMBs can contain erythrocytes, implying that not all CMBs are chronic in nature [5]. Some microaneurysms or pseudoaneurysms, which are widely believed to be the origin of spontaneous intracerebral hemorrhage (ICH), can also give rise to the appearance of CMBs on MRI [6, 7]. Paramagnetic-sensitive MR sequences consistently overestimate the diameter of small lesions, in what has previously been termed the 'blooming effect'. For example, signal voids on susceptibility-weighted imaging (SWI) averaged 1.6 times the size of the associated lesion in one study [8]. Importantly, histopathological specimens can contain MR-negative hemosiderin deposits that tend to be smaller and that consist of only a few perivascular, hemosiderin-laden macrophages [4]. Thus, MR-visible CMBs should be considered as just one small aspect of microbleeding in the brain parenchyma.

Detection of Cerebral Microbleeds

Magnetic Resonance Imaging Parameters

Conventionally, CMBs have been investigated using GRE T2*-weighted sequences. The optimal detection of CMBs depends on MRI parameters, including the pulse sequence, spatial resolution, echo time, slice thickness, flip angle and field strength [9]. SWI sequences typically employ a high-resolution 3D GRE sequence with a long echo time (greater than 40 ms does not seem to usefully increase the detection of CMBs),

Table 1. Standard criteria for cerebral microbleed identification on MRI and their rationale [3, 9] (Elsevier and Springer permitted the reuse)

Criterion	Rationale
1. Black on T_2*-weighted MRI	To ensure that the lesion is paramagnetic and likely to contain blood degradation products
2. Round or ovoid lesions (rather than linear)	To exclude blood vessels and to distinguish microbleeds from subarachnoid blood (the latter may have separate relevance for diagnosing small vessel arteriopathies)
3. Blooming effect on T_2*-weighted MRI	Ensures that the lesion has a susceptibility effect
4. Devoid of signal hyperintensity on T_1-weighted or T_2-weighted sequences	To avoid misclassifying some mimics, including cavernous malformations (bright on T_2) and metastatic melanoma (bright on T_1)
5. At least half of the lesion surrounded by brain parenchyma	To include very superficial cortical lesions, which may be seen in cerebral amyloid angiopathy
6. Distinct from other potential mimics such as iron or calcium deposits, bone, or vessel flow voids	A reminder to consider these mimics
7. Clinical history excluding traumatic diffuse axonal injury	To avoid mixing secondary traumatic microbleeds with spontaneous CMBs caused by cerebrovascular disease

CMBs = Cerebral microbleeds; MRI = magnetic resonance imaging.

making them more sensitive in detecting CMBs than GRE T2* sequences are [9, 10]. As susceptibility effects and the signal-to-noise ratio increase with field strength, visualization of CMBs is improved at 3 T (or 7 T) compared with that at 1.5 T [10, 11]. Thus, SWI using a magnetic field strength increased to 3 T or higher is currently the most sensitive technique to visualize CMBs clinically, but its ability to detect CMBs is still under investigation [9].

Morphology and Cerebral Microbleed Mimics

In general, CMBs are defined as small, rounded (or ovoid), homogenous, hypointense areas of signal void with associated blooming (table 1) [3, 9]. Various size cut-off points have been used to classify CMBs, with a maximum diameter of 5–10 mm and, in some studies, a minimum diameter of 2 mm [3]. A recent study analyzed the volumes of hypointense foci seen on routine clinical T2*-weighted MRI (1.5 T, 5-mm slice thickness) among probable cerebral amyloid angiopathy (CAA) patients and demonstrated a distinctly bimodal distribution, with separate widely spaced peaks, for microbleeds and macrobleeds. The cut-off point that best divided the microbleed and macrobleed peaks was a diameter of 5.7 mm [12]. However, because there are

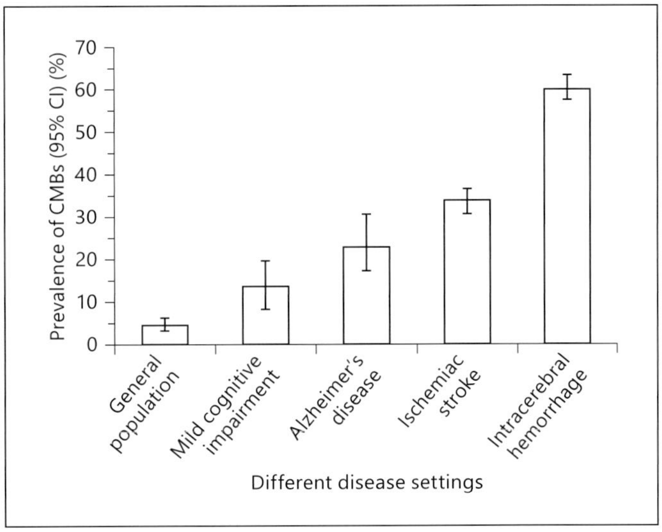

Fig. 1. The prevalence of cerebral microbleeds (CMBs) in different disease settings. The graph was generated from the data of Cordonnier and van der Flier WM [16], with permission for reuse from Oxford University Press. The error bars indicate 95% confidence intervals.

various settings for MRI parameters among different institutes, precise size criteria should not be emphasized [3]. Recognition of 'CMB mimics' is essential to correctly rate CMBs on MRI. These CMB mimics have similar morphologies and signal properties to CMBs on T_1- and T_2-weighted spin echo and GRE MRI sequences. The mimics form two types, including those that contain blood products and those that do not [13]. The CMB mimics that do not contain blood products include partial volume artifacts, blood vessels (vascular flow void), paramagnetic substances (i.e., calcium, manganese, and iron), air embolisms, iatrogenic devices and metallic embolisms. The CMB mimics containing blood products include cavernous malformations, traumatic microbleeds, hemorrhagic metastases, and hemorrhagic transformation of cerebral infarcts.

Prevalence

Around 5.0% (95% confidence interval (CI) 3.9–6.2%) of healthy adults are estimated to have CMBs on conventional GRE T2*-weighted sequences [14]. Using more sensitive imaging sequences, this figure rises to 24% among elderly people [15]. The prevalence of CMBs is also different depending on the specific disease setting (fig. 1) [16]. Among patients with dementia, CMBs are detected in 14% (95% CI 9–20%) of patients with mild cognitive impairment and in 23% (95% CI 17–20%) of patients with Alzheimer's disease [16, 17]. Among patients with stroke, CMBs are detected in 34% (95% CI 31–36%) of ischemic stroke patients and in 60% (95% CI 57–64%) of ICH patients [14]. These data imply an association of CMBs with hypertension as well as with arteriopathy, such as CAA, in Alzheimer's disease.

Distribution and Associations

The topography of CMBs might indicate the presence, type, and severity of underlying SVD. Although risk factors for CMBs have been extensively investigated, aging, hypertension and the apolipoprotein E (ApoE) genotype show the most consistent associations with CMBs across different studies [9]. The association between aging and CMBs might partly reflect the increasing prevalences of hypertension and CAA. Among preventable factors, hypertension has the strongest association with CMBs, both in the general population (odds ratio [OR] 3.9; 95% CI 2.4–6.4) and in stroke patients (OR 2.3; 95% CI 1.7–3.0) [14]. Ambulatory blood pressure monitoring confirmed this association [18, 19] and demonstrated that the likelihood of CMBs was 5- to 6-fold higher in subjects with nocturnal hypertension [18]. Blood pressure is significantly higher in subjects with deep or infratentorial CMBs than in subjects with strictly lobar CMBs [15, 19, 20]. As for the ApoE genotype, the Rotterdam Scan Study found an association with the ApoE e4 allele pertaining only to a subgroup with strictly lobar CMBs and provided evidence that strictly lobar CMBs often reflect the presence of advanced CAA [15]. Thus, recent consensus divides the topographical distribution of CMBs into 'deep or infratentorial' and 'strictly lobar CMBs' (fig. 2). Some subjects with deep or infratentorial CMBs also display (not strictly) lobar CMBs (1.1% in the healthy population; 15% in first-ever stroke patients) [19, 20]. These CMBs are further classified as 'diffuse' or 'mixed' CMBs (fig. 2e, f), for which the association with hypertension is stronger compared with that for 'strictly' deep or infratentorial CMBs [19, 20]. The pathological evidence suggesting the distributional concept of CMBs will be shown in the next section (Pathological Features (2): Vascular Burden). To date, two CMB rating scales have been published: the Microbleed Anatomical Rating Scale [21] and the Brain Observer Micro Bleed Scale [22]. Both scales provide guidance for use, definition criteria for CMBs and CMB mimics, and a table for the anatomical categorization of CMBs (fig. 3).

Pathological Features (2): Vascular Burden

Histopathological studies of the vessels adjacent to CMBs defined on MRI are limited. However, it is accepted that hypertensive arteriopathy (lipofibrohyalinosis) and CAA are the dominant vascular changes associated with CMBs [5]. Fazekas et al. [4] first performed a histopathological analysis of CMBs on MRI among seven ICH patients, including three with deep ICH and four with lobar ICH. MRI showed five deep or infratentorial CMB cases (including four mixed CMB cases) and two strictly lobar CMB cases. All (deep or lobar) ICH patients showed moderate to severe lipofibrohyalinosis, suggesting that lipofibrohyalinosis seems to be the most prominent vascular finding in relation to CMBs. However, in some limited disease settings, CAA could be a specific vascular burden associated with CMBs. Schrag et al. [8] found that most lesions in demented patients contained evidence of CAA with vessel wall thickening

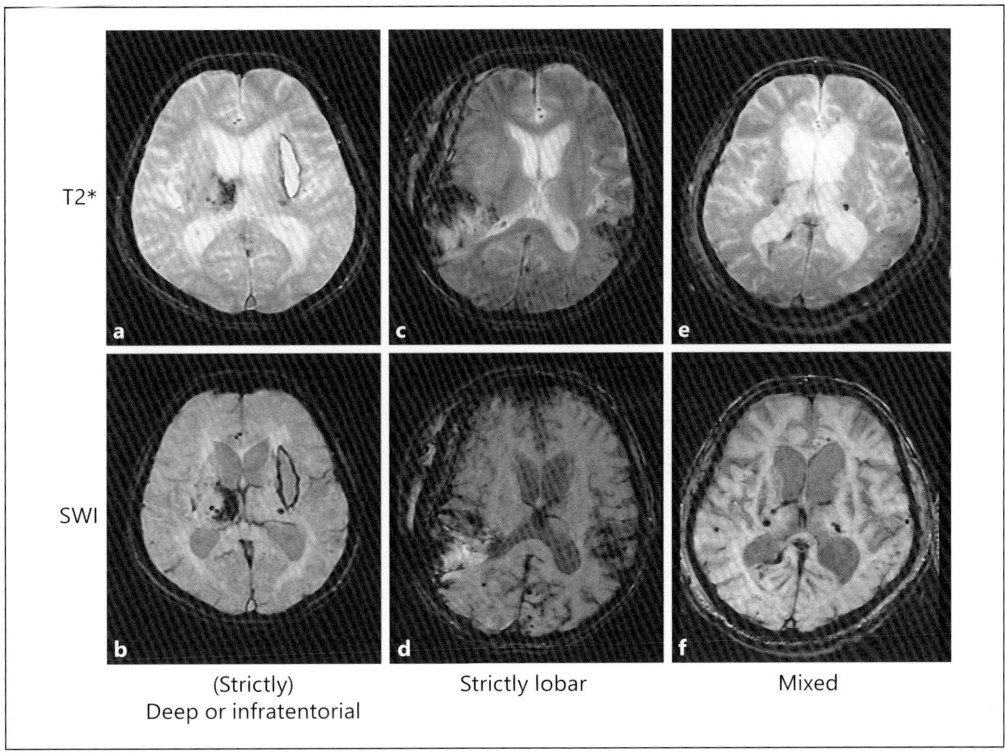

Fig. 2. Representative distributional patterns of CMBs. (Strictly) deep or infratentorial pattern: a gradient-echo (GRE) T2*-weighted image (**a**) and susceptibility-weighted imaging (SWI) (**b**) for a patient with putaminal hemorrhage show multiple CMBs in the bilateral thalamus. Strictly lobar pattern: a GRE T2*-weighted image (**c**) and SWI (**d**) for a patient with lobar hemorrhage show multiple CMBs in the posterior lobes. Hematoma evacuation samples from this patient demonstrate the presence of vascular amyloid beta deposition, suggesting pathological evidence of cerebral amyloid angiopathy (data not shown). Mixed pattern: both images (**e**, **f**) show CMBs in the bilateral thalamus. A right temporal lobar CMB is clearly seen on SWI (**f**) but is faint on the GRE T2*-weighted image (**e**).

and amyloid replacement of vascular smooth muscle. The collected histopathological data and two major factors (hypertension and CAA) lead to hypotheses regarding the topographical distribution of CMBs and their underlying SVD: deep or infratentorial CMBs imply hypertensive arteriopathy, and strictly lobar CMBs share risk factors with CAA. These hypotheses provide further avenues of investigation of the clinical relevance of the CMB distributional pattern.

Coexisting Small Vessel Disease Markers

Cerebral small vessels cannot currently be easily visualized in vivo, but the following associated cerebral parenchymal lesions are useful as SVD-related MRI markers: lacunae, white-matter changes (periventricular hyperintensities and white-matter

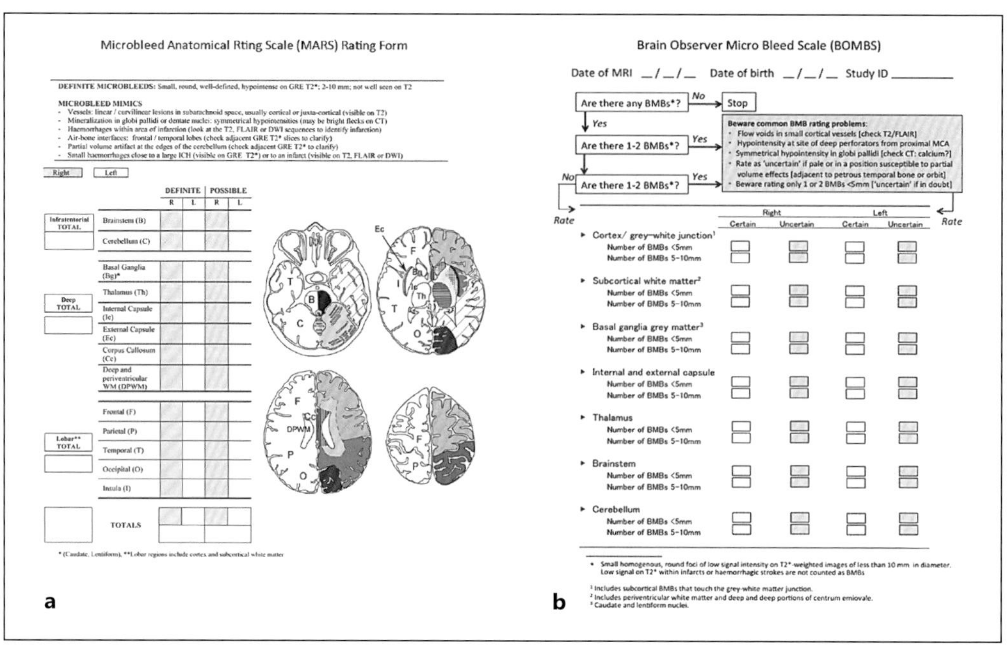
Microbleed Anatomical Rting Scale (MARS) Rating Form

DEFINITE MICROBLEEDS: Small, round, well-defined, hypointense on GRE T2*; 2-10 mm; not well seen on T2

MICROBLEED MIMICS
- Vessels: linear / curvilinear lesions in subarachnoid space, usually cortical or juxta-cortical (visible on T2)
- Mineralization in globi pallidi or dentate nuclei: symmetrical hypointensities (may be bright flecks on CT)
- Haemorrhages within area of infarction (look at the T2, FLAIR or DWI sequences to identify infarction)
- Air-bone interfaces: frontal / temporal lobes (check adjacent GRE T2* slices to clarify)
- Partial volume artifact at the edges of the cerebellum (check adjacent GRE T2* to clarify)
- Small haemorrhages close to a large ICH (visible on GRE T2*) or to an infarct (visible on T2, FLAIR or DWI)

Right Left

		DEFINITE R	DEFINITE L	POSSIBLE R	POSSIBLE L
Infratentorial TOTAL	Brainstem (B)				
	Cerebellum (C)				
Deep TOTAL	Basal Ganglia (Bg)*				
	Thalamus (Th)				
	Internal Capsule (Ic)				
	External Capsule (Ec)				
	Corpus Callosum (Cc)				
	Deep and periventricular WM (DPWM)				
Lobar** TOTAL	Frontal (F)				
	Parietal (P)				
	Temporal (T)				
	Occipital (O)				
	Insula (I)				
	TOTALS				

* (Caudate, Lentiform), **Lobar regions include cortex and subcortical white matter

a

Brain Observer Micro Bleed Scale (BOMBS)

Date of MRI __/__/__ Date of birth __/__/__ Study ID __________

Are there any BMBs*? — No → Stop
↓ Yes
Are there 1-2 BMBs*? — Yes →
↓
Are there 1-2 BMBs*? — Yes →; No → Rate

Beware common BMB rating problems:
- Flow voids in small cortical vessels [check T2/FLAIR]
- Hypointensity at site of deep perforators from proximal MCA
- Symmetrical hypointensity in globi pallidi [check CT: calcium?]
- Rate as 'uncertain' if pale or in a position susceptible to partial volume effects [adjacent to petrous temporal bone or orbit]
- Beware rating only 1 or 2 BMBs <5mm ['uncertain' if in doubt]

→ Rate

	Right Certain	Right Uncertain	Left Certain	Left Uncertain
▸ Cortex/ grey–white junction[1]				
Number of BMBs <5mm				
Number of BMBs 5–10mm				
▸ Subcortical white matter[2]				
Number of BMBs <5mm				
Number of BMBs 5–10mm				
▸ Basal ganglia grey matter[3]				
Number of BMBs <5mm				
Number of BMBs 5–10mm				
▸ Internal and external capsule				
Number of BMBs <5mm				
Number of BMBs 5–10mm				
▸ Thalamus				
Number of BMBs <5mm				
Number of BMBs 5–10mm				
▸ Brainstem				
Number of BMBs <5mm				
Number of BMBs 5–10mm				
▸ Cerebellum				
Number of BMBs <5mm				
Number of BMBs 5–10mm				

* Small homogenous, round foci of low signal intensity on T2*-weighted images of less than 10 mm in diameter. Low signal on T2* within infarcts or haemorrhagic strokes are not counted as BMBs

[1] Includes subcortical BMBs that touch the grey-white matter junction.
[2] Includes periventricular white matter and deep and deep portions of centrum emiovale.
[3] Caudate and lentiform nuclei.

b

Fig. 3. Rating scales for cerebral microbleeds. **a** Microbleed Anatomical Rating Scale: the figure is reproduced from the figure of Gregoire et al. [21]. **b** The Brain Observer Micro Bleed Scale: generated from the figure of Cordonnier et al. [22]. Reuse of the figures has been permitted by Wolters Kluwer Health.

hyperintensities), perivascular spaces (PVSs), and CMBs. CMBs are strongly associated with the other SVD markers, but few studies have simultaneously evaluated all of these MRI markers. Recent data from the Kashima Scan Study (the current author is the chief leader of that study), an ongoing Japanese population-based cohort study investigating age-related brain changes on MRI, included these markers: lacunae, severe periventricular hyperintensities (Fazekas grade 2 or higher), severe white-matter hyperintensities (Fazekas grade 2 or higher), severe basal ganglia (BG) PVSs (11 or more), and severe centrum semiovale PVSs (21 or more) [23]. That study included 1,575 neurologically healthy adults (mean age 57.1 years, standard deviation 9.7; 47% male) and revealed that each marker was significantly associated with CMBs, even after adjusting for age and sex, as follows: lacunae (OR 3.88, 95% CI 2.15–7.02, $p < 0.001$), severe periventricular hyperintensities (OR 5.53, 95% CI 2.87–10.64, $p < 0.001$), severe white-matter hyperintensities (OR 3.28, 95% CI 2.10–5.13, $p < 0.001$), severe BG PVSs (OR 3.46, 95% CI 2.14–5.57, $p < 0.001$), and severe centrum semiovale PVSs (OR 1.93, 95% CI 1.26–2.97, $p < 0.003$) (unpublished data from binary logistic regression analyses). As described above, there are two main sporadic forms of SVD: hypertensive arteriopathy, which typically affects the small perforating end-arteries of the deep gray nuclei and deep white matter, and CAA, a common age-related condition characterized by the progressive deposition of amyloid beta in the media and adventitia of small arteries, arterioles and capillaries in the cerebral cortex, overlying the leptomeninges and gray-white matter junction [24]. Among the ratings of SVD markers, observation of the topographical distribution of CMBs and PVSs could be a specific tool to identify the underlying pathogenesis of SVD; 'deep or infratentorial' CMBs and severe BG PVSs seem to be associated with hypertensive arteriopathy, while strictly lobar CMBs and severe centrum semiovale PVSs share risk factors with CAA [15, 20, 23], suggesting that the combination rating of the topographies of CMBs and PVSs might be useful for further understanding a patient's SVD condition. Recently, an interesting conception of the total SVD score [25], composed of the above-described major MRI markers of SVD, has been proposed as a comprehensive index of SVD severity in the brain. The validity of this score is still unknown, but such a concept might be useful for future observational or interventional clinical studies of stroke or dementia prevention in SVD.

Disease and Cerebral Microbleeds

Stroke

CMBs can appear in any subtypes of stroke, but there are differences in their prevalence; among first-ever stroke patients, the prevalence of CMBs is the highest in spontaneous ICH (79%), followed by atherothrombotic brain infarction (46%), other types of infarction (39%), lacunar infarction (36%), cardioembolic infarction (30%), and transient ischemic attack (TIA) (8%) [19]. Thus, CMBs are common in hemorrhagic or ischemic stroke but rare in TIA, which suggests that the severity of the underlying SVD might be higher in stroke patients than in TIA patients [26].

Spontaneous Intracerebral Hemorrhage

Among all patterns of CMB topography, the strictly lobar CMB type is the most established specific pattern for an SVD that is CAA, which is commonly seen in lobar ICH in the elderly. Similar to lobar ICH, CMBs in CAA have a posterior cortical predominance (favoring the temporal and occipital lobes) (fig. 2c, d), and they also tend to cluster in the same lobe [27]. The Boston criteria (table 1) have been established to make a clinical diagnosis of CAA [28]. The specificity of the Boston criteria has been validated against the established gold standard of neuropathological diagnosis based on autopsy, hematoma evacuation or cortical biopsy. Recently, application of the Boston criteria with the use of T2*-GRE MRI in Dutch-type hereditary CAA yielded a specificity approaching 100% and a much improved sensitivity when lobar CMBs were included in the criteria [29]. A neuroimaging study of clinically probable CAA using noninvasive amyloid imaging with 11C-Pittsburgh Compound B found that lobar CMBs correspond to areas with a high concentration of amyloid [30]. Thus, additional consideration of the location of macro/microhemorrhage on computed tomography and MRI may suggest a diagnosis of CAA-related ICH. In contrast to CAA-related ICH, there are no definite criteria for the diagnosis of hypertensive ICH. However, in addition to the 'deep or infratentorial CMBs', the presence of other hypertensive target organ damage (i.e., cardiomegaly, hypertensive retinopathy, chronic kidney disease) would improve the accuracy of the diagnosis of hypertensive ICH.

Alzheimer's Disease

In Alzheimer's disease, CMBs are of special interest, as they may have a crucial role in the pathophysiology of the disease. In a pooled population, the CMB prevalence was estimated as 23% (95% CI 17–31%) in Alzheimer's disease (fig. 1) [16]. Pathologically, the majority of the lesions appeared in a cortico-subcortical location, and amyloid beta deposition was present in the vessel walls adjacent to the bleeds, suggesting that cortico-subcortical CMBs are a consequence of underlying CAA [8]. Specifically in Alzheimer's disease, it is conceivable that CMBs can develop through both pathways, as CAA and cerebrovascular pathology (i.e., arterial hypertension) both play a role in the pathophysiology of the disease [16]. In the Honolulu Asia Aging Study, mid-life elevated blood pressure was hypothesized to compromise vascular integrity, leading to CAA, implying that long-term hypertension exposure might aggravate or interact with CAA [31].

Cerebral Autosomal Dominant Arteriopathy with Subcortical Infarcts and Leukoencephalopathy

Cerebral autosomal dominant arteriopathy with subcortical infarcts and leukoencephalopathy (CADASIL) is an inherited cerebrovascular disease that results from a mutation in the NOTCH3 gene, which has been mapped to chromosome 19q12. The main clinical manifestations of the disease are migraines with aura, mood disturbances, recurrent ischemic strokes, and progressive cognitive decline. The typical MRI features include white-matter changes on T2-weighted images, lacunar infarcts on T1-weighted images, and CMBs on paramagnetic-sensitive MR sequences. CMBs have been reported to occur in 25–69% of patients with CADASIL. 'Deep or infratentorial CMBs' or 'mixed' patterns seem to be common in CADASIL. In the Dutch series, CMBs were most commonly found in the thalamus (61%), followed by the subcortical white matter (26%), while in the German cohort, they most commonly occurred at the cortical-subcortical junction (38%), followed by the cerebral white matter (20%), the thalamus and BG (20%), and the brain stem (14%) [32]. An autopsy-based CADASIL study found evidence of hemosiderin-laden macrophages in the vicinity of 100- to 300-μm blood vessels, the vessel walls of which showed characteristic degenerative changes, which are considered as representing the involvement of CADASIL-related ultrastructural modifications of the vessel wall [33].

Moyamoya Disease

Moyamoya disease is a chronic progressive, occlusive cerebrovascular disorder in which intracranial internal carotid arteries and their proximal branches become occluded. The name comes from the Japanese word for 'puff of smoke', which refers to

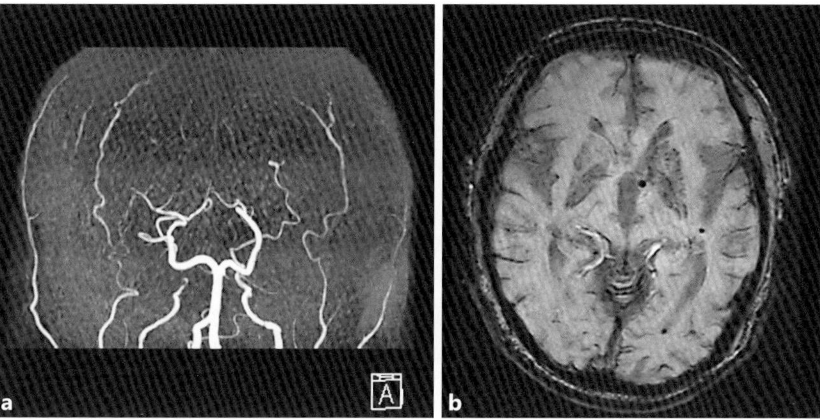

Fig. 4. Images of definite adult-onset moyamoya disease with previous intraventricular hemorrhage. **a** Magnetic resonance angiography shows bilateral occlusions in the terminal portion of the internal carotid artery. **b** SWI shows three CMBs in the periventricular deep white matter (the left hemisphere).

the characteristic appearance of fine tortuous collateral vessels as compensation for the compromise of carotid flow. TIA, ischemic stroke and ICH are recognized complications of the disorder. In a hospitalized patient cohort study, CMBs were seen in 44% of patients with symptomatic moyamoya disease (44% of ischemic nature and 43% of hemorrhagic nature) [34]. Similarly to CMBs with hypertensive pathology, CMBs in moyamoya disease were commonly observed in deep brain areas but were predominantly located in the periventricular deep white matter (fig. 4) [34]. This finding is consistent with the fact that intraventricular hemorrhage is common in patients with hemorrhagic moyamoya disease associated with an increased hemodynamic load in the vessels supplying the walls of the ventricles or the periventricular region.

Neurological Dysfunction and Cerebral Microbleeds

Cognitive Impairment

SVD, particularly that of an ischemic nature (i.e., lacunae, white-matter changes), has been generally accepted as a major risk factor for vascular cognitive impairment. Recently, increasing attention has been paid to the relevance of CMBs with regard to cognition. This interesting association was first reported from a hospital-based stroke patient cohort study, showing that executive dysfunction was more common in the group with CMBs than in the control group [35]. This provisional concept was supported by a subsequent healthy population-based study, which demonstrated that global cognitive dysfunction was independently associated with both the presence and the number of CMBs [36]. One question is whether different effects on global cognitive function might be seen with different distributions (i.e., lobar areas or deep areas) of CMBs. Two large studies of a healthy cohort investigated this issue, but the results of these studies conflicted with each another. The Rotterdam Scan Study indicated that the presence of numerous CMBs, particularly in a strictly lobar location (with relevance to CAA), was associated with cognitive decline in the general population [37]. In contrast, a Japanese healthy population-based study demonstrated that CMB-related global cognitive dysfunction seems to occur based on 'deep or infratentorial' CMBs (which are considered as hypertensive in nature) [20]. Differences in ethnic background (Asian versus non-Asian) could be considered as potential contributors to such contradictory findings. The main CMB-related cognitive domains seemed to be executive functions, including attention and calculation, but not memory [20, 35–37]. The mechanisms underlying pathological associations between CMBs and such cognitive domains remain unclear, but the Kashima Scan Study reported that BG CMBs (but not thalamic or infratentorial CMBs) are significantly associated with global cognitive dysfunction, particularly affecting attention and calculation, implying that a direct or indirect effect of BG CMBs could affect the function of cortico-BG circuits [38]. At present, according to a recent systematic review including seven studies, it can be concluded that CMBs might have some association with cognitive dysfunction, but these findings are tentative in light of the fact that all of the included studies were cross-sectional in nature [39]. To adequately address this question, high-quality prospective longitudinal studies are needed.

Gait Disturbance

Classical SVDs, including lacunae or white-matter changes, adversely affect gait, but little is known about the impact of CMBs on gait disturbance. A Dutch group first indicated the association between CMBs and gait disturbances, independently of other coexisting markers of SVD [40]. The authors reported that those relationships seemed to be mainly explained by CMBs in the frontal lobe and BG (including the thalamus), which are areas involved in the control of gait. The Tasmanian Study of Cognition and Gait (TASCOG) included a population-based sample of older people and investigated the associations between CMBs and pleiotropic variables for gait disturbances (i.e., gait speed, cadence, step length, step width, double support time, and fall risk) [41]. Among those factors, CMBs were associated with only cadence, even after adjustment for other SVD findings. Similar to the issue of CMB-related cognitive impairment, prospective longitudinal studies are needed clarify this issue.

Clinical Relevance of Cerebral Microbleeds

Subsequent Stroke

The strong association between CMBs and stroke raises the question of whether CMBs can predict future stroke. A Japanese longitudinal study of a healthy cohort (mean follow-up interval of 3.6 years) reported that the presence of CMBs at baseline is a strong independent risk factor for subsequent ischemic stroke (hazard ratio [HR], 4.48; 95% CI 2.20–12.2) and subsequent hemorrhagic stroke (deep brain hemorrhage) (HR 50.2; 95% CI 16.7–150.2), even in stroke-free subjects [42]. These surprising results imply that the detection of CMBs on MRI could be an indication for primary preventative measures for stroke, but this notion must be confirmed in other cohorts. A European hospitalized ischemic stroke patient cohort study (median follow-up interval of 2.2 years) revealed that all CMBs were not independent predictors of recurrent stroke but that strictly lobar CMBs (HR 2.3; 95% CI 1.02–5.19) or mixed CMBs (combined lobar and deep CMBs) (HR 2.7; 95% CI 1.2–6.4) were independently associated with recurrent stroke, and especially ischemic stroke [43]. In patients with symptomatic moyamoya disease, the presence of two or more CMBs appeared to be a predictor of subsequent ICH (HR 2.89; 95% CI 1.00–13.24) [44].

Cerebral Microbleeds and Antithrombotic Drug-Related Intracerebral Hemorrhage
Increasing use of antiplatelet or anticoagulant agents for the secondary prevention of ischemic stroke or cardiovascular diseases increases the risk of subsequent ICH, especially in elderly patients. It is a challenge to demonstrate whether CMBs are associated with the development of ICH in patients receiving antithrombotic agent(s) because the necessity of antithrombotic therapy commonly reflects the patient's high vascular burden (including CMBs), which is also strongly associated with ICH. A meta-analysis showed that CMBs are more common in warfarin-related ICH than in spontaneous ICH [45]. Additionally, based on pooled follow-up data for patients treated with antithrombotics (anticoagulant or antiplatelet drugs), the presence of CMBs at baseline was associated with subsequent ICH (OR, 12.1; 95% CI 3.4–42.5) [45]. CAA might be a risk factor for antithrombotic drug-related ICH, so the reliable detection of multiple strictly lobar CMBs could be a promising indictor of the need for anticoagulation therapy [46]. To clarify these issues, one large prospective multicenter MRI study is currently underway in the UK (Clinical Relevance of Microbleeds in Stroke: CROMIS-2; http://www.ucl.ac.uk/cromis-2/).

Cerebral Microbleeds and Post-Thrombolysis Intracerebral Hemorrhage
It would be interesting to determine whether CMBs on pre-thrombolysis MRI can predict subsequent symptomatic ICH. Recently published meta-analysis data suggest a trend toward an increased risk of symptomatic ICH in thrombolyzed ischemic stroke patients with CMBs [47, 48]. CAA might be associated with post-thrombolysis ICH because spontaneous CAA-related ICH and thrombolysis-related ICH share some features, including a predilection for lobar brain regions, a multiplicity of hemorrhages, age dependency and associations with dementia and leukoaraiosis [49].

Conclusions and Future Directions

Evidence suggests that CMBs should not be considered to be clinically 'silent'. When CMBs are detected in healthy adults, physicians should recognize that subclinical SVD might have developed in these adults' brains. At present, we have only antihypertensive treatments as a potential strategy for patients with CMBs to avoid CMB expansion and subsequent ICH. The associations of CMBs with hypertension and with antithrombotic drugs suggest that CMBs are warning signs of inappropriate blood pressure control and antithrombotic drug use. In the field of CAA, new therapeutic approaches, including monoclonal antibodies against vascular amyloid, are being developed. The identification of novel mechanisms may allow therapeutic targeting of amyloid deposition [50]. Thus, CMBs will be important components of future studies investigating how SVD influences neurodegeneration via neurovascular units in elderly populations and in demented persons.

References

1 Offenbacher H, Fazekas F, Schmidt R, Koch M, Fazekas G, Kapeller P: MR of cerebral abnormalities concomitant with primary intracerebral hematomas. AJNR Am J Neuroradiol 1996;17:573–578.
2 Wardlaw JM, Smith EE, Biessels GJ, Cordonnier C, Fazekas F, Frayne R, et al: Neuroimaging standards for research into small vessel disease and its contribution to aging and neurodegeneration. Lancet Neurol 2013;12:822–838.
3 Greenberg SM, Vernooij MW, Cordonnier C, Viswanathan A, Al-Shahi Salman R, Warach S, et al: Cerebral microbleeds: A guide to detection and interpretation. Lancet Neurol 2009;8:165–174.
4 Fazekas F, Kleinert R, Roob G, Kleinert G, Kapeller P, Schmidt R, et al: Histopathologic analysis of foci of signal loss on gradient-echo T2*-weighted MR images in patients with spontaneous intracerebral hemorrhage: evidence of microangiopathy-related microbleeds. AJNR Am J Neuroradiol 1999;20:637–642.
5 Shoamanesh A, Kwok CS, Benavente O: Cerebral microbleeds: histopathological correlation of neuroimaging. Cerebrovasc Dis 2011;32:528–534.
6 Tanaka A, Ueno Y, Nakayama Y, Takano K, Takebayashi S: Small chronic hemorrhages and ischemic lesions in association with spontaneous intracerebral hematomas. Stroke 1999;30:1637–1642.
7 Tatsumi S, Shinohara M, Yamamoto T: Direct comparison of histology of microbleeds with postmortem MR images: a case report. Cerebrovasc Dis 2008; 26:142–146.
8 Schrag M, McAuley G, Pomakian J, Jiffry A, Tung S, Mueller C, et al: Correlation of hypointensities in susceptibility-weighted images to tissue histology in dementia patients with cerebral amyloid angiopathy: a postmortem MRI study. Acta Neuropathol 2010; 119:291–302.
9 Charidimou A, Krishnan A, Werring DJ, Rolf Jager H: Cerebral microbleeds: a guide to detection and clinical relevance in different disease settings. Neuroradiology 2013;55:655–674.
10 Nandigam RN, Viswanathan A, Delgado P, Skehan ME, Smith EE, Rosand J, et al: MR imaging detection of cerebral microbleeds: effect of susceptibility-weighted imaging, section thickness, and field strength. AJNR Am J Neuroradiol 2009;30:338–343.
11 Conijn MM, Geerlings MI, Biessels GJ, Takahara T, Witkamp TD, Zwanenburg JJ, et al: Cerebral microbleeds on MR imaging: comparison between 1.5 and 7T. AJNR Am J Neuroradiol 2011;32:1043–1049.
12 Greenberg SM, Nandigam RN, Delgado P, Betensky RA, Rosand J, Viswanathan A, et al: Microbleeds versus macrobleeds: evidence for distinct entities. Stroke 2009;40:2382–2386.
13 Neshika Samarasekera GP, Al-Shahi Salman R: Cerebral microbleed mimics, in Werring DJ (ed): Cerebral Microbleeds. Cambridge, Cambridge University Press, 2011, pp 44–48.
14 Cordonnier C, Al-Shahi Salman R, Wardlaw J: Spontaneous brain microbleeds: systematic review, subgroup analyses and standards for study design and reporting. Brain 2007;130:1988–2003.

15 Vernooij MW, van der Lugt A, Ikram MA, Wielopolski PA, Niessen WJ, Hofman A, et al: Prevalence and risk factors of cerebral microbleeds: the Rotterdam scan study. Neurology 2008;70:1208–1214.
16 Cordonnier C, van der Flier WM: Brain microbleeds and Alzheimer's disease: innocent observation or key player? Brain 2011;134:335–344.
17 Staekenborg SS, Koedam EL, Henneman WJ, Stokman P, Barkhof F, Scheltens P, et al: Progression of mild cognitive impairment to dementia: contribution of cerebrovascular disease compared with medial temporal lobe atrophy. Stroke 2009;40:1269–1274.
18 Henskens LH, van Oostenbrugge RJ, Kroon AA, de Leeuw PW, Lodder J: Brain microbleeds are associated with ambulatory blood pressure levels in a hypertensive population. Hypertension 2008;51:62–68.
19 Yakushiji Y, Yokota C, Yamada N, Kuroda Y, Minematsu K: Clinical characteristics by topographical distribution of brain microbleeds, with a particular emphasis on diffuse microbleeds. J Stroke Cerebrovasc Dis 2011;20:214–221.
20 Yakushiji Y, Noguchi T, Hara M, Nishihara M, Eriguchi M, Nanri Y, et al. Distributional impact of brain microbleeds on global cognitive function in adults without neurological disorder. Stroke 2012;43:1800–1805.
21 Gregoire SM, Chaudhary UJ, Brown MM, Yousry TA, Kallis C, Jager HR, et al: The microbleed anatomical rating scale (MARS): reliability of a tool to map brain microbleeds. Neurology 2009;73:1759–1766.
22 Cordonnier C, Potter GM, Jackson CA, Doubal F, Keir S, Sudlow CL, et al: Improving interrater agreement about brain microbleeds: development of the brain observer microbleed scale (BOMBS). Stroke 2009;40:94–99.
23 Yakushiji Y, Charidimou A, Hara M, Noguchi T, Nishihara M, Eriguchi M, et al: Topography and associations of perivascular spaces in healthy adults: the Kashima scan study. Neurology 2014;83:2116–2123.
24 Pantoni L: Cerebral small vessel disease: from pathogenesis and clinical characteristics to therapeutic challenges. Lancet Neurol 2010;9:689–701.
25 Staals J, Makin SD, Doubal FN, Dennis MS, Wardlaw JM: Stroke subtype, vascular risk factors, and total MRI brain small-vessel disease burden. Neurology 2014;83:1228–1234.
26 Werring DJ, Coward LJ, Losseff NA, Jager HR, Brown MM: Cerebral microbleeds are common in ischemic stroke but rare in TIA. Neurology 2005;65:1914–1918.
27 Rosand J, Muzikansky A, Kumar A, Wisco JJ, Smith EE, Betensky RA, et al. Spatial clustering of hemorrhages in probable cerebral amyloid angiopathy. Ann Neurol 2005;58:459–462.
28 Knudsen KA, Rosand J, Karluk D, Greenberg SM: Clinical diagnosis of cerebral amyloid angiopathy: validation of the Boston criteria. Neurology 2001;56:537–539.
29 van Rooden S, van der Grond J, van den Boom R, Haan J, Linn J, Greenberg SM, et al: Descriptive analysis of the Boston criteria applied to a Dutch-type cerebral amyloid angiopathy population. Stroke 2009;40:3022–3027.
30 Park JH, Seo SW, Kim C, Kim GH, Noh HJ, Kim ST, et al: Pathogenesis of cerebral microbleeds: in vivo imaging of amyloid and subcortical ischemic small vessel disease in 226 individuals with cognitive impairment. Ann Neurol 2013;73:584–593.
31 Shah NS, Vidal JS, Masaki K, Petrovitch H, Ross GW, Tilley C, et al: Midlife blood pressure, plasma beta-amyloid, and the risk for Alzheimer disease: the Honolulu Asia aging study. Hypertension 2012;59:780–786.
32 Viswanathan A, Chabriat H: Cerebral microhemorrhage. Stroke 2006;37:550–555.
33 Dichgans M, Holtmannspotter M, Herzog J, Peters N, Bergmann M, Yousry TA: Cerebral microbleeds in CADASIL: a gradient-echo magnetic resonance imaging and autopsy study. Stroke 2002;33:67–71.
34 Kikuta K, Takagi Y, Nozaki K, Hanakawa T, Okada T, Mikuni N, et al: Asymptomatic microbleeds in moyamoya disease: T2*-weighted gradient-echo magnetic resonance imaging study. J Neurosurg 2005;102:470–475.
35 Werring DJ, Frazer DW, Coward LJ, Losseff NA, Watt H, Cipolotti L, et al: Cognitive dysfunction in patients with cerebral microbleeds on T2*-weighted gradient-echo MRI. Brain 2004;127:2265–2275.
36 Yakushiji Y, Nishiyama M, Yakushiji S, Hirotsu T, Uchino A, Nakajima J, et al: Brain microbleeds and global cognitive function in adults without neurological disorder. Stroke 2008;39:3323–3328.
37 Poels MM, Ikram MA, van der Lugt A, Hofman A, Niessen WJ, Krestin GP, et al: Cerebral microbleeds are associated with worse cognitive function: the Rotterdam scan study. Neurology 2012;78:326–333.
38 Yakushiji Y, Noguchi T, Charidimou A, Eriguchi M, Nishihara M, Hara M, et al: Basal ganglia cerebral microbleeds and global cognitive function: the Kashima scan study. J Stroke Cerebrovasc Dis 2015;24:431–439.
39 Lei C, Lin S, Tao W, Hao Z, Liu M, Wu B: Association between cerebral microbleeds and cognitive function: a systematic review. J Neurol Neurosurg Psychiatry 2013;84:693–697.
40 de Laat KF, van den Berg HA, van Norden AG, Gons RA, Olde Rikkert MG, de Leeuw FE: Microbleeds are independently related to gait disturbances in elderly individuals with cerebral small vessel disease. Stroke 2011;42:494–497.

41 Choi P, Ren M, Phan TG, Callisaya M, Ly JV, Beare R, et al: Silent infarcts and cerebral microbleeds modify the associations of white matter lesions with gait and postural stability: population-based study. Stroke 2012;43:1505–1510.
42 Bokura H, Saika R, Yamaguchi T, Nagai A, Oguro H, Kobayashi S, et al: Microbleeds are associated with subsequent hemorrhagic and ischemic stroke in healthy elderly individuals. Stroke 2011;42:1867–1871.
43 Thijs V, Lemmens R, Schoofs C, Gorner A, Van Damme P, Schrooten M, et al: Microbleeds and the risk of recurrent stroke. Stroke 2010;41:2005–2009.
44 Kikuta K, Takagi Y, Nozaki K, Sawamoto N, Fukuyama H, Hashimoto N: The presence of multiple microbleeds as a predictor of subsequent cerebral hemorrhage in patients with moyamoya disease. Neurosurgery 2008;62:104–112.
45 Lovelock CE, Cordonnier C, Naka H, Al-Shahi Salman R, Sudlow CL, Edinburgh Stroke Study Group, et al: Antithrombotic drug use, cerebral microbleeds, and intracerebral hemorrhage: a systematic review of published and unpublished studies. Stroke 2010;41:1222–1228.
46 Charidimou A, Gang Q, Werring DJ: Sporadic cerebral amyloid angiopathy revisited: recent insights into pathophysiology and clinical spectrum. J Neurol Neurosurg Psychiatry 2012;83:124–137.
47 Shoamanesh A, Kwok CS, Lim PA, Benavente OR: Postthrombolysis intracranial hemorrhage risk of cerebral microbleeds in acute stroke patients: a systematic review and meta-analysis. Int J Stroke 2013; 8:348–356.
48 Charidimou A, Kakar P, Fox Z, Werring DJ: Cerebral microbleeds and the risk of intracerebral haemorrhage after thrombolysis for acute ischaemic stroke: systematic review and meta-analysis. J Neurol Neurosurg Psychiatry 2013;84:277–280.
49 McCarron MO, Nicoll JA: Cerebral amyloid angiopathy and thrombolysis-related intracerebral haemorrhage. Lancet Neurol 2004;3:484–492.
50 Wilson D, Charidimou A, Werring DJ: Advances in understanding spontaneous intracerebral hemorrhage: insights from neuroimaging. Expert Rev Neurother 2014;14:661–678.

Dr. Yusuke Yakushiji
Division of Neurology, Department of Internal Medicine
Saga University Faculty of Medicine
5-1-1 Nabeshima, Saga, 849-8501 (Japan)
E-Mail yakushij@cc.saga-u.ac.jp

Toyoda K, Anderson CS, Mayer SA (eds): New Insights in Intracerebral Hemorrhage.
Front Neurol Neurosci. Basel, Karger, 2016, vol 37, pp 93–106 (DOI: 10.1159/000437116)

New Insights into Nonvitamin K Antagonist Oral Anticoagulants' Reversal of Intracerebral Hemorrhage

Masahiro Yasaka

Department of Cerebrovascular Medicine and Neurology, National Hospital Organization, Kyushu Medical Center, Fukuoka, Japan

Abstract

The nonvitamin K antagonist oral anticoagulants (NOACs) dabigatran, rivaroxaban, apixaban, and edoxaban are associated with an equal or lower incidence of stroke and systemic embolism and a much lower incidence of intracranial hemorrhage and hemorrhagic stroke than warfarin is, without the need for routine laboratory monitoring. However, reversal strategies are not currently established in the case of NOAC-related hemorrhagic stroke. In emergency situations, well-defined management for NOAC-related hemorrhagic stroke may improve clinical outcomes. Thus, in this chapter, general measures initially required to prevent the expansion of intracerebral hematomas, charcoal administration to reduce NOAC absorption from the gastrointestinal tract, application of hemodialysis to remove dabigatran, and coagulation factor therapy including 4-factor prothrombin complex concentrate and recombinant activated factor VII are reviewed. The specific reversal agents idarucizumab, which is a monoclonal antibody against dabigatran; andexanet alfa, a recombinant human factor Xa decoy for Xa inhibitors; and PER977, a small synthetic molecule for reversal of both Xa and thrombin inhibitors, are currently under development. These agents will facilitate the clinical management of NOAC-associated hemorrhagic stroke and other severe bleeding.

© 2016 S. Karger AG, Basel

Introduction

Since nonvitamin K antagonist oral anticoagulants (NOACs) appeared, the features of intracerebral hemorrhage (ICH) have been noted to differ markedly between warfarin and NOAC treatment, and the superiority of NOACs over warfarin has been

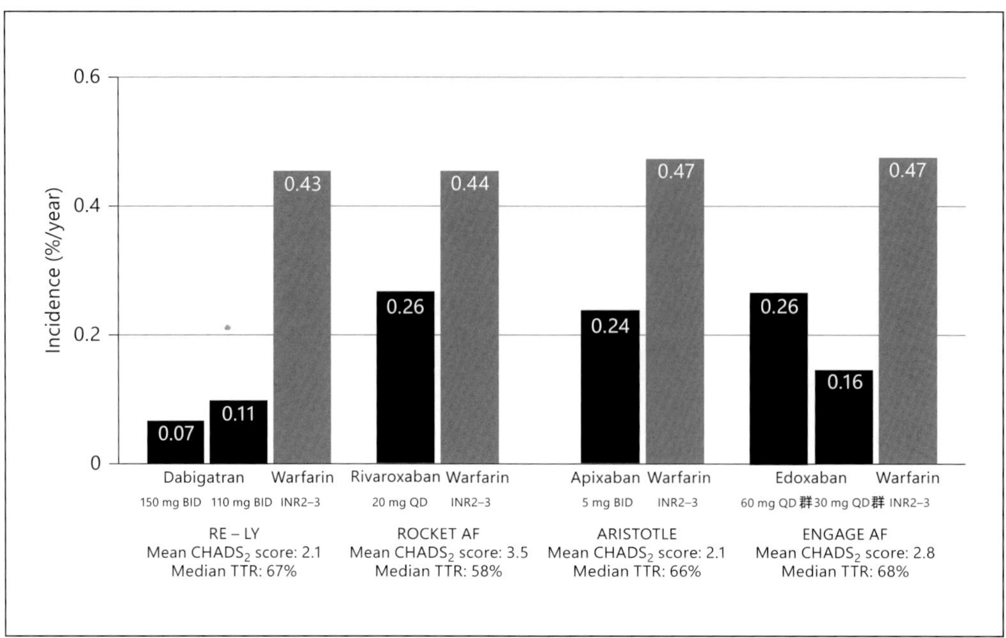

Fig. 1. Incidence of hemorrhagic stroke in phase III trials of nonvitamin K antagonist oral anticoagulants. The incidence of hemorrhagic stroke is based on an on-treatment analysis of each phase III trial, drawn from references [1–4, 6].

clearly shown. However, ICH can occur even during NOAC treatment. This chapter summarizes the features of ICH with NOACs compared with warfarin, describes what actions should be taken and what factors to consider when intracerebral bleeding arises, and refers to the development of antidotes to NOACs.

Features of Intracerebral Hemorrhage during Nonvitamin K Antagonist Oral Anticoagulant Treatment

Phase III trials of NOACs have demonstrated a much lower incidence of intracranial hemorrhage or hemorrhagic stroke in patients treated with NOACs compared with those treated with warfarin [1–6]. The incidence of hemorrhagic stroke, including ICH and subarachnoid hemorrhage, due to NOACs has been reported as 16.3–59.1% of the incidence due to warfarin (fig. 1). Graham et al. [7] investigated the comparative safety of dabigatran and warfarin in a general practice setting using Medicare data from the United States and found that dabigatran was associated with a reduced risk of intracranial hemorrhage. Hagii et al. [8] studied the characteristics of ICH during rivaroxaban treatment in comparison with ICH during warfarin treatment. They compared ICH between 5 patients treated with rivaroxaban and 56 treated with warfarin and found that patients with rivaroxaban-associated

ICH developed relatively small hematomas, showed no expansion of the hematomas, and had favorable functional outcomes compared with patients with warfarin-associated ICH. This may be attributable to the characteristics of NOACs, which have a short half-life of around half a day and which do not affect plasma concentrations of factor VII or the complexes of tissue factor and factor VIIa that are essential for the first reaction in the coagulation cascade, whereas warfarin suppresses factor VII production, even within the therapeutic range of prothrombin time (PT)-international normalized ratios (PT-INRs), resulting in a higher rate of ICH [9–12].

Comparative data on ICH with NOACs and warfarin show an outstandingly low incidence of ICH with dabigatran compared with warfarin (fig. 1). Komori et al. [13] retrospectively reviewed the clinical data and treatment summaries of nine intracranial bleeds (including two intracerebral bleeds) that developed during dabigatran treatment in eight patients with nonvalvular atrial fibrillation and found that hematomas arising due to acute intracranial bleeding during dabigatran treatment seemed to remain small to moderate, tended not to expand much, and were manageable. This phenomenon may be due to not only the short half-life and constant plasma level of VII but also the presence of thrombin-activatable fibrinolysis inhibitor. Dabigatran interacts selectively and reversibly with the active site of the thrombin molecule but does not inhibit thrombin-activatable fibrinolysis inhibitor generation, leading to down-regulation of fibrinolysis [1, 14–16]. Won et al. [15] used dual-energy CT in experimental mouse models of ICH treated with dabigatran or warfarin and found that dabigatran induced less extravasation of contrast medium, a marker of ongoing bleeding, than warfarin did. Lauer et al. [16] demonstrated that in contrast with warfarin, pre-treatment with dabigatran did not increase the hematoma volume in experimental mouse models of ICH.

Hylek et al. [17] investigated the Apixaban for Reduction in Stroke and Other Thromboembolic Events in Atrial Fibrillation (ARISTOTLE) trial data for mortality in patients with major hemorrhage and found that compared with warfarin, apixaban was associated with fewer intracranial hemorrhages, less severe adverse consequences following extracranial hemorrhages, and a 50% reduction in fatal consequences at 30 days in cases of major hemorrhage. One of the reasons for the favorable outcomes in patients with major hemorrhage during apixaban treatment may be that hematomas occurring during apixaban treatment tend to show limited expansion (fig. 2).

In contrast, some reports have indicated unfavorable outcomes of intracranial hemorrhage or ICH in patients treated with NOACs. Hart et al. [6] investigated aspects of intracranial hemorrhage using data from the Randomized Evaluation of Long-Term Anticoagulation Therapy (RE-LY) trial and found that the clinical spectrum of intracranial hemorrhage was similar for patients given warfarin and dabigatran, while absolute rates at all sites of both fatal and traumatic intracranial hemorrhages were lower with dabigatran than with warfarin. However, mortality rates for intracranial hemorrhage during dabigatran treatment were comparable to those

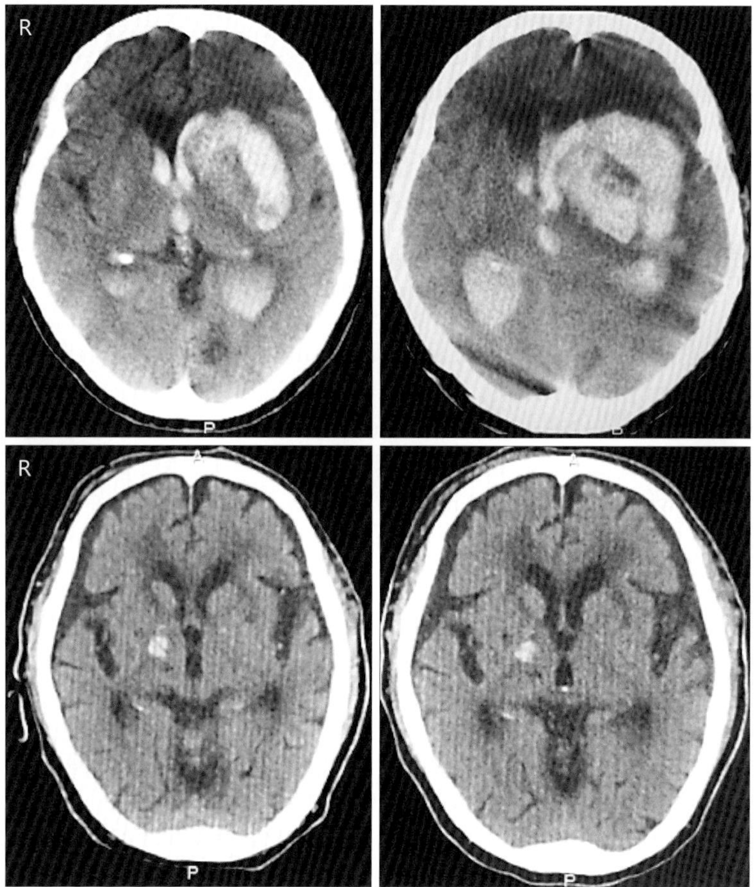

Fig. 2. Intracerebral hemorrhage (ICH) during treatment with warfarin and nonvitamin K antagonist oral anticoagulants. Upper: Brain CT images of an ICH in an 80-year-old woman treated with warfarin. The prothrombin time-international normalized ratio at onset was 2.0. The hematoma that had developed 45 min after onset (left) expanded 5 h and 30 min afterward (right). Lower: Brain CT images indicate that an ICH in an 81-year-old man receiving apixaban treatment did not expanded at all. Left: 1 h after onset. Right: 7 h after onset. R = Right.

during warfarin treatment. Likewise, using a market research database, Alonso et al. [18] found no difference in in-hospital mortality rates between patients with acute intracranial bleeding during treatment with dabigatran and warfarin, and the researchers concluded that reluctance to use dabigatran because of a lack of approved reversal agents was not supported. Shoji et al. [19] reported five cases of intracranial hemorrhage related to dabigatran administration. Outcomes were poor for all but one patient. Debata et al. [20] reported three cases of ICH during rivaroxaban treatment, with two patients showing hematoma expansion on CT and fatal deterioration after admission.

The incidence of ICH during NOAC treatment is obviously much lower than that during warfarin treatment, and some reports have indicated that hematomas arising due to acute ICH during NOAC treatment seem to remain small to moderate, less likely to expand, and manageable. Mortality from intracranial hemorrhage was not increased in NOAC-treated patients compared with those given warfarin. This observation, coupled with the substantially lower absolute rates of intracranial hemorrhage with NOACs, explains why the likelihood of dying from intracranial bleeding is significantly lower during anticoagulation with NOACs compared with warfarin [6]. However, there remains concern that patients with intracranial hemorrhage during treatment with NOACs could show a worse prognosis than those treated with warfarin due to the absence of proven treatments to emergently reverse the antithrombotic effect. It seems quite important both to understand the general measures initially required to prevent the expansion of intracerebral hematoma, the usefulness of charcoal administration to reduce NOAC absorption from the gastrointestinal tract, the application of hemodialysis to remove dabigatran, and the efficacy of coagulation factor therapy including 4-factor prothrombin complex concentrate (PCC) and recombinant activated factor VII (rVIIa) and to develop antidotes for each NOAC.

What Should Be Done When Intracerebral Hemorrhage Occurs?

In the event of an anticoagulant-associated major bleed, besides specific antidotes or general hemostatic agents, general measures are initially required [21–23]. First, to prevent any increase in the concentration of the anticoagulant, anticoagulants must be withheld. Second, if possible, the active hemorrhage must be controlled by compressing or ligating the source of bleeding. Third, in order to maintain the blood pressure within the normal range, lost fluids must be replaced using infusion of intravenous fluids so that the anticoagulant can be efficiently metabolized and excreted from the body; the half-life of NOACs is usually about half a day. Fourth, if hemorrhagic stroke develops, the systolic blood pressure needs to be kept under 140 mm Hg [24].

What Can Be Considered When Intracerebral Hemorrhage Occurs?

Hemostatic measures for reversal of the anticoagulant effects induced by each NOAC are summarized in table 1.

Evaluating the Anticoagulant Effect

A major advantage of NOACs is that routine monitoring of the anticoagulant effect is not required, unlike for warfarin [23]. However, a precise quantitative assessment of anticoagulation would be helpful in a number of clinical settings. Currently, it is known that some laboratory tests are associated with serum concentrations of

Table 1. Hemostatic measures for reversal of the anticoagulant effects induced by each NOAC

	Dabigatran	Rivaroxaban	Apixaban	Edoxaban
Oral activated charcoal	yes	yes	yes	yes
Hemodialysis	yes	no	no	no
Hemoperfusion with activated charcoal	possible	unclear	unclear	unclear
4-factor PCC	possible	possible	possible	possible
Recombinant VIIa	probable	probable	probable	probable
Activated factor VIIa	probable	probable	probable	probable
3-factor PCC	unclear	unclear	unclear	unclear
FFP	no	no	no	no

NOACs, including the activated partial thromboplastin time (aPTT) and the thrombin clotting time in general, the ecarin clotting time for dabigatran, the PT-INRs for rivaroxaban and edoxaban, and anti-Xa activity for all Xa inhibitors. However, there are no widely available, specific laboratory tests to rapidly and precisely assess the degree of real-time anticoagulation in a patient treated with NOACs [23]. Further studies are needed to understand the relationships between laboratory test results and the anticoagulant effect of each NOAC. Standardizing laboratory tests for a better and more precise understanding of these relationships is also required.

Charcoal Administration

T-max, which is the time to the peak serum concentration after taking an NOAC, is usually 1–4 h. The serum concentration may increase after the onset of ICH if ICH happens within 4 h of NOAC administration. In such cases, activated charcoal administration, a therapy with limited side effects, may be strongly indicated to minimize further NOAC absorption. Activated charcoal is a processed form of carbon with a very fine network of pores and a large internal surface area that is available for binding to oral drugs, reducing their absorption from the gastrointestinal tract [25–28]. Limited data have been published on the use of oral activated charcoal in the setting of dabigatran ingestion, but an in vitro study by van Ryn et al. [29] demonstrated that dabigatran can be successfully adsorbed by activated charcoal. Activated charcoal was administered to a 57-year-old woman via gastric lavage after ingestion of 11.25 g dabigatran in a suicide attempt, and major bleeding was successfully avoided [30, 31]. The Food and Drug Administration's advisory committee reported a rat model that showed a 65% decrease in the area under the concentration curve when charcoal was administered 15 min after rivaroxaban ingestion [26, 32].

Hemodialysis

Dabigatran has relatively low plasma protein binding, or 35%, making removal by hemodialysis possible [33]. A single-center report of six patients who had been administered blood product and hemodialysis for dabigatran removal for the treatment of acute life-threatening bleeding demonstrated that dabigatran concentrations decreased by 52–77% during intermittent hemodialysis but rebounded up to 87% within 2 h after completion of dialysis [33]. Initiation of continuous renal replacement therapy after intermittent hemodialysis attenuated the rebound effect in one patient and contributed to an 81% reduction in dabigatran concentrations over 30 h. The authors of the study concluded that hemodialysis removed the dabigatran and may effectively accelerate total clearance. In another study of six volunteers undergoing hemodialysis for end-stage renal disease, 62 and 68% of the drug were removed after 2 and 4 h, respectively [34].

No reports indicating the usefulness of hemodialysis for Xa inhibitor reversal have been published. The plasma protein binding of Xa inhibitors is so high that it may be impossible to remove them effectively with hemodialysis.

Hemoperfusion with Activated Charcoal

The utility of charcoal hemoperfusion was successfully tested in an in vitro study that demonstrated the effective removal of dabigatran through charcoal hemoperfusion from a solution of a mixture of dabigatran and bovine plasma [35]. However, there have been no reports of the use of charcoal hemoperfusion in humans in vivo.

Coagulation Factor Therapy

Prothrombin Complex Concentrate

In a murine model of ICH, either saline or dabigatran at 4.5 or 9.0 mg/kg was administered, and then the mice underwent ICH induction, followed by treatment with saline, murine fresh frozen plasma (FFP), nonactivated 4-factor PCC, or recombinant human VIIa [36]. The mice were sacrificed 24 h later, and the size of their brain hematoma was measured. The researchers showed that 4-factor PCC reversed prolongation of the bleeding time, prevented excess hematoma expansion in a dose-dependent manner, and was associated with improved survival. The reversed prolongation of the bleeding time was observed with the highest dose of PCC (100 U/kg), but not with two lower doses (25 and 50 U/kg). However, a significant reduction in the hematoma volume was obtained not only with the highest dose of PCC but also with the middle dose (50 U/kg), suggesting that the reversal effect of PCC may be manifested without the correction of laboratory tests.

Furthermore, van Ryn et al. investigated six coagulant factor concentrates, including 3-factor PCC (Profilnine, Bebulin), 4-factor PCC (Beriplex, Octaplex), activated PCC (aPCC) (factor VIII inhibitor-bypassing activity (FEIBA)), and recombinant VIIa (NovoSeven), for their ability to reduce bleeding induced by oral dabigatran etexilate (30 mg/kg) in a rat-tail bleeding model. They found that bleeding could be reduced by the six coagulants but that routine coagulant assays did not predict the effect [37]. Other experimental studies also demonstrated the efficacy of 4-factor PCC for reversal of the dabigatran effect, as evaluated based on blood loss and bleeding time, although the aPTT was not corrected [30, 38]. Eerenberg et al. [39] performed a randomized, double-blind, placebo-controlled study in which 12 healthy male volunteers received rivaroxaban at 20 mg twice daily (n = 6) or dabigatran at 150 mg twice daily (n = 6) for 2.5 days, followed by either a single bolus of 50 IU/kg 4-factor PCC (Cofact) or a similar volume of saline. After a washout period, this procedure was repeated with treatment with the other anticoagulant. Rivaroxaban induced a significant prolongation of the PT (15.8 ± 1.3 vs. 12.3 ± 0.7 s at baseline; $p < 0.001$) that was immediately and completely reversed by PCC (12.8 ± 1.0; $p < 0.001$). The endogenous thrombin potential was inhibited by rivaroxaban (51 ± 22%; baseline, 92 ± 22%; $p < 0.002$) and normalized with PCC (114 ± 26%; $p < 0.001$), whereas saline had no effect. Dabigatran increased the aPTT, ecarin clotting time, and thrombin time. Administration of PCC did not restore these coagulation results. It was concluded that PCC immediately and completely reverses the anticoagulant effect of rivaroxaban in healthy individuals but has no effect on the anticoagulant action of dabigatran, although bleeding was not evaluated in the participants.

Recently, reversal of apixaban anticoagulation by 4-factor PCCs in healthy subjects has been reported [40]. Perstein et al. performed an open-label, randomized, placebo-controlled, three-period crossover study in 15 healthy subjects administered apixaban at 10 mg twice daily for 3 days to attain steady-state concentrations. The subjects then received a 30-min infusion of either 50 IU/kg Cofact or Beriplex or saline separately in three different periods. The study clearly demonstrated that both Cofact and Beriplex reversed the steady-state pharmacodynamic effects of apixaban in several coagulation assessments, including a thrombin generation assay. However, the efficacy of the 4-factor PCCs in reducing bleeding events in the subjects was not assessed.

Zahir et al. [41] evaluated the effects of edoxaban (60 mg) on bleeding following punch biopsy and reversal by a 4-factor PCC (Beriplex) in a randomized, double-blind, placebo-controlled, two-way crossover study in 110 healthy subjects. The researchers found that the 4-factor PCC dose-dependently reversed the effects of edoxaban, with complete reversal of the bleeding duration and endogenous thrombin potential and partial reversal of the PT following intravenous administration of 50 IU/kg 4-factor PCC. These results suggest that a 4-factor PCC dose of 50 IU/kg is appropriate to reverse the effect of a therapeutic dose of edoxaban in the case of clinically relevant bleeding or an urgent need for surgery.

Recombinant Activated Factor VII and Activated Prothrombin Complex Concentrate (Factor VIII Inhibitor-Bypassing Activity)

A randomized study investigating the efficacy and safety of rVIIa for acute ICH in patients not treated with any anticoagulants demonstrated that hemostatic therapy with rVIIa reduces enlargement of the hematoma but does not improve survival or functional outcomes after ICH [42]. The experimental study using the murine model of ICH mentioned above showed a negative result for rVIIa-mediated inhibition of hematoma expansion [36]. However, other experiments supported the efficacy of rVIIa in suppressing excess bleeding due to dabigatran [37]. A case report of spontaneous ICH during dabigatran treatment showed that a single dose of rVIIa at 90 μg/kg temporarily normalized the aPTT and increased the endogenous thrombin potential, suggesting that multiple doses may be needed [43].

An in vivo mouse-tail transection model was used to test nonactivated 4-factor PCC (14.3 IU/kg), aPCC (100 U/kg), and rVIIa (3 mg/kg) in animals treated with 60 mg/kg dabigatran etexilate by gavage. Bleeding times were not decreased with rVIIa or nonactivated 4-factor PCC alone, but they were decreased with a combination of nonactivated 4-factor PCC and rVIIa or aPCC [44]. In an ex vivo human study, volunteers were given a single dose of 150 mg dabigatran or 20 mg rivaroxaban, and their blood was drawn 2 h later (peak plasma level). Nonactivated 4-factor PCC (Kanokad), aPCC (FEIBA), or rVIIa (NovoSeven) was added to the test tube, and thrombin generation was measured at baseline, at peak anticoagulant level, and after addition of clotting factor formulations. rVIIa reversed the small decrease in peak thrombin generation induced by dabigatran [45]. Other experimental studies investigating rivaroxaban and rVIIa also demonstrated the efficacy of rVIIa for reversal of the effects of rivaroxaban [46].

Fukuda et al. [47] examined reversal of the anticoagulant effects of edoxaban on PT prolongation in vitro and on bleeding time prolongation in vivo in rats. They found that 4-factor PCC (PPSB-HT), aPCC (FEIBA), and rVIIa significantly reversed the anticoagulant effects of edoxaban in vitro and that rVIIa and FEIBA significantly reversed edoxaban-induced prolongation of the bleeding time in rats.

Fresh Frozen Plasma

In the murine model of ICH mentioned above, FFP was shown to be effective in preventing hematoma expansion with a low, but not a high, dose of dabigatran [36]. The usefulness of FFP administration for acute ICH associated with NOACs in humans in vivo has not been reported.

Antidotes

Through the management of acute ICH in patients treated with warfarin, we have learned that not only blood pressure management and vitamin K administration but also immediate reversal of an elevated PT-INR by PCC administration is quite important to suppress hematoma expansion and to obtain good outcomes [48, 49]. Although NOACs have favorable profiles, such as a much lower incidence of hemorrhagic stroke and a hematoma size that is small to moderate and hard to expand, compared with warfarin, antidotes for NOACs are still required for acute ICH because hematomas arising during NOAC treatment might expand and have poor outcomes. There are three potential antidotes for NOACs in development: idarucizumab, andexanet alfa, and PER977 (table 2).

Table 2. Antidotes

	Idarucizumab (BI 655075) aDabi-Fab	Andexanet alfa (PRT064445 or PRT4445)	PER977
Company	Boehringer Ingelheim	Portola	Perosphere
Characteristic	Monoclonal antibody/Fab	Recombinant factor Xa decoy	Synthetic small molecule
Administration	Intravenous	Intravenous	Intravenous
Studied Anticoagulant(s)	Dabigatran	Rivaroxaban; Apixaban; Edoxaban; LMWH	Dabigatran; Rivaroxaban; Apixaban; Edoxaban; LMWH; UFH
Stage of development	Phase III	Phase III for rivaroxaban and apixaban	Phase III for edoxaban

LMWH = Low-molecular-weight heparin; UFH = unfractionated heparin.

Idarucizumab

Idarucizumab is a dabigatran-specific reversal agent consisting of a fully humanized mouse monoclonal antibody fragment (Fab) [50, 51]. The binding pattern of the Fab seems similar to the pattern of dabigatran binding to thrombin. The affinity of the Fab for thrombin is 350 times stronger than that of dabigatran, and the Fab has no effect on coagulation or platelet activity.

Using healthy volunteers, Schiele et al. [52–54] performed the first clinical study that demonstrated the potential of the Fab as a specific antidote for immediate, complete, and sustained reversal of dabigatran-induced anticoagulation. This clinical study examined the safety, tolerability, pharmacokinetics, and pharmacodynamics of the Fab antidote via a randomized, double-blind, placebo-controlled study design involving 145 healthy male volunteers. In the first step, the tolerability of the Fab was tested by intravenous infusion of increasing doses (up to 8 g). In the second step, the potential for reversal of dabigatran-induced anticoagulation was evaluated, with 5-min infusions using three different doses (1, 2, and 4 g) administered following dabigatran pre-treatment (220 mg twice daily for 3 days). All administered doses of the Fab antidote were well tolerated. A 5-min infusion of the antidote following dabigatran pre-treatment was able to achieve immediate, complete, and sustained reversal of the anticoagulant effect of dabigatran. For the 2 and 4 g doses, the reversal effect was maintained for more than 12 h after the end of infusion (fig. 3).

Idarucizumab is currently being tested in a phase III prospective cohort study evaluating 5 g idarucizumab in patients with dabigatran-associated bleeding [51]. Recently, interim analysis of the study included 90 patients who received idarucizumab has been performed and indicated that idarucizumab completely reversed the anticoagulant effect of dabigatran within minutes [55].

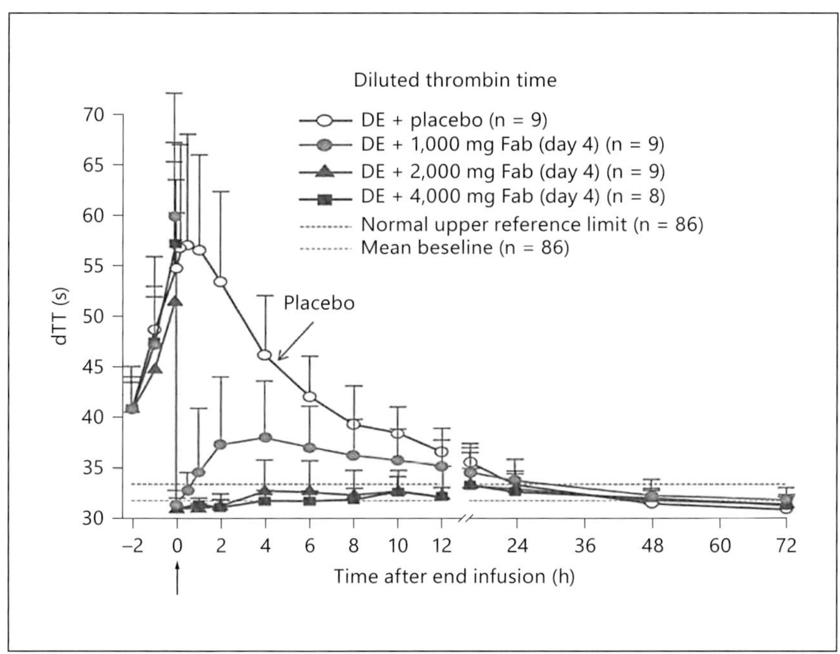

Fig. 3. Reversal of dabigatran-induced anticoagulation with an antibody fragment, as measured based on the diluted thrombin time. dTT = Diluted thrombin time; DE = dabigatran etexilate. Arrow: start of the administration of the antibody fragment. Image: Boehringer Ingelheim GmbH, from http://www.boehringer-ingelheim.com/news/news_releases/press_releases/2013/18_november_2013dabigatranetexilate.html.

Andexanet Alfa

Andexanet alfa is a recombinant human coagulation factor Xa decoy that is produced in Chinese hamster ovary cells [50, 51, 56]. It is similar to native factor Xa but lacks the gamma-carboxyglutamic acid domain required for efficient incorporation into the thrombinase complex. This decoy has the ability to bind to the factor Xa inhibitors rivaroxaban, apixaban, and edoxaban and to reverse their anticoagulant effects. It does not reverse the anticoagulant activity of dabigatran or unfractionated heparin but may reverse that of low-molecular-weight heparins. Andexanet alfa is currently being tested in a phase III randomized, double-blind, placebo-controlled trial to evaluate the reversal of the effect of rivaroxaban or apixaban in healthy volunteers.

PER977

PER977 is a small, synthetic, water-soluble molecular substance directly binding to unfractionated heparin, low-molecular-weight heparin, dabigatran, rivaroxaban, apixaban, and edoxaban, and it reverses their anticoagulant effects through noncovalent hydrogen bonding and charge-charge interactions [51, 57]. The pharmacokinetic and pharmacodynamic effects of escalating, single intravenous doses of PER977

(5–300 mg) administered alone and after a 60-mg oral dose of edoxaban were studied in a double-blind, placebo-controlled trial involving 80 healthy persons [51]. After the administration of edoxaban, the mean whole-blood clotting time increased to 37% above the baseline value. In patients receiving a single intravenous dose of PER977 (100–300 mg) 3 h after the administration of edoxaban, the whole-blood clotting time decreased to within 10% above the baseline value in 10 min or less, whereas in patients receiving placebo, the time to reach that level was much longer (approximately 12–15 h). The whole-blood clotting time remained within 10% above or below the baseline value for 24 h after the administration of a single dose of PER977. Additional phase II clinical trials have been performed, and phase III trials were scheduled to start in 2015 or 2016.

References

1 Connolly SJ, Ezekowitz MD, Yusuf S, et al: Dabigatran versus warfarin in patients with atrial fibrillation. N Engl J Med 2009;361:1139–1151 and Erratum in: N Engl J Med 2010;363:1877.

2 Patel MR, Mahaffey KW, Garg J, et al: Rivaroxaban versus warfarin in nonvalvular atrial fibrillation. N Engl J Med 2011;365:883–891.

3 Granger CB, Alexander JH, McMurray JJ, et al: Apixaban versus warfarin in patients with atrial fibrillation. N Engl J Med 2011;365:981–992.

4 Giugliano RP, Ruff CT, Braunwald E, et al: Edoxaban versus warfarin in patients with atrial fibrillation. N Engl J Med 2013;369:2093–2104.

5 Hori M, Matsumoto M, Tanahashi N, et al: Rivaroxaban vs warfarin in Japanese patients with atrial fibrillation – the J-ROCKET AF study –. Circ J 2012; 76:2104–2111.

6 Hart RG, Diener HC, Yang S, et al: Intracranial hemorrhage in atrial fibrillation patients during anticoagulation with warfarin or dabigatran: the RE-LY trial. Stroke 2012;43:1511–1517.

7 Graham DJ, Reichman ME, Wernecke M, et al: Cardiovascular, bleeding, and mortality risks in elderly Medicare patients treated with dabigatran or warfarin for nonvalvular atrial fibrillation. Circulation 2015;131:157–164.

8 Hagii J, Tomita H, Metoki N, et al: Characteristics of intracerebral hemorrhage during rivaroxaban treatment: comparison with those during warfarin. Stroke 2014;45:2805–2807.

9 Yasaka M: J-ROCKET AF trial increased expectation of lower-dose rivaroxaban made for Japan. Circ J 2012;76:2086–2087.

10 Wong KS, Hu D, Oomman A, et al: Rivaroxaban for stroke prevention in East Asia patients from the ROCKET AF trial. Stroke 2014;45:1739–1749.

11 Yasaka M, Lip GY: Stroke prevention in Asian patients with atrial fibrillation. Stroke 2014;45:1608–1609.

12 Yasaka M, Lip GY: Impact of non-vitamin k antagonist oral anticoagulants on intracranial bleeding in Asian patients with non-valvular atrial fibrillation. Circ J 2014;78:2367–2372.

13 Komori M, Yasaka M, Kokuba K, et al: Intracranial hemorrhage during dabigatran treatment. Circ J 2014;78:1335–1341.

14 Hirano T: New era of oral anticoagulation for Japanese non-valvular atrial fibrillation patients. Circ J 2014;78:1317–1319.

15 Won SY, Schlunk F, Dinkel J, et al: Imaging of contrast medium extravasation in anticoagulation-associated intracerebral hemorrhage with dual-energy computed tomography. Stroke 2013;44:2883–2890.

16 Lauer A, Cianchetti FA, Van Cott EM, et al: Anticoagulation with the oral direct thrombin inhibitor dabigatran does not enlarge hematoma volume in experimental intracerebral hemorrhage. Circulation 2011;124:1654–1662.

17 Hylek EM, Held C, Alexander JH, et al: Major bleeding in patients with atrial fibrillation receiving apixaban or warfarin: the ARISTOTLE Trial (Apixaban for Reduction in Stroke and Other Thromboembolic Events in Atrial Fibrillation): predictors, characteristics, and clinical outcomes. J Am Coll Cardiol 2014; 63:2141–2147.

18 Alonso A, Bengtson LG, MacLehose RF, et al: Intracranial hemorrhage mortality in atrial fibrillation patients treated with dabigatran or warfarin. Stroke 2014;45:2286–2291.

19 Shoji A, Satoh K, Nakano Y, et al: Dabigatran related intracranial hemorrhage, five cases report. Jpn J Stroke 2014;36:186–190.

20 Debata A, Tateishi Y, Hamabe J, et al: Three cases of spontaneous intracerebral hemorrhage under rivaroxaban. Jpn J Stroke 2015;37:41–46.
21 Kaatz S, Kouides PA, Garcia DA, et al: Guidance on the emergent reversal of oral thrombin and factor Xa inhibitors. Am J Hematol 2012;87(suppl 1):S141–S145.
22 Hankey GJ: Unanswered questions and research priorities to optimise stroke prevention in atrial fibrillation with the new oral anticoagulants. Thromb Haemost 2014;111:808–816.
23 Miller MP, Trujillo TC, Nordenholz KE: Practical considerations in emergency management of bleeding in the setting of target-specific oral anticoagulants. Am J Emerg Med 2014;32:375–382.
24 Anderson CS, Huang Y, Wang JG, et al: Intensive blood pressure reduction in acute cerebral haemorrhage trial (INTERACT): a randomised pilot trial. Lancet Neurol 2008;7:391–399.
25 Alikhan R, Rayment R, Keeling D, et al: The acute management of haemorrhage, surgery and overdose in patients receiving dabigatran. Emerg Med J 2014;31:163–168.
26 Hankey GJ: Unanswered questions and research priorities to optimise stroke prevention in atrial fibrillation with the new oral anticoagulants. Thromb Haemost 2014;111:808–816.
27 Labrador J, Franciso S, Lozano FS, et al: Management of bleeding complications of dabigatran. J Hematol Thromb Dis 2014;2:127.
28 Kumar R, Henry BL, Smith RE: Management of dabigatran associated hemorrhage. J Hematol Transfus 2013;1:1010.
29 van Ryn J, Sieger P, Kink-Eiband M, et al: Adsorption of dabigatran etexilate in water or dabigatran in pooled human plasma by activated charcoal in vitro. 51st ASH Annual Meeting and Exposition, New Orleans, LA, 2009. ASH Annual Meeting Abstracts 114: 1065.
30 Kaatz S, Crowther M: Reversal of target-specific oral anticoagulants. J Thromb Thrombolysis 2013;36: 195–202.
31 Woo JS, Kapadia N, Phanco SE, et al: Positive outcome after intentional overdose of dabigatran. J Med Toxicol 2013;9:192–195.
32 Gruber A, Marzec U, Holcomb J: Potential of activated prothrombin complex concentrate and activated factor VII to reverse the anticoagulant effects of rivaroxaban in primates. 50th ASH Annual Meeting and Exposition, San Francisco, CA, 2008.
33 Singh T, Maw TT, Henry BL, et al: Extracorporeal therapy for dabigatran removal in the treatment of acute bleeding: a single center experience. Clin J Am Soc Nephurol 2013;8:1533–1539.
34 Stangier J, Rathgen K, Stahle H, et al: Influence of renal impairment on the pharmacokinetics and pharmacodynamics of oral dabigatran etexilate: an open-label, parallel-group, single-centre study. Clin Pharmacokinet 2010;49:259–268.
35 Van Ryn J, Neubauer M, Flieg R, et al: Successful removal of dabigatran in flowing blood with an activated charcoal hemoperfusion column in an in vitro test system. Haematologica 2010;95:293.
36 Zhou W, Schwarting S, Illanes S, et al: Hemostatic therapy in experimental intracerebral hemorrhage associated with the direct thrombin inhibitor dabigatran. Stroke 2011;42:3594–3599.
37 van Ryn J, Schurer J, Kink-Eiband M, et al: Reversal of dabigatran-induced bleeding by coagulation factor concentrates in a rat-tail bleeding model and lack of effect on assays of coagulation. Anesthesiology 2014;120:1429–1440.
38 Pragst I, Zeitler SH, Doerr B, et al: Reversal of dabigatran anticoagulation by prothrombin complex concentrate (Beriplex P/N) in a rabbit model. J Thromb Haemost 2012;10:1841–1848.
39 Eerenberg ES, Kamphuisen PW, Sijpkens MK, et al: Reversal of rivaroxaban and dabigatran by prothrombin complex concentrate. A randomized, placebo-controlled, crossover study in healthy subjects. Circulation 2011;124:1573–1579.
40 Perlstein I, Wang Z, Yan Song Y, et al: Reversal of apixaban anticoagulation by 4-factor prothrombin complex concentrates in healthy subjects. 56th American Society of Hematology Annual Meeting and Exposition, San Francisco, CA, 2014.
41 Zahir H, Brown KS, Vandell A, et al: Edoxaban effects on bleeding following punch biopsy and reversal by a 4-factor prothrombin complex concentrate. Circulation 2015;131:82–90.
42 Mayer SA, Brun NC, Begtrup K, et al: Efficacy and safety of recombinant activated factor VII for acute intracerebral hemorrhage. N Engl J Med 2008;358: 2127–2137.
43 Aron JL, Gosselin R, Moll S, et al: Effects of recombinant factor VIIa on thrombin generation and thromboelastography in a patient with dabigatran-associated intracranial hemorrhage. J Thromb Thrombolysis 2014;37:76–79.
44 Lambourne MD, Eltringham-Smith LJ, Gataiance S, et al: Prothrombin complex concentrates reduce blood loss in mice rendered coagulopathic by warfarin but not dabigatran etexilate. Transfusion 2012; 52:56A–57A.
45 Marlu R, Hodaj E, Paris A, et al: Effect of non-specific reversal agents on anticoagulant activity of dabigatran and rivaroxaban: a randomised crossover ex vivo study in healthy volunteers. Thromb Haemost 2012;108:217–224.

46 Godier A, Miclot A, Le Bonniec B, et al: Evaluation of prothrombin complex concentrate and recombinant activated factor VII to reverse rivaroxaban in a rabbit model. Anesthesiology 2012;116:94–102.
47 Fukuda T, Honda Y, Kamisato C, et al: Reversal of anticoagulant effects of edoxaban, an oral, direct factor Xa inhibitor, with haemostatic agents. Thromb Haemost 2012;107:253–259.
48 Kuwashiro T, Yasaka M, Itabashi R, et al: Enlargement of acute intracerebral hematomas in patients on long-term warfarin treatment. Cerebrovasc Dis 2010;29:446–453.
49 Aguilar MI, Hart RG, Kase CS, et al: Treatment of warfarin-associated intracerebral hemorrhage: literature review and expert opinion. Mayo Clin Proc 2007;82:82–92.
50 Vanden Daelen S, Peetermans M, Vanassche T, et al: Monitoring and reversal strategies for new oral anticoagulants. Expert Rev Cardiovasc Ther 2015;13:95–103.
51 Costin J, Ansell J, Laulicht B, et al: Reversal agents in development for the new oral anticoagulants. Postgrad Med 2014;126:19–24.
52 Schiele F, van Ryn J, Manada K, et al: A specific antidote for dabigatran: functional and structural characterization. Blood 2013;121:3554–3562.
53 Glund S, Stangier J, Shmohl M, et al: A specific antidote for dabigatran: immediate complete and sustained reversal of dabigatran induced anticoagulation in healthy male volunteers [abstract]. Circulation 2013;128:A17765.
54 Boehringer Ingelheim: First human data show promise of Boehringer Ingelheim's specific antidote for immediate, complete and sustained reversal of Pradaxa®-induced anticoagulation. 2013. http://www.boehringer-ingelheim.com/news/news_releases/press_releases/2013/18_november_2013dabigatranetexilate.html (accessed December 24, 2014).
55 Pollack CV Jr, Reilly PA, Eikelboom J, et al: Idarucizumab for dabigatran reversal. N Engl J Med 2015;373:511–520.
56 Lu G, DeGuzman FR, Hollenbach SJ, et al: A specific antidote for reversal of anticoagulation by direct and indirect inhibitors of coagulation factor Xa. Nat Med 2013;19:446–451.
57 Ansell JE, Bakhru SH, Laulicht BE, et al: Use of PER977 to reverse the anticoagulant effect of edoxaban. N Engl J Med 2014;371:2141–2142.

Dr. Masahiro Yasaka
Department of Cerebrovascular Medicine and Neurology
National Hospital Organization, Kyushu Medical Center
1-8-1 Jigyohama, Chuo-ku
Fukuoka 810-8563 (Japan)
E-Mail yasaka@kyumed.jp

Toyoda K, Anderson CS, Mayer SA (eds): New Insights in Intracerebral Hemorrhage.
Front Neurol Neurosci. Basel, Karger, 2016, vol 37, pp 107–129 (DOI: 10.1159/000437117)

Ultra-Early Hemostatic Therapy for Intracerebral Hemorrhage: Future Directions

Katja E. Wartenberg[a] • Stephan A. Mayer[b]

[a]Neurocritical Care Unit, Department of Neurology, Martin-Luther-University Halle-Wittenberg, Halle, Germany; [b]Institute for Critical Care Medicine, The Mount Sinai Hospital, New York, N.Y., USA

Abstract

Hematoma expansion after initial bleeding is associated with many risk factors, such as anticoagulation, diagnosis by computed tomography (CT) shortly after symptom onset, liver disease, and a high initial blood pressure, among others, and with increased mortality and poor long-term functional outcomes. Contrast extravasation on CT angiogram, termed 'the spot sign', and on delayed-contrast CT scans (13–59%) may help to identify impending intracerebral hemorrhage growth and may open a window of opportunity for therapeutic interventions. The spot sign score, the prediction score for hematoma expansion, and the BRAIN score were developed to assess the probability of hematoma expansion at 24 h. Therapeutic interventions to promote hemostasis are currently limited to intensive blood pressure control and antagonization of the effect of antiplatelets and anticoagulation. Ultra-early hemostasis for ICH not associated with coagulopathy may include administration of recombinant factor VIIa and tranexamic acid to selected patients based on the presence of a spot sign on the CT angiogram is currently under investigation. © 2016 S. Karger AG, Basel

Scope of the Problem: Hematoma Growth

Hematoma volume was identified as the single most powerful predictor of poor functional outcomes and mortality after intracerebral hemorrhage (ICH), followed by the presence of intraventricular hemorrhage (IVH), a depressed level of consciousness, age, and an infratentorial location [1–8].

Moreover, retrospective observational studies revealed that ICHs undergo progressive growth within the first 24 h [9] (fig. 1). In the first prospective study of this phenomenon, at least 38% of 103 patients experienced >33% growth in the ICH volume during the first 24 h after symptom onset. In 26% of patients, ICH growth had already occurred within the first hour, and in 12%, growth had occurred between

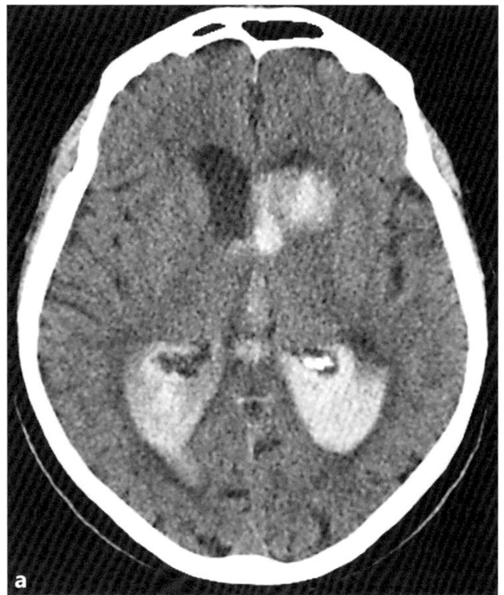

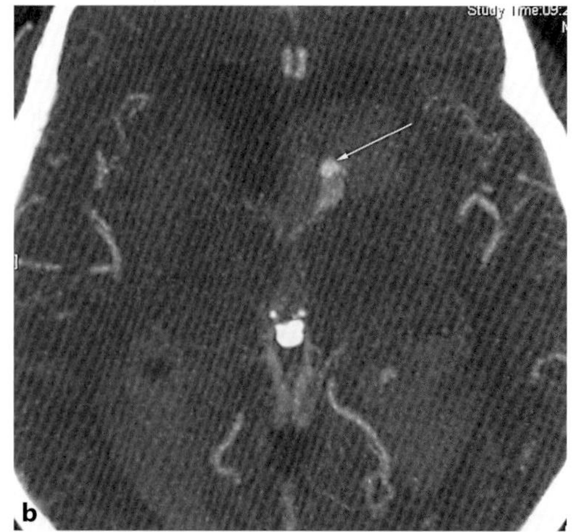

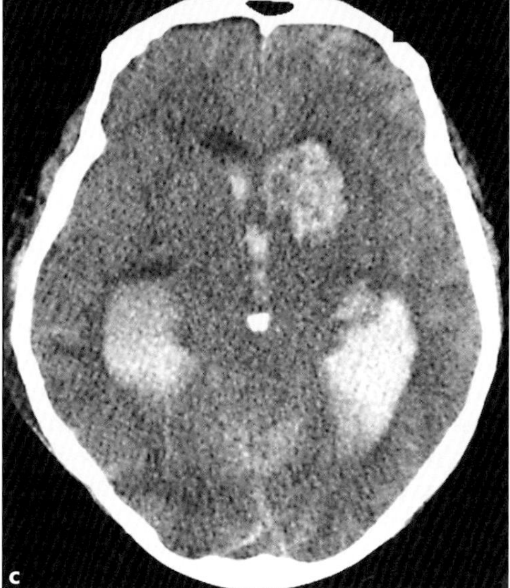

Fig. 1. A computed tomography scan demonstrates a left caudate hemorrhage with extension into the ventricles (**a**) and the spot sign (see arrow) on the source images of the angiogram (**b**). On follow-up imaging after 24 h, the caudate hemorrhage had doubled in size, and the amount of ventricular hemorrhage had increased as well (**c**).

1 and 20 h. ICH growth was accompanied by neurological deterioration, as detected based on concurrent National Institutes of Health Stroke Scale and Glasgow Coma Scale scores, in one third of patients within 1 h of the first computed tomography (CT) image and in an additional 25% of patients within the next 20 h [10]. Although all studies examining early ICH growth have found the highest rates within 6 h of onset [10–25], the finding of neurological deterioration with hematoma growth between 6 and 48 h has been substantiated by other studies [11, 13, 17, 18]. Several multivariate analyses have identified factors associated with hematoma enlargement and early neurological deterioration after ICH (table 1).

Patients with hematoma expansion were found to have an increased frequency of neurological deterioration (66 vs. 14%) and higher ICH-related mortality rates

Table 1. Risk factors for hematoma growth

1.	Shorter time from symptom onset to first CT [12, 15, 21, 26, 38, 51, 62, 133]
2.	Large hematoma size [30, 51, 62, 133]; hematoma volume on first CT <25 mm^3 [26]
3.	Irregular hematoma shape and heterogeneous lesions [12, 134]
4.	MAP >120 mm Hg [30]; SBP ≥200 mm Hg [26]; highest SBP [135, 136]; history of hypertension [38]
5.	GCS score ≤8 [30]; presence of consciousness disturbance [12]; higher NIHSS score [21]
6.	History of cerebral infarction [26]
7.	Liver disease [26]
8.	Fasting plasma glucose ≥141 mg/dl and hemoglobin A_{1c} ≥5.1% [26]; hyperglycemia [62, 133, 137]
9.	Hypocholesterolemia [137] or hypercholesteremia [133]
10.	Alcohol consumption (46.3 g/day) [12]
11.	Reduced fibrinogen level (<87 mg/dl) [12]; elevated serum fibrinogen level (>523 mg/dl) [135]
12.	Body temperature >37.5°C [135]
13.	Neutrophil count (by 1,000-unit increase) [135]
14.	IVH [135]
15.	Admission cellular fibronectin level >6 μg/ml and admission interleukin-6 level >24 pg/ml [138]
16.	Oral anticoagulation [15, 21, 23, 38, 51]; increased INR 2 h after presentation [22]; INR >2 before treatment or ≥24 h after PCC administration [24]
17.	Use of antithrombotic agents prior to hemorrhage [21, 133]
18.	Baseline weight [133]
19.	Increased serum creatinine [133]
20.	White-matter hyperintensities on MRI [139]

CT = Computed tomography; MAP = mean arterial blood pressure; SBP = systolic blood pressure; GCS = Glasgow Coma Scale; NIHSS = National Institutes of Health Stroke Scale; IVH = intraventricular hemorrhage; INR = international normalized ratio; PCC = prothrombin complex concentrate; MRI = magnetic resonance imaging.

(29% vs. 3%) compared with those without expansion [13, 15, 26]. For every 1 ml increase in the baseline ICH volume, the hazard ratio of dying increased by 1% [18]. For every 10% increase in the ICH volume at 24 h, the patients were 16% more likely to exhibit a one-point increase on the modified Rankin scale (mRS) for outcomes and 18% more likely to worsen from independence to assisted independence or from assisted independence to a poor outcome [18]. Ultra-early hematoma growth, defined as the relationship between the baseline ICH volume and an ICH onset-to-imaging-time >10.2 ml/h, represents the most powerful predictor of hematoma growth, neurological deterioration, a poor long-term outcome, and mortality [27]. Therefore, it seems reasonable that therapy directed at stopping bleeding as early as possible could potentially decrease mortality and improve functional neurological outcomes. The most interesting questions that remain are as follows: Which type of hemorrhage will expand further after first presentation? Which therapeutic agent is most effective in stopping the bleeding, outweighing all risks associated with its administration?

Prediction of Intracerebral Hemorrhage Growth: The Spot Sign

Contrast-enhanced imaging studies may indicate an active bleeding process during the acute phase of ICH. Leakage of contrast dye during cerebral angiography was reported in 12.5–42% of patients whose initial CT scan was taken within 5 h of ICH onset [28, 29]. CT angiography (CTA) performed within 12 h of onset showed contrast extravasation in 46% of 113 patients [30]. The patients with contrast leakage were more likely to have been imaged earlier and were significantly more likely to die (64 vs. 16%) [30]. A gadolinium-enhanced magnetic resonance imaging (MRI) study confirmed that 36% of patients had active extravasation of contrast, and in half of these cases, contrast extravasation was also documented on cerebral angiography [16].

Further evidence indicating that bleeding is a dynamic and active process in the first few hours after ICH onset was found in early ICH surgery trials. A pilot study of ultra-early ICH evacuation within 4 h of onset was associated with fatal postoperative bleeding in 3 of 11 patients, which led to termination of the study [31]. Another study included 100 patients treated with surgical evacuation within 7 h of symptom onset and found an association between postsurgical rebleeding and poor outcomes [32].

With the application of CTA as a routine diagnostic tool in cerebrovascular disease, contrast extravasation is seen more commonly in the arterial phase of CTA, which is termed 'the spot sign', and on delayed-contrast imaging (table 2).

The spot sign is defined as tiny enhancing foci within a hematoma, with or without clear contrast extravasation seen in the arterial phase of the CT angiogram, that occur in 13–57% of patients imaged within 24 h of symptom onset [33–60]. Given an inter-rater variability of kappa 0.80–0.94, this sign can be easily recognized [33, 61, 62].

The following criteria were proposed to define the spot sign:

(1) ≥1 focus of contrast pooling within the ICH

(2) Attenuation of ≥120 Hounsfield Units

(3) Discontinuity from normal or abnormal vasculature adjacent to the ICH

(4) Any size or morphology [63]

or

(1) Serpiginous and/or spot-like appearance

Table 2. Prediction of hematoma expansion based on the spot sign and delayed contrast extravasation on CTA

Study	Hematoma expansion	Spot sign						Delayed contrast extravasation				
		number of patients	frequency	sensitivity	specificity	PPV	NPV	frequency	sensitivity	specificity	PPV	NPV
Becker et al., 1999 [30]	N/A	113	52 (46%)									
Goldstein et al., 2007* [61]	<48 h 14 (13%)	104	58 (56%) Central 38% Peripheral 38% Mixed 13%	93%	50%	24%	98%					
Wada et al., 2007§ [33]	<48 h 11 (28%)	39	13 (33%)	91%	89%	77%	96%	6 (15%)	45%	96%	83%	81%
Kim et al., 2008& [35]	<60 h 42 ml with extravasation 23 ml without extravasation	56	10 (18%) 1–2 foci					13 (23%) 1–7 foci				
Ederies et al., 2009§ [64]	<24 h Volume change ~26%	61	21 (34%)	78%	84%	67%	90%	11 (18%)	Combined with spot sign 94%	Combined with spot sign 79%	Combined with spot sign 65%	Combined with spot sign 97%
Hallevi et al., 2010# [34]	<24 h 16 (57%)	28	11 (41%)	73%	100%	100%	75%	13 (59%)	100% Combined with spot sign 100%	100% Combined with spot sign 100%	100% Combined with spot sign 100%	100% Combined with spot sign 100%

Table 2. Continued

Study	Hematoma expansion	Spot sign						Delayed contrast extravasation				
		number of patients	frequency	sensitivity	specificity	PPV	NPV	frequency	sensitivity	specificity	PPV	NPV
Delgado Almandoz et al., 2009§ [62]	<48 h 56 (15%)	367	65 (18%)	88%	93%	69%	98%	24/75 (32%)			67%	
Delgado Almandoz et al., 2010§ [63]	<48 h	573	122 (21%)					45/116 (39%)				
Evans et al., 2010§ [68]	Unknown	59	17 (29%)									
Park et al., 2010§ [36]	<48 h	110	19 (17%)	81%	83%	55%	97%					
Wang et al., 2011§ [37]	<24 h	321	76 (24%)	78%	93%	79%	93%					
Demchuk et al., 2012° [66] First prospective trial	<24 h	228	61 (27%)	63%	90%	73%	84%					
Brouwers et al., 2012° [38]	<48 h	391	74 (19%)	46%	87%	45%	88%					
Li et al., 2011^ [39]	<24 h	139	30 (22%)	72%	94%	79%	92%					

Table 2. Continued

Study	Hematoma expansion	Spot sign						Delayed contrast extravasation				
		number of patients	frequency	sensitivity	specificity	PPV	NPV	frequency	sensitivity	specificity	PPV	NPV
Koculym et al., 2013§ [40]	<24 h	28	CTA 8 (29%) CTP 14 (50%)	CTA 44% CTP 78%	CTA 69% CTP 69%	CTA 63% CTP 77%	CTA 50% CTP 71%	9 (32%)	50%	69%	66%	53%
Sun et al., 2013§ [41]	<24 h	112	CTA 24 (21%) CTP 30 (27%)	CTA 61% CTP 89%	CTA 92% CTP 94%	CTA 71% CTP 83%	CTA 86% CTP 96%					
Sorimachi et al., 2013^ [42]	Unknown	141	30 (21%)									
Romero et al., 2013§ [43]	<48 h	131	31 (24%)	64%	86%	52%	91%					
Dowlatshahi et al., 2014 [44]		35	13 (37%)									
Brouwers et al., 2014° [51]	<24 h	817	160 (20%)									
Havsteen et al., 2014 [45]	<24 h	138	40 (29%)									
Chakraborty et al., 2014 [46]	N/A	34	Whole-brain dynamic CTA 13 (42%)									

Table 2. Continued

Study	Hematoma expansion	Spot sign						Delayed contrast extravasation				
		number of patients	frequency	sensitivity	specificity	PPV	NPV	frequency	sensitivity	specificity	PPV	NPV
Hotta et al., 2014^ [47]	<24 h	323	80 (24.7%)									
D'Esterre et al., 2011§ [48]	<24 h	16	4 (25%)					6 (38%)				
Thompson et al., 2009 [49]	N/A	36	12 (33%)									
Radmanesh et al., 2014° [50]	<72 h	741	178 (24%)									
Brouwers et al., 2014 [52]	<24 h	95	32 (34%)									
Tsukabe et al., 2014§ [53]	<24 h	83	20 (24%)	48%	87.5%	65%	77.8%	44 (53%)	92.6%	66%	56.8%	94.9%
Hou and Gao, 2014 [54]		53	13 (24.5%)	80%	97.4%	92.3%	92.5%					
Kim et al., 2014§ [55]	<24 h	316	47 (15%)									
Moon et al., 2014 [56]	<24–72 h	287	40 (14%)									
Han et al., 2014^ [57]		187	61 (32.6%)									

Table 2. Continued

Study	Hematoma expansion	Spot sign						Delayed contrast extravasation				
		number of patients	frequency	sensitivity	specificity	PPV	NPV	frequency	sensitivity	specificity	PPV	NPV
Rosa Júnior et al., 2013° [58]	N/A	65	19 (29%)	67%	91%							
Rizos et al., 2013° [59]	<24 h	101	27 (26.7%)	50%	84%							
Ciura et al., 2014° [60]	<24 h	74	10 (13.5%)	55%	94%	60%	92%	14 (18.9%)	55%	87%	43%	92%

Hematoma expansion defined as * >33%, § >30% or 6 ml, ° >33% or 6 ml, & continuous growth, # >20% from baseline, and ^ >33% or 12.5 ml. PPV = Positive predictive value; NPV = negative predictive value; CTA = computed tomography angiography; CTP = computed tomography perfusion.

(2) Location within the margin of the parenchymal hematoma, without connection to an outside vessel

(3) Size of >1.5 mm in diameter in the maximal axial dimension

(4) At least double the density (in Hounsfield Units) compared with background hematoma

(5) Single or multiple lesions [49].

The suggested underlying pathophysiology includes the following:

- Manifestation of early but slow parenchymal leakage from blood vessels feeding the hematoma [33, 34, 64]
- Saccular or asymmetric fusiform aneurysms involving penetrating arteries, amyloid-related microaneurysms, vascular tortuosity, lipohyalinotic (Charcot-Bouchard) aneurysms (red-cell extravasation demonstrated in chronic lesions), and focal ruptures of elongated aneurismal dilatations [33, 49]
- Fibrin globes or pseudoaneurysms with enclosure of red cells in concentric rings of fibrin adjacent to the arteriolar defect and disruption and shearing of the adjacent vasculature due to hematoma expansion followed by ischemia of the vessel wall, with an increase in permeability [16, 34, 49, 65] in the later phase [44]
- Primary bleeding from described aneurysms, contributing to hematoma expansion or causing a domino effect, with progressive rupture of the vascular source with continued bleeding [49, 61]
- Active ongoing bleeding from a ruptured vascular source, as listed above [16, 33, 34, 61, 64], in the early phase [44]
- Pooling of contrast within a collapsed vein trapped within the hematoma [61].

The spot sign tends to be central in the blood clot, which indicates bleeding from a vascular source, rather from necrotic or edematous tissue [30]. The 'Predicting hEmatoma growth anD outcome in Intracerebral hemorrhage using contrast bolus CT' (PREDICT) study was one of the first prospective multicenter studies that validated the spot sign as an independent predictor of hematoma growth, neurological deterioration, and long-term functional outcomes [66]. The sensitivity and specificity for the prediction of hematoma growth in the presence of the spot sign on CTA are highly variable and range around 53 and 88%, respectively [67]. The accuracy of diagnosing hematoma growth based on the presence of the spot sign is 92% [62]. Patients with ICH without evidence of chronic hypertension or cerebral amyloid angiopathy on MRI were shown to have a higher incidence of the spot sign compared with patients with imaging signs of chronic hypertension or cerebral amyloid angiopathy associated with a higher risk of hematoma expansion [68].

In addition, further contrast extravasation or enlargement of the contrast density was seen on delayed postcontrast images (2–3 min) following the original CTA (frequency 15–59%, table 2). The interrater variability for this finding was even higher (kappa 0.94–0.97) [62, 63].

The original spot sign and delayed contrast extravasation are not often seen in the same place [34]. In relation to bolus injection, CTA images may be obtained too

Table 3. The spot sign score

Characteristic	PPV for hematoma expansion	Number of points	Spot sign score	Hematoma expansion
Number of spot signs			0	2%
1–2		1	1	33%
≥3	96%	2	2	50%
Maximum axial dimension			3	94%
1–4 mm		0	4	100%
≥5	91%	1		
Maximum attenuation				
120–179 HU		0		
≥180 HU	84%	1		

The spot sign score is obtained during the arterial phase of the CT angiogram. Hematoma expansion is defined as >30% or 6 ml on a follow-up CT scan within 48 h after the CT angiogram. PPV = Positive predictive value; HU = Hounsfield Units. Modified from [62, 63].

quickly, with insufficient time for contrast accumulation. Therefore, contrast extravasation on delayed postcontrast images is seen more often than the spot sign is seen on CTA and is noted up to 48 h after symptom onset [34, 35, 64].

The spot sign and delayed contrast extravasation on CTA are the most powerful predictors of hematoma expansion [33, 34, 61, 62]. If CTA was done earlier in relation to the index hemorrhage, the likelihood of detecting the spot sign and the delayed contrast extravasation increases [30, 62], as does the spot sign score [62]. Later image acquisition by CTA in the venous phase increases the frequency of spot sign detection [69], as does three-dimensional assessment by dynamic CTA [46].

The spot sign score was developed to quantify contrast extravasation after ICH and IVH growth (table 3) [62, 63]. This score was found to be a significant predictor of hematoma expansion, independent of the time from symptom onset to CTA and independent of anticoagulation, the mean arterial blood pressure, the blood glucose level, and the initial ICH volume [43, 70], as well as of in-hospital mortality and a poor functional outcome [43]. However, the number of spot signs on CTA was found to be equally accurate in the prediction of hematoma growth, with near-perfect interobserver agreement [71]. Another prediction score was developed in a large prospective ICH cohort, encompassing use of a vitamin K antagonist, the time to the initial CT scan, the baseline ICH volume, and the presence of the spot sign on CTA (table 4) [51].

Important spot sign mimics to consider encompass the following:

- Punctuate or irregularly shaped calcifications (due to choroid plexus compression, a tumor, infection, or inflammation or physiological) → compare with noncontrast CT
- Aneurysms that are partially thrombosed or at bifurcations → review CTA

Table 4. Prediction score for hematoma expansion at 24 h

Score component	Points	Total points	Probability of ICH growth (%)
Use of vitamin K antagonist			
No	0	0	5.7
Yes	2	1	11.1
Time to initial CT in h			
≤6	2	2	7.7
>6	0	3	17.9
Baseline ICH volume in ml			
<30	0	4	29.6
30–60	1	5	35.4
>60	2	6	53.6
CTA spot sign			
Absent	0	7	45.5
Present	3	8	0
Unavailable	1	9	80

ICH = Intracerebral hemorrhage; CT = computed tomography; CTA = CT angiography. Modified after [51].

- Microarteriovenous malformations → review CTA, linear densities extend beyond the hematoma margin
- Pseudoaneurysms, such as in Moya Moya disease → review CTA [72].

If hematoma expansion can be anticipated with nearly 100% accuracy, more patients may benefit from targeting reduction of hematoma growth by reversing the effect of antiplatelets, anticoagulation, and high blood pressure. Ongoing trials, such as 'The SpoT sign fOr Predicting and treating ICH growth study with activated factor VII' (STOP-IT; http://www.clinicaltrials.gov/ct2/show/NCT00810888) and the 'Spot Sign' Selection of Intracerebral Hemorrhage to Guide Hemostatic Therapy (SPOTLIGHT; https://clinicaltrials.gov/ct2/show/NCT01359202), have selected patients with ICH to be randomized to recombinant factor VIIa or placebo to reduce ICH expansion based on the presence of the spot sign on CTA. The 'Spot Sign and Tranexamic Acid On Preventing ICH Growth – AUStralasia Trial' (STOP-AUST; https://clinicaltrials.gov/ct2/show/NCT01702636) is investigating the effect of tranexamic acid on hematoma growth in ICH patients with contrast extravasation on CTA [73]. In the 'Spot Sign Score in Restricting ICH Growth' (SCORE-IT) trial, a substudy of the 'Antihypertensive Treatment of Cerebral Hemorrhage' (ATACH)-II trial, validation of the spot sign score as a predictor of hemorrhage growth and prediction of clinical benefit from intensive blood pressure control in patients with the spot sign will be explored [74].

If the application of contrast media is contraindicated, hematoma expansion can be predicted by quantitative CT densitometry demonstrating heterogeneous ICH attenuation within 3 h of onset, which may reflect an active bleeding process [75]. A

Table 5. BRAIN score for prediction of hematoma expansion at 24 h

BRAIN score component	Points	Total points	Probability of ICH growth (%)
Baseline ICH volume			
≤10 ml	0	0	3.4
10–20 ml	5	1	4.2
≥20 ml	7	2	5.1
Recurrent ICH			
No	0	3	6.3
Yes	4	4	7.7
Anticoagulation with vitamin K antagonist			
No	0	5	9.4
Yes	6	6	11.3
Intraventricular extension			
No	0	7	13.7
Yes	2	8	16.4
Numbers of hours to baseline CT scan from symptom onset			
≤1	5	9	19.5
1–2	4	10	23.1
2–3	3	11	27.2
3–4	2	12	31.6
4–5	1	13	36.4
>5	0	14	41.5
		15	46.7
		16	52.1
		17	57.4
		18	62.5
		19	67.4
		20	71.9
		21	76.0
		22	79.7
		23	83.0
		24	85.8

ICH = Intracerebral hemorrhage; CT = computed tomography. Modified from [76].

subanalysis of the 'Intensive Blood Pressure Reduction in Acute Cerebral Haemorrhage 2' (INTERACT2) trial introduced a 24-point BRAIN score to assess the probability of ICH growth (see table 5) [76].

Pathophysiology of Early Hematoma Growth

In the absence of any animal models, most clinicians believe that early hematoma growth represents ongoing bleeding and rebleeding from one or more ruptured arteries or arterioles. Following abrupt arterial rupture, rapid accumulation of blood within the brain parenchyma increases the local tissue pressure. A degree of physical destruction is plausible and may be explained by the shearing forces of the expanding hematoma and by the ischemia induced by the increased local tissue pressure. In addition to the relative mass effect, the hematoma itself causes (a) neuronal and glial cell death due to apoptosis and inflammation, (b) vasogenic edema, and (c) breakdown of the blood-brain barrier. Evidence from pathological and neuroimaging studies demonstrated secondary multifocal bleeding into the tissue surrounding the initial hematoma. Multiple micro- and macroscopic hemorrhages were discovered at the periphery of fatal hemorrhages in a histopathological analysis; these were thought to result from ruptured arterioles and venules [77]. Secondary confluent hemorrhages into the congested and hypoperfused perilesional tissue of an existing clot were demonstrated by simultaneous CT and single-photon emission CT studies [78].

These findings were confirmed by MRI and CTA studies showing contrast extravasation, as mentioned above [30, 33–35, 38, 60–64, 79]. Ongoing hemorrhage from lenticulostriate arteries has been observed immediately after ICH during cerebral angiography [28, 80–83]. Furthermore, early hematoma growth was reported to be associated with irregular clot morphology, presumably due to multifocal hemorrhages from multiple arterioles [12, 84].

These observations suggest that early hemorrhage growth may result from bleeding into congested and damaged tissue surrounding a hematoma [85]. Tissue necrosis and the presence of ischemia around the blood clot were confirmed in pathological and biochemical models of ICH, but the extent of ischemic damage is probably negligible [85, 86]. Multiple studies utilizing positron emission tomography and diffusion-weighted imaging in humans have failed to demonstrate true ischemia in the hypoperfused brain tissue surrounding the initial hematoma as early as 6 h after onset. Perihematomal hypoperfusion seems to result from a reduction in metabolic demand [87–91].

Postulated mechanisms for secondary bleeding after ICH include increased intravascular hydrostatic pressure; increased local tissue pressure and shear forces, resulting in mechanical injury; reduced cerebral blood flow; plasma protein induction, resulting in secondary inflammation; ischemia; and fluid extravasation [92, 93]. Thrombin, fibrin degradation products, and plasmin concentrated within the hematoma [93] elicit an inflammatory response [94–98], metalloprotease induction [94, 99], alterations in the blood-brain barrier's permeability [86, 92], and localized coagulopathy [100] in the surrounding brain tissue.

Hemostatic Therapy

Rapid induction of hemostasis would be the logical therapeutic step to counteract hematoma growth immediately after presentation. Given the risk factors for hematoma expansion (table 1), options to decrease hematoma growth encompass blood pressure control [17, 19, 101], antagonization of the effect of antiplatelets and anticoagulation [102–104], and administration of a drug to facilitate hemostasis in general. A useful hemostatic agent should inhibit fibrinolysis and activate coagulation locally, without causing systemic thrombotic events.

Aminocaproic Acid, Tranexamic Acid, and Aprotinin

The synthetic derivatives of the amino acid lysine, aminocaproic acid, and tranexamic acid and the polypeptide aprotinin initiate hemostasis in the absence of any coagulopathy [105]. Aminocaproic acid and tranexamic acid enter the extracellular space and reversibly attach to plasminogen, which results in blockade of its activation by fibrin and prevents its conversion to plasmin. These acids inhibit clot fibrinolysis and stabilize clots but do not activate coagulation, thrombin generation, or clot formation. Tranexamic acid (trans-4-(aminomethyl) cyclohexanecarboxylic acid) is also a competitive inhibitor of tissue plasminogen activator and a direct inhibitor of plasmin activity. Tranexamic acid is about 10 times more potent than ε-aminocaproic acid, binds more strongly to the receptor sites of the plasminogen molecule, and has a longer half-life [105]. Lysine derivatives are effective in the treatment of primary menorrhagia [106], upper gastrointestinal bleeding [107], and mucosal bleeding in patients with coagulation disorders or thrombocytopenia [108]. These drugs are useful for clot stabilization, rather than for the promotion of clot formation, as they principally inhibit fibrinolysis.

In patients with subarachnoid hemorrhage, aminocaproic acid decreased the incidence of rebleeding but resulted in a higher frequency of delayed cerebral ischemia and other thrombotic complications [109–112]. A pilot study examined the potential effect of aminocaproic acid on the prevention of early hematoma growth after ICH [113]. Three of the first five patients who were given a 5-g intravenous (IV) loading dose of aminocaproic acid followed by an infusion of 1 g/h for 23 h experienced significant hematoma expansion compared with 2 of 9 control patients. The 80% confidence interval for the frequency of hematoma growth in the patients treated with aminocaproic acid was 32–88%. The authors concluded that the rate of hematoma expansion in patients given aminocaproic acid within 12 h of ICH is probably no less than the natural history rate, although this treatment appears to be safe [113].

Aprotinin, an inhibitor of serine proteases such as trypsin, chymotrypsin, plasmin, and kallikrein, disrupts anticoagulation by indirect inhibition of factor XII formation through its action against kallikrein. Aprotinin primarily interferes with both the coagulation and the fibrinolysis induced by the contact of blood with a foreign surface but has no effect on platelet function [105]. The main indication is reduction of perioperative bleeding, especially during cardiac surgery [114] and orthotopic liver transplantation [115]. The use of aprotinin is not associated with an increased risk of thromboembolic complications [105]. To date, there are no data on the effect of aprotinin on hemorrhage expansion in patients with ICH.

Tranexamic acid (1 g IV bolus, followed by 1 g over 8 h), given over 8 h in patients with trauma at risk of bleeding, significantly reduced all-cause mortality (mainly head injury, multiorgan failure, and vaso-occlusive complications) and mortality due to hemorrhage if given within 3 h of injury [116, 117]. The drug has been further applied to decrease the requirement for blood transfusions during surgical procedures [107, 118] and to decrease blood loss and maternal morbidity in postpartum hemorrhage [119]. In subarachnoid hemorrhage, the risk of rebleeding was diminished with tranexamic acid at the expense of an increased risk of delayed cerebral ischemia [120]. Short-term application (72 h) in subarachnoid hemorrhage patients was associated with a trend toward an improved outcome [121]. In a case series, patients with ICH underwent strict blood pressure control (<150 mm Hg systolic) in combination with administration of 1 g tranexamic acid over 6 h or 2 g tranexamic acid over 10 min. Hematoma growth was significantly reduced with rapid antifibrinolytic therapy compared with prolonged administration of tranexamic acid [122]. In a single-center, randomized, placebo-controlled, blinded-endpoint pilot trial, 24 patients with acute ICH were randomized to 1 g IV tranexamic acid over 10 min followed by an infusion of 1 g over 8 h or to placebo within 24 h of onset. The intervention was safe and feasible [123]. The phase II randomized, placebo-controlled, double-blind trial STOP-AUST is currently recruiting patients with ICH with the spot sign on CTA to receive either 1 g IV tranexamic acid over 10 min followed by an infusion of 1 g over 8 h or placebo within 4.5 h of ICH [73].

Recombinant Factor VIIa

Activated factor VII initiates hemostasis by forming a complex with tissue factor in the circulating blood following trauma through activation of factor X and conversion of prothrombin into thrombin. Recombinant activated factor VII (rFVIIa) was found to facilitate hemostasis during spontaneous and surgical bleeds in patients with hemophilia A or B receiving inhibitors of factors VIII and IX, respectively [124]. Exogenous rFVIIa binds to the activated platelet surface with low affinity and mediates both the conversion of factor X into activated factor Xa and platelet surface thrombin generation, independent of tissue factor and factors VIII and IX [125]. Therefore, rFVIIa enhances local hemostasis after binding to exposed tissue factor, even in the absence of coagulopathy. Internal, retroperitoneal, and central nervous system hemorrhages (76–91% efficacy rate) were effectively terminated by rFVIIa in patients with normal coagulation [126]. Furthermore, rFVIIa at a dose of 80–100 μg/kg was shown to promote hemostasis of central nervous system bleeds in patients with hemophilia, resulting in cessation of bleeding in 84% of patients, without the occurrence of any adverse events [127]. The half-life of rFVIIa is short, or 2.3 h, and its onset of action is rapid and localized to the site of bleeding [126]. Given its potential, rFVIIa was tested in two randomized, double-blind, placebo-controlled trials as ultra-early hemostatic intervention in ICH in the absence of coagulopathy, as well as in the NovoSeven® ICH trial and the 'Factor Seven for Acute Hemorrhagic Stroke' (FAST) trial [20, 128].

In the NovoSeven® ICH trial, which was a phase II study, 399 patients with spontaneous ICH received treatment with rFVIIa at a dose of 40, 80, or 160 μg/kg or with placebo within 4 h after ICH onset. The primary outcome was alteration in the hematoma volume at 24 h. The mean percentage increase in the ICH volume was 29% in the placebo group and 16%, 14%, and 11% in the groups that received 40, 80, or 160 μg/kg, respectively. The difference was statistically significant when comparing the placebo group with all rFVIIa treatment groups combined ($p = 0.01$) or with the 160 μg/kg rFVIIa group alone ($p = 0.02$). The absolute increase in the ICH volume was 4.4 ml in the rFVIIa group and 10.7 ml in the placebo arm ($p = 0.009$). The effect of rFVIIa on hemostasis was greatest when rFVIIa was given within 3 h after symptom onset (269 patients), resulting in a mean percentage increase in the ICH volume of 13% in patients treated with rFVIIa, compared with 34% in the placebo group ($p = 0.004$). The administration of rFVIIa was associated with a 38% reduction in mortality and significantly improved functional outcomes (based on the mRS) at 90 days, despite a 5% rate of arterial thromboembolic adverse events, such as non-ST-elevation myocardial events and cerebral ischemic infarctions, within 4 days of administration of rFVIIa [128].

The FAST trial, which was a phase III study, compared doses of 80 and 20 μg/kg rFVIIa with placebo in 841 patients with ICH. No significant difference was found in the main outcome measure, which was the proportion of patients with death or severe disability according to the mRS at 90 days (score of 5 or 6), but the hemostatic effect (hematoma growth in the placebo group, 26%; rFVIIa at 20 μg/kg, 18%; and rFVIIa at 80 μg/kg, 11%) and side effect profiles (arterial thrombosis in the placebo group, 4%; rFVIIa at 20 μg/kg, 5%; and rFVIIa at 80 μg/kg, 8%; especially including ischemic stroke and myocardial infarction) were confirmed [20]. Based on this trial, routine administration of rFVIIa as hemostatic therapy for all patients with ICH within a 4-h time window cannot be recommended. The lack of effect of rFVIIa in ICH, despite this therapy's ability to limit hematoma growth, suggests that targeting this therapy to subgroups of patients may impact the functional outcome after ICH. In a FAST trial subgroup analysis, a potential effect of rFVIIa was seen in patients aged <70 years with a baseline hematoma volume <60 ml, a baseline IVH volume <5 ml and a time from onset <2.5 h [129].

Patients with ICH who received rFVIIa at 40–90 μg/kg prior to hematoma evacuation and within 5 h of symptom onset had minimal residual or recurrent hematoma volumes [130]. However, in a randomized phase II study of patients with ICH undergoing early hematoma evacuation, postsurgical hematoma volumes and thrombotic events were not significantly different [131]. In a pooled safety analysis of 4,468 patients (one third with ICH) evaluating off-label treatment with high doses of rFVIIa, the rate of arterial thromboembolic events was 9.0% in patients who received rFVIIa and were older than 65 years (placebo, 3.8%; p = 0.003) [132]. This risk of increased deep vein thrombosis and arterial thrombosis after application of rFVIIa in patients with ICH and traumatic brain injury was confirmed in another meta-analysis [131].

Ongoing trials aimed at improved patient selection based on the presence of the spot sign on CTA, including STOP-IT and SPOTLIGHT, are currently reinvestigating the role of rFVIIa as potential hemostatic therapy in the acute phase of ICH.

References

1 Broderick JP, Brott TG, Duldner JE, Tomsick T, Huster G: Volume of intracerebral hemorrhage. A powerful and easy-to-use predictor of 30-day mortality. Stroke 1993;24:987–993.

2 Gebel JM Jr, Jauch EC, Brott TG, Khoury J, Sauerbeck L, Salisbury S, et al: Relative edema volume is a predictor of outcome in patients with hyperacute spontaneous intracerebral hemorrhage. Stroke 2002; 33:2636–2641.

3 Juvela S: Risk factors for impaired outcome after spontaneous intracerebral hemorrhage. Arch Neurol 1995;52:1193–1200.

4 Tuhrim S, Dambrosia JM, Price TR, Mohr JP, Wolf PA, Hier DB, et al: Intracerebral hemorrhage: external validation and extension of a model for prediction of 30-day survival. Ann Neurol 1991;29:658–663.

5 Daverat P, Castel JP, Dartigues JF, Orgogozo JM: Death and functional outcome after spontaneous intracerebral hemorrhage. A prospective study of 166 cases using multivariate analysis. Stroke 1991;22: 1–6.

6 Portenoy RK, Lipton RB, Berger AR, Lesser ML, Lantos G: Intracerebral haemorrhage: a model for the prediction of outcome. J Neurol Neurosurg Psychiatry 1987;50:976–979.

7 Qureshi AI, Safdar K, Weil J, Barch C, Bliwise DL, Colohan AR, et al: Predictors of early deterioration and mortality in black Americans with spontaneous intracerebral hemorrhage. Stroke 1995;26:1764–1767.

8 Hallevy C, Ifergane G, Kordysh E, Herishanu Y: Spontaneous supratentorial intracerebral hemorrhage. Criteria for short-term functional outcome prediction. J Neurol 2002;249:1704–1709.

9 Chen ST, Chen SD, Hsu CY, Hogan EL: Progression of hypertensive intracerebral hemorrhage. Neurology 1989;39:1509–1514.

10 Brott T, Broderick J, Kothari R, Barsan W, Tomsick T, Sauerbeck L, et al: Early hemorrhage growth in patients with intracerebral hemorrhage. Stroke 1997; 28:1–5.

11 Fujitsu K, Muramoto M, Ikeda Y, Inada Y, Kim I, Kuwabara T: Indications for surgical treatment of putaminal hemorrhage. Comparative study based on serial CT and time-course analysis. J Neurosurg 1990;73:518–525.

12 Fujii Y, Takeuchi S, Sasaki O, Minakawa T, Tanaka R: Multivariate analysis of predictors of hematoma enlargement in spontaneous intracerebral hemorrhage. Stroke 1998;29:1160–1166.

13 Kazui S, Naritomi H, Yamamoto H, Sawada T, Yamaguchi T: Enlargement of spontaneous intracerebral hemorrhage. Incidence and time course. Stroke 1996;27:1783–1787.

14 Jauch EC, Lindsell CJ, Adeoye O, Khoury J, Barsan W, Broderick J, et al: Lack of evidence for an association between hemodynamic variables and hematoma growth in spontaneous intracerebral hemorrhage. Stroke 2006;37:2061–2065.

15 Cucchiara B, Messe S, Sansing L, Kasner S, Lyden P: Hematoma growth in oral anticoagulant related intracerebral hemorrhage. Stroke 2008;39:2993–2996.

16 Murai Y, Ikeda Y, Teramoto A, Tsuji Y: Magnetic resonance imaging-documented extravasation as an indicator of acute hypertensive intracerebral hemorrhage. J Neurosurg 1998;88:650–655.

17 Qureshi AI, Palesch YY, Martin R, Novitzke J, Cruz-Flores S, Ehtisham A, et al: Effect of systolic blood pressure reduction on hematoma expansion, perihematomal edema, and 3-month outcome among patients with intracerebral hemorrhage: results from the antihypertensive treatment of acute cerebral hemorrhage study. Arch Neurol 2010;67:570–576.

18 Davis SM, Broderick J, Hennerici M, Brun NC, Diringer MN, Mayer SA, et al: Hematoma growth is a determinant of mortality and poor outcome after intracerebral hemorrhage. Neurology 2006;66:1175–1181.

19 Anderson CS, Huang Y, Wang JG, Arima H, Neal B, Peng B, et al: Intensive blood pressure reduction in acute cerebral haemorrhage trial (INTERACT): a randomised pilot trial. Lancet Neurol 2008;7:391–399.

20 Mayer SA, Brun NC, Begtrup K, Broderick J, Davis S, Diringer MN, et al: Efficacy and safety of recombinant activated factor VII for acute intracerebral hemorrhage. N Engl J Med 2008;358:2127–2137.
21 Toyoda K, Yasaka M, Nagata K, Nagao T, Gotoh J, Sakamoto T, et al: Antithrombotic therapy influences location, enlargement, and mortality from intracerebral hemorrhage. The Bleeding with Antithrombotic Therapy (BAT) Retrospective Study. Cerebrovasc Dis 2009;27:151–159.
22 Huttner HB, Schellinger PD, Hartmann M, Kohrmann M, Juettler E, Wikner J, et al: Hematoma growth and outcome in treated neurocritical care patients with intracerebral hemorrhage related to oral anticoagulant therapy: comparison of acute treatment strategies using vitamin K, fresh frozen plasma, and prothrombin complex concentrates. Stroke 2006;37:1465–1470.
23 Flibotte JJ, Hagan N, O'Donnell J, Greenberg SM, Rosand J: Warfarin, hematoma expansion, and outcome of intracerebral hemorrhage. Neurology 2004;63:1059–1064.
24 Yasaka M, Minematsu K, Naritomi H, Sakata T, Yamaguchi T: Predisposing factors for enlargement of intracerebral hemorrhage in patients treated with warfarin. Thromb Haemost 2003;89:278–283.
25 Lee SB, Manno EM, Layton KF, Wijdicks EF: Progression of warfarin-associated intracerebral hemorrhage after INR normalization with FFP. Neurology 2006;67:1272–1274.
26 Kazui S, Minematsu K, Yamamoto H, Sawada T, Yamaguchi T: Predisposing factors to enlargement of spontaneous intracerebral hematoma. Stroke 1997;28:2370–2375.
27 Rodriguez-Luna D, Rubiera M, Ribo M, Coscojuela P, Pineiro S, Pagola J, et al: Ultraearly hematoma growth predicts poor outcome after acute intracerebral hemorrhage. Neurology 2011;77:1599–1604.
28 Huckman MS, Weinberg PE, Kim KS, Davis DO: Angiographic and clinico-pathologic correlates in basal ganglionic hemorrhage. Radiology 1970;95:79–92.
29 Yamaguchi K, Uemura K, Takahashi H, Kowada M, Kutsuzawa T: Intracerebral leakage of contrast medium in apoplexy. Br J Radiol 1971;44:689–691.
30 Becker KJ, Baxter AB, Bybee HM, Tirschwell DL, Abouelsaad T, Cohen WA: Extravasation of radiographic contrast is an independent predictor of death in primary intracerebral hemorrhage. Stroke 1999;30:2025–2032.
31 Morgenstern LB, Demchuk AM, Kim DH, Frankowski RF, Grotta JC: Rebleeding leads to poor outcome in ultra-early craniotomy for intracerebral hemorrhage. Neurology 2001;56:1294–1299.
32 Kaneko M, Tanaka K, Shimada T, Sato K, Uemura K: Long-term evaluation of ultra-early operation for hypertensive intracerebral hemorrhage in 100 cases. J Neurosurg 1983;58:838–842.
33 Wada R, Aviv RI, Fox AJ, Sahlas DJ, Gladstone DJ, Tomlinson G, et al: CT angiography 'spot sign' predicts hematoma expansion in acute intracerebral hemorrhage. Stroke 2007;38:1257–1262.
34 Hallevi H, Abraham AT, Barreto AD, Grotta JC, Savitz SI: The spot sign in intracerebral hemorrhage: the importance of looking for contrast extravasation. Cerebrovasc Dis 2010;29:217–220.
35 Kim J, Smith A, Hemphill JC, 3rd, Smith WS, Lu Y, Dillon WP, et al: Contrast extravasation on CT predicts mortality in primary intracerebral hemorrhage. AJNR Am J Neuroradiol 2008;29:520–525.
36 Park SY, Kong MH, Kim JH, Kang DS, Song KY, Huh SK: Role of 'spot sign' on CT angiography to predict hematoma expansion in spontaneous intracerebral hemorrhage. J Korean Neurosurg Soc 2010;48:399–405.
37 Wang YH, Fan JY, Luo GD, Lin T, Xie DX, Ji FY, et al: Hematoma volume affects the accuracy of computed tomographic angiography 'spot sign' in predicting hematoma expansion after acute intracerebral hemorrhage. Eur Neurol 2011;65:150–155.
38 Brouwers HB, Falcone GJ, McNamara KA, Ayres AM, Oleinik A, Schwab K, et al: CTA spot sign predicts hematoma expansion in patients with delayed presentation after intracerebral hemorrhage. Neurocrit Care 2012;17:421–428.
39 Li N, Wang Y, Wang W, Ma L, Xue J, Weissenborn K, et al: Contrast extravasation on computed tomography angiography predicts clinical outcome in primary intracerebral hemorrhage: a prospective study of 139 cases. Stroke 2011;42:3441–3446.
40 Koculym A, Huynh TJ, Jakubovic R, Zhang L, Aviv RI: CT perfusion spot sign improves sensitivity for prediction of outcome compared with CTA and postcontrast CT. AJNR Am J Neuroradiol 2013;34:965–970.S1.
41 Sun SJ, Gao PY, Sui BB, Hou XY, Lin Y, Xue J, et al: 'Dynamic spot sign' on CT perfusion source images predicts haematoma expansion in acute intracerebral haemorrhage. Eur Radiol 2013;23:1846–1854.
42 Sorimachi T, Osada T, Baba T, Inoue G, Atsumi H, Ishizaka H, et al: The striate artery, hematoma, and spot sign on coronal images of computed tomography angiography in putaminal intracerebral hemorrhage. Stroke 2013;44:1830–1832.
43 Romero JM, Brouwers HB, Lu J, Delgado Almandoz JE, Kelly H, Heit J, et al: Prospective validation of the computed tomographic angiography spot sign score for intracerebral hemorrhage. Stroke 2013;44:3097–3102.
44 Dowlatshahi D, Wasserman JK, Momoli F, Petrcich W, Stotts G, Hogan M, et al: Evolution of computed tomography angiography spot sign is consistent with a site of active hemorrhage in acute intracerebral hemorrhage. Stroke 2014;45:277–280.

45 Havsteen I, Ovesen C, Christensen AF, Hansen CK, Nielsen JK, Christensen H: Showing no spot sign is a strong predictor of independent living after intracerebral haemorrhage. Cerebrovasc Dis 2014;37:164–170.
46 Chakraborty S, Alhazzaa M, Wasserman JK, Sun YY, Stotts G, Hogan MJ, et al: Dynamic characterization of the CT angiographic 'spot sign'. PLoS One 2014;9:e90431.
47 Hotta K, Sorimachi T, Osada T, Baba T, Inoue G, Atsumi H, et al: Risks and benefits of CT angiography in spontaneous intracerebral hemorrhage. Acta Neurochir (Wien) 2014;156:911–917.
48 d'Esterre CD, Chia TL, Jairath A, Lee TY, Symons SP, Aviv RI: Early rate of contrast extravasation in patients with intracerebral hemorrhage. AJNR Am J Neuroradiol 2011;32:1879–1884.
49 Thompson AL, Kosior JC, Gladstone DJ, Hopyan JJ, Symons SP, Romero F, et al: Defining the CT angiography 'spot sign' in primary intracerebral hemorrhage. Can J Neurol Sci 2009;36:456–461.
50 Radmanesh F, Falcone GJ, Anderson CD, Battey TW, Ayres AM, Vashkevich A, et al: Risk factors for computed tomography angiography spot sign in deep and lobar intracerebral hemorrhage are shared. Stroke 2014;45:1833–1835.
51 Brouwers HB, Chang Y, Falcone GJ, Cai X, Ayres AM, Battey TW, et al: Predicting hematoma expansion after primary intracerebral hemorrhage. JAMA Neurol 2014;71:158–164.
52 Brouwers HB, Raffeld MR, van Nieuwenhuizen KM, Falcone GJ, Ayres AM, McNamara KA, et al: CT angiography spot sign in intracerebral hemorrhage predicts active bleeding during surgery. Neurology 2014;83:883–889.
53 Tsukabe A, Watanabe Y, Tanaka H, Kunitomi Y, Nishizawa M, Arisawa A, et al: Prevalence and diagnostic performance of computed tomography angiography spot sign for intracerebral hematoma expansion depend on scan timing. Neuroradiology 2014;56:1039–1045.
54 Hou XY, Gao PY: Perihematomal perfusion typing and spot sign of acute intracerebral hemorrhage with multimode computed tomography: a preliminary study. Chin Med Sci J 2014;29:139–143.
55 Kim SH, Jung HH, Whang K, Kim JY, Pyen JS, Oh JW: Which emphasizing factors are most predictive of hematoma expansion in spot sign positive intracerebral hemorrhage? J Korean Neurosurg Soc 2014;56:86–90.
56 Moon BH, Jang DK, Han YM, Jang KS, Huh R, Park YS: Association factors for CT angiography spot sign and hematoma growth in Korean patients with acute spontaneous intracerebral hemorrhage: a single-center cohort study. J Korean Neurosurg Soc 2014;56:295–302.
57 Han JH, Lee JM, Koh EJ, Choi HY: The spot sign predicts hematoma expansion, outcome, and mortality in patients with primary intracerebral hemorrhage. J Korean Neurosurg Soc 2014;56:303–309.
58 Rosa Junior M, Rocha AJ, Saade N, Maia Junior AC, Gagliardi RJ: Active extravasation of contrast within the hemorrhage (spot sign): a multidetector computed tomography finding that predicts growth and a worse prognosis in non-traumatic intracerebral hemorrhage. Arq Neuropsiquiatr 2013;71:791–797.
59 Rizos T, Dorner N, Jenetzky E, Sykora M, Mundiyanapurath S, Horstmann S, et al: Spot signs in intracerebral hemorrhage: useful for identifying patients at risk for hematoma enlargement? Cerebrovasc Dis 2013;35:582–589.
60 Ciura VA, Brouwers HB, Pizzolato R, Ortiz CJ, Rosand J, Goldstein JN, et al: Spot sign on 90-second delayed computed tomography angiography improves sensitivity for hematoma expansion and mortality: prospective study. Stroke 2014;45:3293–3297.
61 Goldstein JN, Fazen LE, Snider R, Schwab K, Greenberg SM, Smith EE, et al: Contrast extravasation on CT angiography predicts hematoma expansion in intracerebral hemorrhage. Neurology 2007;68:889–894.
62 Delgado Almandoz JE, Yoo AJ, Stone MJ, Schaefer PW, Goldstein JN, Rosand J, et al: Systematic characterization of the computed tomography angiography spot sign in primary intracerebral hemorrhage identifies patients at highest risk for hematoma expansion: the spot sign score. Stroke 2009;40:2994–3000.
63 Delgado Almandoz JE, Yoo AJ, Stone MJ, Schaefer PW, Oleinik A, Brouwers HB, et al: The spot sign score in primary intracerebral hemorrhage identifies patients at highest risk of in-hospital mortality and poor outcome among survivors. Stroke 2010;41:54–60.
64 Ederies A, Demchuk A, Chia T, Gladstone DJ, Dowlatshahi D, Bendavit G, et al: Postcontrast CT extravasation is associated with hematoma expansion in CTA spot negative patients. Stroke 2009;40:1672–1676.
65 Boulouis G, Dumas A, Betensky RA, Brouwers HB, Fotiadis P, Vashkevich A, et al: Anatomic pattern of intracerebral hemorrhage expansion: relation to CT angiography spot sign and hematoma center. Stroke 2014;45:1154–1156.
66 Demchuk AM, Dowlatshahi D, Rodriguez-Luna D, Molina CA, Blas YS, Dzialowski I, et al: Prediction of haematoma growth and outcome in patients with intracerebral haemorrhage using the CT-angiography spot sign (PREDICT): a prospective observational study. Lancet Neurol 2012;11:307–314.

67 Du FZ, Jiang R, Gu M, He C, Guan J: The accuracy of spot sign in predicting hematoma expansion after intracerebral hemorrhage: a systematic review and meta-analysis. PLoS One 2014;9:e115777.
68 Evans A, Demchuk A, Symons SP, Dowlatshahi D, Gladstone DJ, Zhang L, et al: The spot sign is more common in the absence of multiple prior microbleeds. Stroke 2010;41:2210–2217.
69 Rodriguez-Luna D, Dowlatshahi D, Aviv RI, Molina CA, Silva Y, Dzialowski I, et al: Venous phase of computed tomography angiography increases spot sign detection, but intracerebral hemorrhage expansion is greater in spot signs detected in arterial phase. Stroke 2014;45:734–739.
70 Romero JM, Heit JJ, Delgado Almandoz JE, Goldstein JN, Lu J, Halpern E, et al: Spot sign score predicts rapid bleeding in spontaneous intracerebral hemorrhage. Emerg Radiol 2012;19:195–202.
71 Huynh TJ, Demchuk AM, Dowlatshahi D, Gladstone DJ, Krischek O, Kiss A, et al: Spot sign number is the most important spot sign characteristic for predicting hematoma expansion using first-pass computed tomography angiography: analysis from the PREDICT study. Stroke 2013;44:972–977.
72 Gazzola S, Aviv RI, Gladstone DJ, Mallia G, Li V, Fox AJ, et al: Vascular and nonvascular mimics of the CT angiography 'spot sign' in patients with secondary intracerebral hemorrhage. Stroke 2008;39:1177–1183.
73 Meretoja A, Churilov L, Campbell BC, Aviv RI, Yassi N, Barras C, et al: The spot sign and tranexamic acid on preventing ICH growth–AUStralasia Trial (STOP-AUST): protocol of a phase II randomized, placebo-controlled, double-blind, multicenter trial. Int J Stroke 2014;9:519–524.
74 Goldstein J, Brouwers H, Romero J, McNamara K, Schwab K, Greenberg S, et al: SCORE-IT: the Spot Sign score in restricting ICH growth horizontal line an Atach-II ancillary study. J Vasc Interv Neurol 2012;5(supp):20–25.
75 Barras CD, Tress BM, Christensen S, Collins M, Desmond PM, Skolnick BE, et al: Quantitative CT densitometry for predicting intracerebral hemorrhage growth. AJNR Am J Neuroradiol 2013;34:1139–1144.
76 Wang X, Arima H, Al-Shahi Salman R, Woodward M, Heeley E, Stapf C, et al: Clinical prediction algorithm (BRAIN) to determine risk of hematoma growth in acute intracerebral hemorrhage. Stroke 2015;46:376–381.
77 Fisher CM: Pathological observations in hypertensive cerebral hemorrhage. J Neuropathol Exp Neurol 1971;30:536–550.
78 Mayer SA, Lignelli A, Fink ME, Kessler DB, Thomas CE, Swarup R, et al: Perilesional blood flow and edema formation in acute intracerebral hemorrhage: a SPECT study. Stroke 1998;29:1791–1798.
79 Murai Y, Takagi R, Ikeda Y, Yamamoto Y, Teramoto A: Three-dimensional computerized tomography angiography in patients with hyperacute intracerebral hemorrhage. J Neurosurg 1999;91:424–431.
80 Mizukami M, Araki G, Mihara H, Tomita T, Fujinaga R: Arteriographically visualized extravasation in hypertensive intracerebral hemorrhage. Report of seven cases. Stroke 1972;3:527–537.
81 Komiyama M, Yasui T, Tamura K, Nagata Y, Fu Y, Yagura H: Simultaneous bleeding from multiple lenticulostriate arteries in hypertensive intracerebral haemorrhage. Neuroradiology 1995;37:129–130.
82 Wolpert SM, Schatzki SC: Extravasation of contrast material in the intracerebral basal ganglia. Radiology 1972;102:83–85.
83 Kowada M, Yamaguchi K, Matsuoka S, Ito Z: Extravasation of angiographic contrast material in hypertensive intracerebral hemorrhage. J Neurosurg 1972;36:471–473.
84 Fujii Y, Tanaka R, Takeuchi S, Koike T, Minakawa T, Sasaki O: Hematoma enlargement in spontaneous intracerebral hemorrhage. J Neurosurg 1994;80:51–57.
85 Takasugi S, Ueda S, Matsumoto K: Chronological changes in spontaneous intracerebral hematoma–an experimental and clinical study. Stroke 1985;16:651–658.
86 Nath FP, Kelly PT, Jenkins A, Mendelow AD, Graham DI, Teasdale GM: Effects of experimental intracerebral hemorrhage on blood flow, capillary permeability, and histochemistry. J Neurosurg 1987;66:555–562.
87 Zazulia AR, Diringer MN, Videen TO, Adams RE, Yundt K, Aiyagari V, et al: Hypoperfusion without ischemia surrounding acute intracerebral hemorrhage. J Cereb Blood Flow Metab 2001;21:804–810.
88 Carhuapoma JR, Wang PY, Beauchamp NJ, Keyl PM, Hanley DF, Barker PB: Diffusion-weighted MRI and proton MR spectroscopic imaging in the study of secondary neuronal injury after intracerebral hemorrhage. Stroke 2000;31:726–732.
89 Qureshi AI, Wilson DA, Hanley DF, Traystman RJ: No evidence for an ischemic penumbra in massive experimental intracerebral hemorrhage. Neurology 1999;52:266–272.
90 Powers WJ, Zazulia AR, Videen TO, Adams RE, Yundt KD, Aiyagari V, et al: Autoregulation of cerebral blood flow surrounding acute (6 to 22 h) intracerebral hemorrhage. Neurology 2001;57:18–24.
91 Adams RE, Diringer MN: Response to external ventricular drainage in spontaneous intracerebral hemorrhage with hydrocephalus. Neurology 1998;50:519–523.
92 Yang GY, Betz AL, Chenevert TL, Brunberg JA, Hoff JT: Experimental intracerebral hemorrhage: relationship between brain edema, blood flow, and blood-brain barrier permeability in rats. J Neurosurg 1994;81:93–102.

93 Wagner KR, Xi G, Hua Y, Kleinholz M, de Courten-Myers GM, Myers RE, et al: Lobar intracerebral hemorrhage model in pigs: rapid edema development in perihematomal white matter. Stroke 1996; 27:490–497.
94 Silva Y, Leira R, Tejada J, Lainez JM, Castillo J, Davalos A: Molecular signatures of vascular injury are associated with early growth of intracerebral hemorrhage. Stroke 2005;36:86–91.
95 Lee KR, Colon GP, Betz AL, Keep RF, Kim S, Hoff JT: Edema from intracerebral hemorrhage: the role of thrombin. J Neurosurg 1996;84:91–96.
96 Gong C, Hoff JT, Keep RF: Acute inflammatory reaction following experimental intracerebral hemorrhage in rat. Brain Res 2000;871:57–65.
97 Xi G, Wagner KR, Keep RF, Hua Y, de Courten-Myers GM, Broderick JP, et al: Role of blood clot formation on early edema development after experimental intracerebral hemorrhage. Stroke 1998; 29:2580–2586.
98 Jenkins A, Mendelow AD, Graham DI, Nath FP, Teasdale GM: Experimental intracerebral haematoma: the role of blood constituents in early ischaemia. Br J Neurosurg 1990;4:45–51.
99 Rosenberg GA, Navratil M: Metalloproteinase inhibition blocks edema in intracerebral hemorrhage in the rat. Neurology 1997;48:921–926.
100 Olson JD: Mechanisms of hemostasis. Effect on intracerebral hemorrhage. Stroke 1993;24(12 suppl): I109–I114.
101 Anderson CS, Heeley E, Huang Y, Wang J, Stapf C, Delcourt C, et al: Rapid blood-pressure lowering in patients with acute intracerebral hemorrhage. N Engl J Med 2013;368:2355–2365.
102 de Gans K, de Haan RJ, Majoie CB, Koopman MM, Brand A, Dijkgraaf MG, et al: PATCH: platelet transfusion in cerebral haemorrhage: study protocol for a multicentre, randomised, controlled trial. BMC Neurol 2010;10:19.
103 Steiner T, Bosel J: Options to restrict hematoma expansion after spontaneous intracerebral hemorrhage. Stroke 2010;41:402–409.
104 Steiner T, Bohm M, Dichgans M, Diener HC, Ell C, Endres M, et al: Recommendations for the emergency management of complications associated with the new direct oral anticoagulants (DOACs), apixaban, dabigatran and rivaroxaban. Clin Res Cardiol 2013;102:399–412.
105 Mannucci PM: Hemostatic drugs. N Engl J Med 1998;339:245–253.
106 Bonnar J, Sheppard BL: Treatment of menorrhagia during menstruation: randomised controlled trial of ethamsylate, mefenamic acid, and tranexamic acid. BMJ 1996;313:579–582.
107 Henry DA, O'Connell DL: Effects of fibrinolytic inhibitors on mortality from upper gastrointestinal haemorrhage. BMJ 1989;298:1142–1146.
108 Walsh PN, Rizza CR, Matthews JM, Eipe J, Kernoff PB, Coles MD, et al: Epsilon-Aminocaproic acid therapy for dental extractions in haemophilia and Christmas disease: a double blind controlled trial. Br J Haematol 1971;20:463–475.
109 Kassell NF, Torner JC, Adams HP Jr: Antifibrinolytic therapy in the acute period following aneurysmal subarachnoid hemorrhage. Preliminary observations from the Cooperative Aneurysm Study. J Neurosurg 1984;61:225–230.
110 Vermeulen M, Lindsay KW, Murray GD, Cheah F, Hijdra A, Muizelaar JP, et al: Antifibrinolytic treatment in subarachnoid hemorrhage. N Engl J Med 1984;311:432–437.
111 Tsementzis SA, Hitchcock ER, Meyer CH: Benefits and risks of antifibrinolytic therapy in the management of ruptured intracranial aneurysms. A double-blind placebo-controlled study. Acta Neurochir (Wien) 1990;102:1–10.
112 Starke RM, Kim GH, Fernandez A, Komotar RJ, Hickman ZL, Otten ML, et al: Impact of a protocol for acute antifibrinolytic therapy on aneurysm rebleeding after subarachnoid hemorrhage. Stroke 2008;39:2617–2621.
113 Piriyawat P, Morgenstern LB, Yawn DH, Hall CE, Grotta JC: Treatment of acute intracerebral hemorrhage with epsilon-aminocaproic acid: a pilot study. Neurocrit Care 2004;1:47–51.
114 Royston D, Bidstrup BP, Taylor KM, Sapsford RN: Effect of aprotinin on need for blood transfusion after repeat open-heart surgery. Lancet 1987;2: 1289–1291.
115 Neuhaus P, Bechstein WO, Lefebre B, Blumhardt G, Slama K: Effect of aprotinin on intraoperative bleeding and fibrinolysis in liver transplantation. Lancet 1989;2:924–925.
116 CRASH-2 Collaborators, Roberts I, Shakur H, Afolabi A, Brohi K, Coats T, et al: The importance of early treatment with tranexamic acid in bleeding trauma patients: an exploratory analysis of the CRASH-2 randomised controlled trial. Lancet 2011;377:1096–1101.e1–e2.
117 CRASH-2 Trial Collaborators, Shakur H, Roberts I, Bautista R, Caballero J, Coats T, et al: Effects of tranexamic acid on death, vascular occlusive events, and blood transfusion in trauma patients with significant haemorrhage (CRASH-2): a randomised, placebo-controlled trial. Lancet 2010; 376:23–32.
118 Ker K, Edwards P, Perel P, Shakur H, Roberts I: Effect of tranexamic acid on surgical bleeding: systematic review and cumulative meta-analysis. BMJ 2012;344:e3054.
119 Ducloy-Bouthors AS, Jude B, Duhamel A, Broisin F, Huissoud C, Keita-Meyer H, et al: High-dose tranexamic acid reduces blood loss in postpartum haemorrhage. Crit Care 2011;15:R117.

120 Roos Y, Rinkel G, Vermeulen M, Algra A, van Gijn J: Antifibrinolytic therapy for aneurysmal subarachnoid hemorrhage: a major update of a cochrane review. Stroke 2003;34:2308–2309.
121 Hillman J, Fridriksson S, Nilsson O, Yu Z, Saveland H, Jakobsson KE: Immediate administration of tranexamic acid and reduced incidence of early rebleeding after aneurysmal subarachnoid hemorrhage: a prospective randomized study. J Neurosurg 2002;97:771–778.
122 Sorimachi T, Fujii Y, Morita K, Tanaka R: Rapid administration of antifibrinolytics and strict blood pressure control for intracerebral hemorrhage. Neurosurgery 2005;57:837–844.
123 Sprigg N, Renton CJ, Dineen RA, Kwong Y, Bath PM: Tranexamic acid for spontaneous intracerebral hemorrhage: a randomized controlled pilot trial (ISRCTN50867461). J Stroke Cerebrovasc Dis 2014;23:1312–1318.
124 Key NS, Aledort LM, Beardsley D, Cooper HA, Davignon G, Ewenstein BM, et al: Home treatment of mild to moderate bleeding episodes using recombinant factor VIIa (Novoseven) in haemophiliacs with inhibitors. Thromb Haemost 1998;80:912–918.
125 Hedner U: NovoSeven as a universal haemostatic agent. Blood Coagul Fibrinolysis 2000;11(suppl 1):S107–S111.
126 Hedner U, Ingerslev J: Clinical use of recombinant FVIIa (rFVIIa). Transfus Sci 1998;19:163–176.
127 Rice KM, Savidge GF: NovoSeven (recombinant factor VIIa) in centeral nervous systems bleeds. Haemostasis 1996;26(suppl 1):131–134.
128 Mayer SA, Brun NC, Begtrup K, Broderick J, Davis S, Diringer MN, et al: Recombinant activated factor VII for acute intracerebral hemorrhage. N Engl J Med 2005;352:777–785.
129 Mayer SA, Davis SM, Skolnick BE, Brun NC, Begtrup K, Broderick JP, et al: Can a subset of intracerebral hemorrhage patients benefit from hemostatic therapy with recombinant activated factor VII? Stroke 2009;40:833–840.
130 Sutherland CS, Hill MD, Kaufmann AM, Silvaggio JA, Demchuk AM, Sutherland GR: Recombinant factor VIIa plus surgery for intracerebral hemorrhage. Can J Neurol Sci 2008;35:567–572.
131 Yuan ZH, Jiang JK, Huang WD, Pan J, Zhu JY, Wang JZ: A meta-analysis of the efficacy and safety of recombinant activated factor VII for patients with acute intracerebral hemorrhage without hemophilia. J Clin Neurosci 2010;17:685–693.
132 Levi M, Levy JH, Andersen HF, Truloff D: Safety of recombinant activated factor VII in randomized clinical trials. N Engl J Med 2010;363:1791–1800.
133 Broderick JP, Diringer MN, Hill MD, Brun NC, Mayer SA, Steiner T, et al: Determinants of intracerebral hemorrhage growth: an exploratory analysis. Stroke 2007;38:1072–1075.
134 Barras CD, Tress BM, Christensen S, MacGregor L, Collins M, Desmond PM, et al: Density and shape as CT predictors of intracerebral hemorrhage growth. Stroke 2009;40:1325–1331.
135 Leira R, Davalos A, Silva Y, Gil-Peralta A, Tejada J, Garcia M, et al: Early neurologic deterioration in intracerebral hemorrhage: predictors and associated factors. Neurology 2004;63:461–467.
136 Ohwaki K, Yano E, Nagashima H, Hirata M, Nakagomi T, Tamura A: Blood pressure management in acute intracerebral hemorrhage: relationship between elevated blood pressure and hematoma enlargement. Stroke 2004;35:1364–1367.
137 Broderick J, Mayer S, Brun NC, Begtrup K, Diringer MN, Davis S, et al: Determinants of hemorrhage growth in a randomized trial of recombinant activated factor VII. J Neurol Sci 2005;238(suppl 1): S69.
138 Silva Y, Puigdemont M, Castellanos M, Serena J, Suner RM, Garcia MM, et al: Semi-intensive monitoring in acute stroke and long-term outcome. Cerebrovasc Dis 2005;19:23–30.
139 Lou M, Al-Hazzani A, Goddeau RP Jr, Novak V, Selim M: Relationship between white-matter hyperintensities and hematoma volume and growth in patients with intracerebral hemorrhage. Stroke 2010;41:34–40.

Dr. Katja E. Wartenberg
Neurocritical Care Unit, Department of Neurology
Martin-Luther-University Halle-Wittenberg
Ernst-Grube-Strasse 40, DE–06120 Halle/Saale (Germany)
E-Mail katja.wartenberg@medizin.uni-halle.de

Toyoda K, Anderson CS, Mayer SA (eds): New Insights in Intracerebral Hemorrhage.
Front Neurol Neurosci. Basel, Karger, 2016, vol 37, pp 130–147 (DOI: 10.1159/000437118)

Ventriculostomy and Lytic Therapy for Intracerebral Hemorrhage

Wendy C. Ziai • Paul A. Nyquist • Daniel F. Hanley

Department of Neurology, Divisions of Brain Injury Outcomes and Neurocritical Care, The Johns Hopkins University School of Medicine, Baltimore, Md., USA

Abstract

Intraventricular hemorrhage (IVH) frequently complicates intracranial hemorrhage (ICH) and is a significant independent contributor to morbidity and mortality, yet therapy directed at ameliorating intraventricular clotting has been limited and until recently, has not been subject to systematic evaluation. Thrombolytic therapy with placement of an external ventricular drain for management of severe IVH secondary to ICH has been investigated in multiple observational studies, small randomized controlled trials and several meta-analyses, soon to culminate with the completion of the 500 patient CLEAR IVH randomized controlled trial. We review conventional and lytic therapeutic approaches to severe IVH in the setting of small ICH, articulating the scope of the problem, management issues, and relevant questions for future research.
© 2016 S. Karger AG, Basel

Epidemiology and Pathophysiology

Intraventricular hemorrhage (IVH) is the direct hemorrhage of blood into the ventricles of the brain. Mortality estimates for intracranial hemorrhage (ICH) with significant IVH range from 50 to 80% [1–3]. Approximately 45% of cases of spontaneous ICH and 25% of cases of aneurysmal subarachnoid hemorrhage (SAH) extend into the ventricles [4–7]. Patients with severe IVH are twice as likely to have poor outcomes (modified Rankin scale score of 4–6 at hospital discharge) and are nearly three times more likely to die than ICH cohorts without IVH [8]. Risk factors for IVH in association with spontaneous ICH include old age, a high baseline ICH volume, a mean arterial pressure of greater than 120 mm Hg, and a deep subcortical location of primary ICH in close proximity to the ventricles [1].

Primary IVH, which has a reported incidence of 3–7%, is confined to the ventricular system and ependymal lining of the ventricles and originates from either an intraventricular (IVR) source or a lesion within the ventricular wall (e.g., IVR trauma or an aneurysm, vascular malformation or tumor, usually involving the choroid plexus) [9]. A search for these lesions must be undertaken prior to initiation of IVR thrombolytic therapy. Choroid plexus arteriovenous malformation lesions have been documented in primary IVH in contrast with secondary IVH. Dural arteriovenous malformations have also rarely been described in association with primary IVH, and they are presumed to result from retrograde venous drainage, creating backflow into the subependymal veins and causing their rupture [10]. Secondary IVH results from extension of an intracerebral hemorrhage or SAH into the ventricular system. Vascular rupture into a ventricle due to a parenchymal ICH may occur by two proposed pathogenic mechanisms: erosion of the ventricular wall under the ventricular hemorrhage; or distention of the regional subependymal vessels, with some of the vessels occluded by thrombus [11]. It is not clear, however, if ependymal erosion is the primary event or if it occurs secondary to the presence of IVR blood [12]. Small parenchymal hemorrhagic infarcts at the ventricular edge with presumed secondary rupture through the ependyma have also been described [13]. The implications of these mechanisms of IVH formation in thrombolytic therapy are incompletely understood at this time.

The morbidity of IVH results in large part from acute obstructive hydrocephalus, which elevates intracranial pressure (ICP), decreases cerebral perfusion pressure and, if it is severe enough, results in brain herniation. Controlling ICP with an external ventricular drain (EVD), however, does not usually result in immediate mental status improvement [14]. Thus, the direct mass effect of IVH may be a significant pathophysiologic factor independent of ICP elevation and requiring a specific management approach. Cerebral ischemia and the toxic effects of ventricular blood on adjacent periventricular brain tissue, including the hippocampus, diencephalon and brainstem, likely also play important roles [15]. Vasospasms due to circulation of blood through cerebrospinal fluid (CSF) into the basal cisterns are infrequently investigated but have been frequently reported and may contribute to inflammatory, vasospastic and ischemic injuries [16]. Secondary effects of IVH treatment include bacterial meningitis, which is related to EVD usage, and more controversially, toxicity related to IVR thrombolysis with tissue plasminogen activator (tPA), which may also worsen edema and inflammation. Finally, permanent occlusion and scarring of arachnoid granulations at CSF absorption sites results in delayed development of communicating hydrocephalus, which necessitates permanent CSF shunt placement in 30–60% of patients and is associated with impairments in cognition, gait, balance, and urinary continence [12, 17–19] (table 1).

Table 1. Differential diagnosis of intraventricular hemorrhage

Primary IVH
Head trauma
Intraventricular vascular malformation, aneurysm, tumor
Bleeding diathesis
Moyamoya disease
Insertion/removal of a ventricular catheter
Secondary IVH
Extension of intracerebral hematoma or subarachnoid hemorrhage caused by:
Hypertension
Cerebral aneurysm
Head trauma
Arteriovenous malformation
Vasculitis
Coagulation disorder
Hemorrhagic transformation of an ischemic infarct
Tumor
Extension of a germinal matrix hematoma (premature infants)

Adapted from Andrews and Engelhard [20].

Prognostication in Spontaneous Intraventricular Hemorrhage

IVH volume is a surrogate for IVH severity, and a larger volume is correlated with a worse prognosis. The Turhim model depicts the contribution of IVH volume to 30-day mortality, with adjustments for the Glasgow Coma Scale (GCS) score and the size of the associated ICH, thus establishing IVH volume as an independent prognostic factor for poor outcome (fig. 1) [21]. Patients with IVH in addition to ICH have a lower initial GCS score and a larger ICH volume. The number of ventricles containing blood and blood in the fourth ventricle also contribute to poor outcome. Young et al. [3] have demonstrated that patients with supratentorial ICH and more than 20 cc of interventricular blood in general have poor outcomes. However, patients with primary IVH can often survive with such a large IVH volume without developing loss of consciousness or hydrocephalus, and they have a good 3-month outcome, indicating the importance of the underlying etiology [22].

Other significant predictors of long-term poor outcome include dilation of both the third and fourth ventricles due to hemorrhage [23, 24]. An IVH scoring system developed for the prediction of 30-day mortality in patients with an EVD has revealed the following independent predictors of outcome: an ICH volume of >60 ml; severe hydrocephalus; a GCS score of ≤8; and an age of ≥70 years (table 2) [25]. This scoring system performed favorably compared to other prognostic models for ICH, especially for prediction of 30-day mortality and functional outcome at 6 months [26].

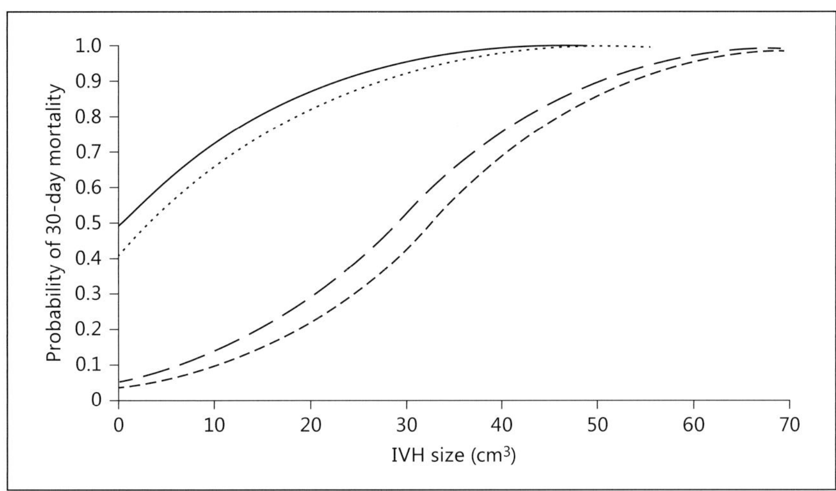

Fig. 1. Effect of increasing intraventricular hemorrhage (IVH) volume on predicted 30-day mortality. The lines represent specific disease severity groupings. In this model, IVH volume accounts for >50% of mortality, independent of the Glasgow Coma Scale (GCS) score or initial intracranial hemorrhage (ICH) size. Adapted from: Tuhrim et al. [21]. —— = GCS score ≤8, ICH size = 80 cc, pulse pressure ≤85, hydrocephalus present. · · · · · = GCS score ≤8, ICH size = 20 cc, pulse pressure ≤85, hydrocephalus present. — — = GCS score >8, ICH size = 80 cc, pulse pressure ≤85, hydrocephalus present. - - - = GCS score >8, ICH size = 20 cc, pulse pressure ≤85, hydrocephalus present.

Table 2. IVH score

Component	Points
GCS score	
≥13	0
9–12	1
≤8	2
ICH volume, ml	
<30	0
≥30	1
≥60	2
Hydrocephalus	
Absent	0
Moderate	1
Severe	2
Age	
<70	0
≥70	1
Total	0–7

GCS = Glasgow Coma Scale; ICH = intracerebral hemorrhage. Thirty-day mortality rates for scores of 2, 3, 4, 5 and 6 were 9.1, 14.3, 46.2, 75 and 100%, respectively [25].

Expansion of IVH within the first 24 h was identified in the FAST trial (recombinant activated factor VII) as an independent predictor of death or severe disability [1, 27]. Risk factors for IVH growth (>2 ml) included a baseline mean arterial pressure of greater than 120 mm Hg, a large baseline ICH volume, IVH present at baseline, a short time from symptom onset to baseline CT scan, and treatment with recombinant activated factor VII (vs. placebo).

Conventional Intraventricular Hemorrhage Therapy and Rationale for Thrombolytics

The standard of care for the management of IVH causing obstructive hydrocephalus remains placement of an EVD for CSF diversion and ICP control. EVDs also assist with removal of blood breakdown products, which may cause chemical meningitis [28]. However, in the absence of a randomized controlled trial (RCT) addressing ventriculostomy usage (an unlikely proposal based on ethical considerations), ICH management guidelines do not make strong recommendations about how, when, and for whom invasive monitoring of ICP or ventriculostomy should be performed [29]. Instead, the clinical benefit of EVD placement is debated [14] despite evidence that obstructive hydrocephalus on admission CT is an independent predictor of increased in-hospital and 30-day mortality [30, 31] and also of 6-month neurologic outcome for caudate ICH [32]. Hydrocephalus occurs in 20–40% of all IVH patients [30]. In both the International Surgical Trial in Intracerebral Hemorrhage (STICH) study [33] and the recombinant activated factor VII for acute intracerebral hemorrhage (NovoSeven) trial [1], however, EVDs were placed in ≤10% of patients with IVH. In the STICH trial, favorable outcomes were less frequent when IVH was present and were significantly lower with accompanying hydrocephalus [34]. In this situation, medical management is often insufficient for reducing ICP, and EVD placement is necessary [35]. Analysis of an IVH cohort from a large prospective randomized study of thrombolysis in IVH has demonstrated that continuous drainage of CSF contributes to the normalization of ICP and that high ICP (>30 mm Hg) is independently predictive of both morbidity and mortality [36]. Huttner et al. [37] has found that the long-term outcomes of patients with pure ganglionic ICH do not differ between those who have received IVH and EVD treatments, suggesting that CSF drainage is beneficial. The general pessimism toward EVD treatment alone is not without evidence. In a systematic review of 22 retrospective studies of IVH in the setting of ICH and SAH, EVD placement improved the mortality but not the morbidity of IVH [38]. The case fatality rate was 78% in conservatively treated patients versus 58% in those treated with EVD, and the unfavorable outcomes (modified Rankin Score of 4 or 5) did not differ (90 vs. 89%, respectively). Adams and Diringer's [14] study of 22 patients with spontaneous ICH and hydrocephalus has found that EVD drainage reduces ventricular volume but does not change the level of consciousness. Shapiro et al. [23] have concluded that the use of ventriculostomy to treat hemorrhagic dilation of the 4th ventricle does not improve outcome. More recently, Staykov et al. [39] have reported a mortality rate of 53% (n = 133) in patients treated with EVD alone compared with 71% (n = 91) in those treated conservatively. In our retrospective cohort of 183 IVH patients, EVD placement was an independent predictor of reduced mortality and a modified Rankin score of 0–3 [40]. Among patients presenting with obstructive hydrocephalus and a GCS score of above 3, after adjustment, EVD was associated with a 98% reduction in the odds of in-hospital death. These findings suggest that EVD assists with ICP control, reducing early mortality, but may have less impact on morbidity due to the previously described inflammatory mechanisms. EVD alone does not alter the rate of blood clot resolution [41] and may even slow the rate of IVH clearance by removing tPA released from the clot into the CSF. EVDs therefore fail to decrease the degree and incidence of communicating hydrocephalus. Moreover, catheter occlusions occur frequently in the setting of a large IVH volume and can result in poor ICP control, requiring repeated catheter exchanges, thus increasing the risks of hemorrhage and infection [42]. It is generally agreed that hydrocephalus and a deteriorating neurologic condition are indications for placement of an EVD; however, its use remains inconsistent. It is unclear whether preemptive ventriculostomy is beneficial.

Injection of thrombolytic agents into the ventricular space has evolved in response to the challenges of catheter obstruction and slow IVH clearance, and it has been shown to be safe and effective in animal studies [43, 44] and in multiple small clinical case series [45–48]. In experimental studies, the thrombolytic-mediated removal of clots has been shown to facilitate their removal and to improve hydrocephalus and inflammation [49–51]. Larger systematic reviews evaluating intraventricular fibrinolysis (IVF) date back to 2000, when a systematic review of 16 retrospective studies (n = 201) of patients with severe IVH (Graeb score of ≥7) secondary to ICH reported that combined therapy with EVD and IVF was associated with a significantly lower mortality rate (9%) and a lower risk of unfavorable outcome (22%) compared with treatment with EVD alone (mortality 56%; poor outcome: 87%) [38]. In 2002, a Cochrane database systematic review of 10 independent studies (8 case series/retrospective studies, 1 quasi-RCT, and 1 RCT) of IVR thrombolytic agents found anecdotal evidence supporting their safety and possible therapeutic value [52]. Nearly a decade later, a systematic review of 4 randomized and 8 observational studies comparing treatments with EVD alone and with EVD combined with IVF in patients with severe IVH due to spontaneous supratentorial ICH reported that the overall mortality risk decreased from 46.7% (EVD alone) to 22.7% (EVD + IVF) (table 2) [53]. IVF was also associated with an increase in good functional outcome, and there were no significant differences between the 2 groups in shunt dependence or complications, although the rebleeding rate was greater in the IVF group (11.4 vs. 6.4% in the EVD group). The mortality results were highly significant with urokinase, but not with recombinant tissue plasminogen activator (rtPA), suggesting that the therapeutic effect could differ

Table 3. Systematic reviews of thrombolytic therapy for intraventricular hemorrhage

Study	Total no. of patients	Total no. of studies	Comparison groups	Odds ratio (95% CI) or relative risk (95% CI) or %
Nieuwkamp et al. [38], 2000	EVD: 33 EVD + IVF: 75	16 retrospective	EVD + IVF vs. EVD	9 vs. 56, mortality 22 vs. 87, poor outcome
Staykov et al. [55], 2010	No EVD: 91 EVD: 133 EVD + IVF: 212	3 randomized 3 prospective 17 retrospective	Cons/EVD/ EVD + IVF	71/53/16, mortality 86/70/45, poor outcome at end of study
Gaberel et al. [53], 2011	EVD: 149 EVD + IVF: 167 EVD: 70 EVD + IVF: 76 EVD: 88 EVD + IVF: 99	4 RCTs 8 observational	EVD + IVF vs. EVD	OR = 0.32 (0.19–0.52), mortality OR = 5.02 (2.07–12.20), good outcome at discharge/1 month OR = 2.35 (0.97–5.69), good outcome at ≥3 months
Khan et al. [54], 2014	Control: 367 EVD + IVF: 418 Control: 199 EVD + IVF: 237	8 RCTs 4 prospective 12 observational	EVD + IVF vs. control	RR = 0.55 (0.42–0.71), mortality at end of study RR = 1.66 (1.27–2.19), good outcome at end of study

Cons = Conservative treatment; CI = confidence interval.

depending on the choice of thrombolytic agent. Staykov et al. [39] performed a systematic review of 23 studies (1993–2010) (n = 436), reporting a mortality rate of 53% (n = 133) for patients treated with EVD alone and 16% (n = 212) for those treated with EVD plus thrombolysis compared to 71% (n = 91) for conservatively treated patients. The incidence of unfavorable outcome was not as low in the IVF group (45 vs. 70%-EVD alone vs. 86%-conservative treatment) compared to the other systematic reviews, but this finding still indicates a potentially significant benefit from IVF. Finally, an updated systematic review including 8 RCTs demonstrated consistent results that IVF reduced mortality in IVH by nearly half (compared to EVD alone), increased the likelihood of good functional outcome by 66%, and decreased the rate of shunt dependence (relative risk = 0.62) [54]. IVF was not associated with an increased rate of ventriculitis or rehemorrhage. All of these reviews have demonstrated that IVF may be an effective strategy for reducing mortality and improving functional outcome, with no significant increase in the complication rate. They are limited by the level of evidence (grades II and III mostly), with considerable heterogeneity among patient populations, dosing regimens, the length of follow-up, and conditions (including both ICH and SAH as etiologies of IVH) (table 3).

A phase III multinational RCT (Clot Lysis Evaluating Accelerated Resolution of IVH [CLEAR III]) recently completed enrollment of 500 patients with primary or secondary spontaneous IVH causing obstructive hydrocephalus requiring EVD and with small ICH (<30 cc) [56]. The patients were randomized (1:1) to receive IVF with rtPA or placebo (http://www.cleariii.com). The results of the CLEAR III study should provide the highest quality evidence of the benefits and complications of IVF and are due sometime in 2016. The phase II clinical trial Clot Lysis Evaluating Accelerated Resolution of IVH (CLEAR IVH), which was completed in 2008 [57], showed that the use of low-dose rtPA (3 mg q12 h) for the treatment of ICH with IVH resulted in lower than expected rates of death and ventriculitis, and bleeding events remained below the prespecified thresholds mortality [18% rtPA; 23% placebo], ventriculitis [8% rtPA; 9% placebo], and symptomatic bleeding [23% rtPA; 5% placebo; $p = 0.1$]. The median duration of dosing was 7.5 days for rtPA and 12 days for placebo. There was a significant beneficial effect of rtPA on the rate of clot resolution ($p < 0.001$).

This trial was followed by dose interval finding studies (CLEAR A and B), which randomized patients 1:1 to receive IVR rtPA, at a dose of either 0.3 or 1.0 mg q12 h ($n = 16$) (CLEAR A) or to receive 1.0 mg q12 h or q8 h ($n = 36$) (CLEAR B). These studies demonstrated dose-specific clot lysis rates of 21.7%/day, 25.1%/day, 24.2%/day, and 19.9%/day for the 3.0 mg, 1.0 mg (q12 h), 0.3 mg, and 1.0 mg (q8 h) groups, respectively, over the first 3 days of treatment. The safety profiles for the two lower doses were numerically superior to that of the 3.0 mg dose, with a symptomatic hemorrhage rate of 5.8% (3/52 patients).

Preliminary data from the CLEAR III trial for the first 250 subjects enrolled demonstrated that all safety endpoints were lower than expected for severe IVH, indicating that the study protocol is safe [58]. Adjudicated safety events totaled three (1.2%) cases of symptomatic hemorrhage within 72 h of receiving the study agent, ten (4.0%) cases of bacterial ventriculitis, 13 (5.2%) cases of nonbacterial ventriculitis and 31 (12.4%) deaths at 30 days. These event rates are the lowest to date in any of the CLEAR IVH trials and rely on strict protocols for stability of hemorrhage and concurrent drug use and careful tracking of adverse events with an adjudication process. Translating this safety to real-world experience is discussed next.

Safety Issues in Thrombolytic Therapy

The most relevant safety considerations for thrombolytic administration are minimization of the risks of hemorrhage, infection and medical comorbidities, which frequently occur in this population. The potential for ongoing intracranial bleeding with IVR rtPA, whether from the ICH, IVH or EVD tract (catheter tract hemorrhage (CTH)), puts patients at risk of further injury. Khan et al.'s [54] meta-analysis did not find an association between IVF and an increased risk of rehemorrhage (relative risk = 1.06; 95% CI, 0.66–1.70; $p = 0.80$). Detailed analysis of the pre-randomization scans of the first 300 patients enrolled in the CLEAR III IVH trial showed that most bleeding events stabilized within 48 h after diagnostic CT [59]. IVH expansion (>5 cc) was significantly more common than ICH expansion in patients with severe IVH (27 vs. 11.0%). CTHs were common, occurring in 22.1% of patients with an EVD, but they rarely expanded during the initial stabilization period (1%). CTHs could be newly detected, however, well beyond 24 h after EVD placement, and they were significantly associated with pre-admission antiplatelet therapy.

The CLEAR IVH trials minimized the risk of rebleeding after IVF using strict selection criteria and a protocolized approach to stabilizing hemorrhage, which included the following: mandatory radiologic investigations to exclude structural lesions prior to randomization [56]; establishing stability of the initial bleed via sequential CTs ≥6 h apart; repeatedly stabilizing any rebleeding of >5 cc in any compartment using serial CTs every 12 h until no further increase in hematoma size was detected; restricting the use of IVF to at least 12 h after symptom onset and 6 h after any EVD insertion; daily head CTs (after every 3rd dose of the study agent) to assess any new bleeding events; and a 12-h suspension in dosing after each EVD change or new EVD insertion until the absence/stabilization of significant CTH was proven by CT. These assessments were supervised by a centralized image reading center in the trial but can be readily performed by treating physicians using a similar approach.

In IVH patients, the risk of EVD-associated infection depends variably on catheter duration and CSF leakage [60, 61]. In the largest reported meta-analysis of the use of IVF to treat IVH, IVF was not found to be associated with an increased rate of ventriculitis (relative risk = 1.46; 95% CI, 0.77–2.76; p = 0.25) [54]. The infection rates in the CLEAR III trial based on preliminary analyses of the first 250 patients are comparable to those previously reported in EVD case series. Meta-analysis of 33 published series of EVD placement in 9,667 cases identified 568 reported infections. The pooled infection incidence rate was 7.9% (6.3%, 9.4%), compared to 4.4% (1.9%, 6.9%) in the CLEAR III trial. These low rates occurred despite multiple daily injections, blood in the ventricles, the use of thrombolysis in half of the cases and generalization to over 60 trial sites. Of interest, all 10 cases of bacterial ventriculitis occurred in 82 patients without an antibiotic-coated EVD who were not taking periprocedural antibiotics.

The use of the prophylactic heparin during and immediately after IVR rtPA dosing is of potential concern. In the first 250 patients treated in CLEAR III, prophylactic anticoagulation was associated with a small, nonsignificant increase in the frequency of intracranial bleeding. However, thrombotic events were significantly more frequent in patients not receiving prophylaxis. Of 80 subjects who were not on prophylactic heparin during the acute study phase, 23% had a thrombotic event, compared to 9% of 170 on prophylactic heparin (p = 0.005). We therefore recommend following AHA guidelines when prescribing low-dose heparin for prophylaxis during IVF therapy. Evaluating the safety of low-dose heparin interactions with IVF therapy will have to await the CLEAR III results.

Genetic and Imaging Predictors of Safety and Outcome of Fibrinolytic Therapy in Intracranial Hemorrhage/Intraventricular Hemorrhage

The risk of secondary bleeding in ICH and IVH in the setting of intravenous thrombolytics may be influenced by preexisting risk factors. A number of studies have used imaging markers such as CT angiography and MRI to identify features associated with an increased risk of rebleeding in primary ICH/IVH. The CT angiography 'spot sign' is a useful marker for prediction of progression of ICH when it is visualized on initial CT angiography in the setting of acute ICH [62]. It also may be a useful marker for potential post-thrombolytic hemorrhage in the setting of thrombolytic use for resolution of primary ICH or IVH.

Ischemic white matter disease or leukoaraiosis on MRI has been associated with increased risks of hemorrhage in general and of rebleeding after primary ICH [63, 64]. It is also a marker of an increased risk for rebleeding with the use of thrombolytics after acute stroke or the use of warfarin for atrial fibrillation [65, 66]. These same risk factors may also be predictive of the risk of secondary bleeding in the setting of thrombolytic therapy in ICH and IVH and may help to predict functional outcomes in this setting [67].

The APOE genotype, which has been associated with an increased risk of white matter disease, has also been associated with increased risks of hemorrhage growth and secondary bleeding and worse outcome in ICH. Thus, its assessment may help to determine risk in patients with high white matter burden who receive thrombolytic therapy [68, 69]. Another genetic characteristic that may be helpful in assigning the risk of rebleeding in the setting of thrombolytic therapy in IVH and ICH is the haptoglobin phenotype. Haptoglobin is a free heme-scavenging protein that exists in two subtypes. Type 1 is the major allele, and type 2 the minor allele, which occurs in approximately 21% of the population. The type 2 allele is known to result in an altered iron binding capacity and to have a more aggressive effect on inflammation via secondary pathways [70–72]. Recently, in a prospective observational study of ICH in humans, the type 2 allele was found to be associated with worse functional outcome [73].

These genetic factors not only may affect rebleeding in response to thrombolytics but also may influence survival and functional outcome in the setting of IVH and ICH in general via inflammatory mechanisms. Presently, studies are underway to better understand the effects of imaging and genetic characteristic on rebleeding in the setting of thrombolytic therapy in ICH and IVH.

Strategies to Improve Fibrinolytic Drug Delivery

Strategies to optimize the delivery of fibrinolytic agents to maximize IVR clot resolution while minimizing unwanted new hemorrhage are focused on dosing, EVD catheter positioning and the use of multiple catheters. Historically, doses of up to 8 mg rtPA in a single bolus have been reported, although the 3 mg rtPA dose used in the CLEAR IVH Safety Trial was associated with a higher than acceptable symptomatic bleeding rate (23 vs. 5% in placebo-treated patients) [74]. A dose-response study found that high-dose IVF (4 mg alteplase every 12 h, maximum of 20 mg) and low-dose IVF (1 mg alteplase every 8 h, maximum of 12 mg) had similar rates of IVH clearance from the third and fourth ventricles and similar safety profiles [75]. The total clot half-life was significantly longer in the low-dose group by 1 day, but the 3-month outcomes were not different between the groups. Evaluation of even lower doses (0.3 mg twice daily) in the dose-finding studies of the CLEAR IVH trials did reveal a dose-response relationship [76]. IVH clearance to 50% of baseline occurred faster with increasing rtPA doses and was the fastest in the midline ventricles, followed by the anterior half of the lateral ventricles, and was the slowest in the posterior half of the lateral ventricles. Once the midline ventricles are open, rtPA may be diverted away from blood in the posterolateral ventricles, potentially limiting the thrombolytic effectiveness in regions distant from the EVD. Thus, clearance of blood from the 3rd and 4th ventricles has been a key endpoint in trials of IVR thrombolysis, with evidence from retrospective studies that IVF may reduce the need for ventriculoperitoneal (VP) shunting [38, 45]. Analysis of IVH clearance rates showed an initial rapid clearance and a subsequent slower clearance phase.

There is experimental evidence that optimal rtPA dosing is also influenced by potential toxicity, at least for the higher doses. Animal studies have demonstrated a dose-dependent effect of rtPA on periventricular and choroid plexus edema in addition to IVR leukocytosis in experimental IVH [77]. Leukocyte recruitment has been attributed to plasmin (the product of the tPA reaction), a potent monocyte chemoattractant [78], and fibrin degradation products, potent neutrophil chemotaxins [79]. Plasmin and neutrophils are associated with an increase in blood-brain barrier permeability [80–82]. Thus, higher doses of tPA may lead to these undesirable phenomena by activating more plasmin and more rapidly producing fibrin degradation products. In clinical IVH, 2 independent studies using computerized volumetric analysis have found no significant increase in perihematomal edema in patient treated with IVR rtPA compared to controls treated only with EVD [83, 84]. Hallevi et al. [28] described development of a cellular inflammatory reaction in approximately half of IVH patients on around day 2, which peaked on days 4–6 and gradually subsided with IVH clearance. The cellular response was attenuated in tPA-treated patients compared to those treated with EVD alone, but it was not significantly different between the groups. The findings of these clinical studies suggest that the use of low-dose rtPA (1 mg every 8 h was used in the CLEAR III trial) with continuous removal of lysed IVR clots may limit these potential toxicities. In a study of experimental ICH, Wagner et al. [51] reported that ultra-early clot aspiration (<4 h) of experimental ICH after lysis with rtPA markedly reduced the occurrence of perihematomal brain edema. Optimal drainage goals in the IVH population require further study.

The choice of fibrinolytic agent, at least in North America, has been limited by unavailability of urokinase since 2000. Compared to urokinase, tPA is far more

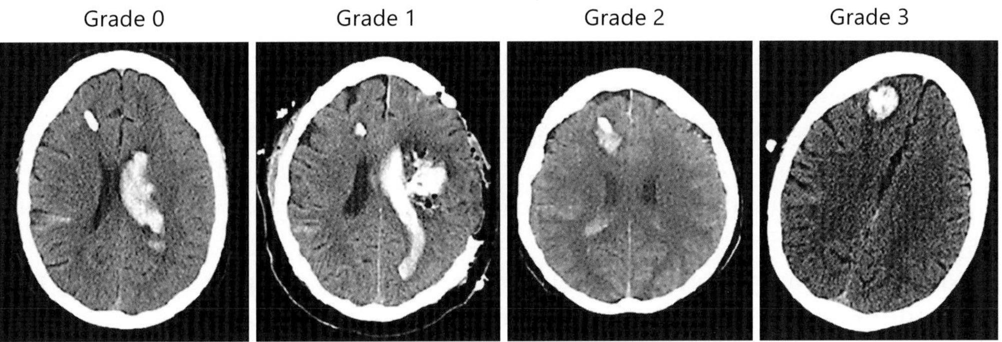

Fig. 2. Catheter Tract Hemorrhage Grading Scale. With permission from Jackson et al. [91].

fibrin-specific and approximately 10 times more effective for *in vitro* fibrinolysis [85, 86]. Gaberel et al. [87] compared urokinase with tPA in a collagenase IVH model and reported improved functional recovery only in the urokinase-treated animals. It was demonstrated that urokinase lacked the pro-inflammatory and pro-excitotoxic effects of tPA, which may have led to the improved outcome and similar lytic efficacy. It is also possible that enhanced finbrinolysis with rtPA caused the release of more blood breakdown products, especially hemoglobin and iron, which are important factors for secondary brain injury after ICH [88]. A clinical trial comparing urokinase with rtPA has not been performed. Safer thrombolytics, such as the recently proposed Optimized tPA, a human tPA containing 2 point mutations that has been reported to lack NMDAR-dependent neurotoxicity and has been proposed (although not yet tested clinically) as an alternative thrombolytic for intracranial applications [89].

Other factors that may improve IVH clot removal are the laterality of EVD placement relative to the side with the greatest IVH volume, the EVD position within the ventricle, and the use of multiple catheters, typically bilateral EVDs. An evaluation of all 100 patients from the CLEAR IVH phase I + II trials showed a trend toward the more rapid clearance of total IVH through an EVD placed on the side with the most IVR blood compared with an EVD placed on the side with less blood ($p = 0.09$) [90]. In this study, two-thirds of the patients had catheters placed on the side with less blood, which is typically favored to reduce the likelihood of EVD obstruction but may not optimize IVH clearance. EVD positioning with all fenestrations on the distal end of the EVD fully inside of the ventricle may prevent catheter-related hemorrhage when using thrombolytics. In a study of 27 patients who received IVR rtPA for IVH (median dose of 2 mg), CTH was evident in 30% of EVDs prior to rtPA injection [91]. After rtPA injection, the worsening of tract hemorrhage (by at least 1 grade) (fig. 2) was seen in 46.7% of the EVD placements, with a significantly higher incidence of incorrectly placed EVDs (with fenestrations outside of the ventricle). EVD placement was correct in 70% of the cases, suggesting an opportunity for improvement. EVD-associated intracranial bleeding has a reported incidence ranging from 6.5 to 20.7%

[92, 93]. Most of these hematomas are thought to be asymptomatic, although the patient condition may be too poor to appreciate subtle findings. Diffusion tract imaging analysis appears to be useful to identify injuries to specific tracts from such hemorrhages. In the first 250 patients treated in the CLEAR III trial, CTHs accounted for 3/6 symptomatic and 48% (n = 48) of asymptomatic hemorrhages on day 30 [58]. They are most likely attributable to direct vascular trauma but may be preventable with an improved placement technique.

Placement of more than one catheter into a ventricular clot may improve the efficiency of clot removal. In the setting of a very large IVH (>40 cc) with casting and mass effect, the use of bilateral simultaneous EVDs compared to that of a single EVD has been shown to increase clot resolution with adjunctive thrombolytic therapy [94]. With dual catheters, it is generally recommended to either alternate sides with each dose or to administer the doses to the side with the greatest IVH volume. In patients with an IVH volume of <40 cc, Staykov et al. [55] found no difference in clot resolution between single vs. dual EVDs, although they reported a trend of a longer EVD duration and higher infection rate in the bilateral EVD group. Pending further study, our current recommendation is to use dual catheters for the management of very large volume IVHs, trapped ventricles, or catheter obstruction. Other indications currently under evaluation are for the treatment of refractory intracranial hypertension and for reducing the mass effect of IVH and the risk of ischemic injury.

Mechanical Strategies to Improve Intraventricular Hemorrhage Removal

Several small studies have focused on the feasibility and safety of minimally invasive techniques to endoscopically evacuate IVH [95–101], including 1 prospective study (n = 42) and a RCT (n = 48) [101]. The procedure utilizes either flexible or rigid endoscopy via a frontal approach, or rarely, an occipital approach, either unilateral or bilateral, with aspiration of ventricular blood clots from the lateral ventricle, followed by the 3rd and 4th ventricles. A variety of irrigation solutions are used, typically Ringer's lactate, and the use of fibrinolytics (after EVD placement), septotomy and third ventriculostomy have all been described. These studies have reported the relatively rapid removal of IVH, although the RCT found no significant difference in the mortality rates or outcomes at 30 and 90 days between endoscopically treated and EVD-treated groups. The need for VP shunting was reduced by half in the endoscopic group, and the intensive care unit length of stay was significantly shorter. A case series of 48 patients treated with endoscopy (vs. 48 historical controls) also reported no significant difference in mortality or neurologic outcome but a significant reduction in shunt-dependent hydrocephalus [100]. The endoscopic procedure appears to be relatively safe, although irrigation can cause prolonged intracranial hypertension [101]. More recently, a systematic review of eleven trials (5 RCTs and 6 ORs) (n = 680) comparing neuroendoscopic surgery (NE) versus EVD alone or with IVF in patients with

IVH secondary to spontaneous supratentorial ICH [102] reported a statistically significant benefit of NE + EVD over EVD + IVF in terms of mortality, the effective hematoma evacuation rate, functional outcome, and the VP shunt dependence rate. The NE approach with EVD could become an alternative to EVD + IVF for the treatment of IVH, although there is insufficient data at this time to recommend one approach over the other.

Lumbar drainage has been used successfully after clearance of the lower ventricular system to shorten EVD duration and to treat communicating hydrocephalus [12, 103–105]. Combining IVR thrombolysis with lumbar drainage may also enhance resolution of IVH. A prospective study of 28 patients with IVH treated with IVR thrombolysis followed by early replacement of an EVD with a lumbar drain reported only 1 required VP shunt at 3 months [105].

External Ventricular Drain Management during Thrombolysis

Managing EVD drainage during thrombolytic therapy depends on the opening pressure and IVH clot burden, although there remains some controversy as to whether the use of an open EVD with continuous drainage of CSF or a closed EVD with intermittent opening as necessary to drain CSF is the best approach. In a study of traumatic brain injury patients requiring EVD, the ICP burden (ICP ≥20 mm Hg) was significantly higher in the intermittent EVD group in comparison with the continuous EVD group [106]. The rationale for continuous drainage in spontaneous IVH is likely similar and may allow for the more rapid clearance of ventricular blood and presumably spasmogenic and irritating contents from bloody CSF.

Conclusions

While the pathophysiology of IVH remains incompletely understood, effective management of nontraumatic IVH requires therapies that rapidly stabilize bleeding sites and clotting, reduce clot volume quickly and minimize exposure to blood products and inflammation within the ventricle. CLEAR III, the first, large, randomized, multicenter, double-blinded, placebo-controlled phase III trial assessing the efficacy of IVR thrombolytic therapy in IVH patients, will provide guidance on thrombolysis as a therapeutic option for acute hemorrhagic stroke treatment in patients with small ICH. Patients with large ICH and IVH may benefit from this type of approach, but there is little available data. Strategies to improve thrombolytic efficacy, including optimizing EVD positioning, targeting lytic agents to regions of high clot volume and strategic 1st and/or 2nd catheter placement are likely to be important considerations. On the horizon are approaches utilizing neuroendoscopy, lumbar drainage and potentially, alternative thrombolytic agents.

References

1 Steiner T, Diringer MN, Schneider D, et al: Dynamics of intraventricular hemorrhage in patients with spontaneous intracerebral hemorrhage: risk factors, clinical impact, and effect of hemostatic therapy with recombinant activated factor VII. Neurosurgery 2006;59:767–773.

2 Tuhrim S, Dambrosia JM, Price TR, et al: Intracerebral hemorrhage: external validation and extension of a model for prediction of 30-day survival. Ann Neurol 1991;29:658–663.

3 Young WB, Lee KP, Passin MS: Prognostic significance of ventricular blood in supratentorial hemorrhage: a volumetric study. Neurology 1990;40:616–619.

4 Broderick JP, Brott T, Tomsick T, et al: Intracerebral hemorrhage more than twice as common as subarachnoid hemorrhage. J Neurosurg 1993;78:188–191.

5 Daverat P, Castel JP, Dartigues JF, et al: Death and functional outcome after spontaneous intracerebral hemorrhage. A prospective study of 166 cases using multivariate analysis. Stroke 1991;22:1–6.

6 Mohr G, Ferguson G, Khan M, et al: Intraventricular hemorrhage from ruptured aneurysm. Retrospective analysis of 91 cases. J Neurosurg 1983;58:482–487.

7 Coplin WM, Vinas FC, Agris JM, et al: A cohort study of the safety and feasibility of intraventricular urokinase for nonaneurysmal spontaneous intraventricular hemorrhage. Stroke 1998;29:1573–1579.

8 Hallevi H, Albright KC, Aronowski J, et al: Intraventricular hemorrhage: anatomic relationships and clinical implications. Neurology 2008;70:848–852.

9 Graeb DA, Robertson WD, Lapointe JS, et al: Computed tomographic diagnosis of intraventricular hemorrhage. Etiology and prognosis. Radiology 1982;143:91–96.

10 Irie F, Fujimoto S, Uda K, et al: Primary intraventricular hemorrhage from dural arteriovenous fistula. J Neurol Sci 2003;215:115–118.

11 Gordon A: Primary ventricular hemorrhage: further contribution to a characteristic symptom group. Arch Neurol Psychiatry 1938;39:1272–1276.

12 Huttner HB, Nagel S, Tognoni E, et al: Intracerebral hemorrhage with severe ventricular involvement: lumbar drainage for communicating hydrocephalus. Stroke 2007;38:183–187.

13 Gates PC, Barnett HJ, Vinters HV, et al: Primary intraventricular hemorrhage in adults. Stroke 1986;17:872–877.

14 Adams RE, Diringer MN: Response to external ventricular drainage in spontaneous intracerebral hemorrhage with hydrocephalus. Neurology 1998;50:519–523.

15 Lee KR, Betz AL, Kim S, et al: The role of the coagulation cascade in brain edema formation after intracerebral hemorrhage. Acta Neurochir 1996;138:396–401.

16 Ziai WC, Triantaphyllopoulou A, Razumovsky AY, et al: Treatment of sympathomimetic induced intraventricular hemorrhage with intraventricular urokinase. J Stroke Cerebrovasc Dis 2003;12:276–279.

17 Ellington E, Margolis G: Block of arachnoid villus by subarachnoid hemorrhage. J Neurosurg 1969;30:651–657.

18 Kibler RF, Couch RSC, Crompton MR: Hydrocephalus in the adult following spontaneous hemorrhage. Brain 1961;84:45–61.

19 Tung MY, Ong PL, Seow WT, et al: A study on the efficacy of intraventricular urokinase in the treatment of intraventricular haemorrhage. Br J Neurosurg 1998;12:234–239.

20 Andrews CO, Engelhard HH: Fibrinolytic therapy in intraventricular hemorrhage. Ann Pharmacother 2001;35:1435–1448.

21 Tuhrim S, Horowitz DR, Sacher M, et al: Volume of ventricular blood is an important determinant of outcome in supratentorial intracerebral hemorrhage. Crit Care Med 1999;27:617–621.

22 Roos YB, Hasan D, Vermeulen M: Outcome in patients with large intraventricular haemorrhages: a volumetric study. J Neurol Neurosurg Psychiatry 1995;58:622–624.

23 Shapiro SA, Campbell RL, Scully T: Hemorrhagic dilation of the fourth ventricle: an ominous predictor. J Neurosurg 1994;80:805–809.

24 Ozdemir O, Calisaneller T, Hasturk A, et al: Prognostic significance of third ventricle dilation in spontaneous intracerebral hemorrhage: a preliminary clinical study. Neurol Res 2008;30:406–410.

25 Stein M, Luecke M, Preuss M, et al: Spontaneous intracerebral hemorrhage with ventricular extension and the grading of obstructive hydrocephalus: the prediction of outcome of a special life-threatening entity. Neurosurgery 2010;67:1243–1251; discussion 1252.

26 Stein M, Luecke M, Preuss M, et al: The prediction of 30-day mortality and functional outcome in spontaneous intracerebral hemorrhage with secondary ventricular hemorrhage: a score comparison. Acta Neurochir Suppl 2011;112:9–11.

27 Broderick JP, Diringer MN, Hill MD, et al: Determinants of intracerebral hemorrhage growth: an exploratory analysis. Stroke 2007;38:1072–1075.

28 Hallevi H, Walker KC, Kasam M, et al: Inflammatory response to intraventricular hemorrhage: time course, magnitude and effect of t-PA. J Neurol Sci 2012;315:93–95.

29 Steiner T, Al-Shahi Salman R, Beer R, et al: European Stroke Organisation (ESO) guidelines for the management of spontaneous intracerebral hemorrhage. Int J Stroke 2014;9:840–855.
30 Diringer MN, Edwards DF, Zazulia AR: Hydrocephalus: a previously unrecognized predictor of poor outcome from supratentorial intracerebral hemorrhage. Stroke 1998;29:1352–1357.
31 Phan TG, Koh M, Vierkant RA, et al: Hydrocephalus is a determinant of early mortality in putaminal hemorrhage. Stroke 2000;31:2157–2162.
32 Liliang PC, Liang CL, Lu CH, et al: Hypertensive caudate hemorrhage prognostic predictor, outcome, and role of external ventricular drainage. Stroke 2001;32:1195–1200.
33 Mendelow AD, Gregson BA, Fernandes HM, et al: Early surgery versus initial conservative treatment in patients with spontaneous supratentorial intracerebral haematomas in the International Surgical Trial in Intracerebral Haemorrhage (STICH): a randomised trial. Lancet 2005;365:387–397.
34 Bhattathiri PS, Gregson B, Prasad KS, et al: Intraventricular hemorrhage and hydrocephalus after spontaneous intracerebral hemorrhage: results from the STICH trial. Acta Neurochir Suppl 2006;96:65–68.
35 Ronning P, Sorteberg W, Nakstad P, et al: Aspects of intracerebral hematomas – an update. Acta Neurol Scand 2008;118:347–361.
36 Ziai WC, Melnychuk E, Thompson CB, et al: Occurrence and impact of intracranial pressure elevation during treatment of severe intraventricular hemorrhage. Crit Care Med 2012;40:1601–1608.
37 Huttner HB, Kohrmann M, Berger C, et al: Influence of intraventricular hemorrhage and occlusive hydrocephalus on the long-term outcome of treated patients with basal ganglia hemorrhage: a case-control study. J Neurosurg 2006;105:412–417.
38 Nieuwkamp DJ, de Gans K, Rinkel GJ, et al: Treatment and outcome of severe intraventricular extension in patients with subarachnoid or intracerebral hemorrhage: a systematic review of the literature. J Neurol 2000;247:117–121.
39 Staykov D, Bardutzky J, Buttner HB, et al: Intraventricular fibrinolysis for intracerebral hemorrhage with severe ventricular involvement. Neurocrit Care 2011;15:194–209.
40 Herrick DB, Ullman N, Nekoovaght-Tak S, et al: Determinants of intraventricular catheter placement in patients with intraventricular hemorrhage. Neurocrit Care 2014;21:426–434.
41 Naff NJ, Williams MA, Rigamonti D, et al: Blood clot resolution in human cerebrospinal fluid: evidence of first-order kinetics. Neurosurgery 2001;49:614–619.
42 Carhuapoma JR: Thrombolytic therapy after intraventricular hemorrhage: do we know enough? J Neurol Sci 2002;202:1–3.
43 Pang D, Sclabassi RJ, Horton JA: Lysis of intraventricular blood clot with urokinase in a canine model: part 3. Effects of intraventricular urokinase on clot lysis and posthemorrhagic hydrocephalus. Neurosurgery 1986;19:553–572.
44 Shen PH, Matsuoka Y, Kawajiri K, et al: Treatment of intraventricular hemorrhage using urokinase. Neurol Med Chir (Tokyo) 1990;30:329–333.
45 Huttner HB, Tognoni E, Bardutzky J, et al: Influence of intraventricular fibrinolytic therapy with rt-PA on the long-term outcome of treated patients with spontaneous basal ganglia hemorrhage: a case-control study. Eur J Neurol 2008;15:342–349.
46 Vereecken KK, Van Havenbergh T, De Beuckelaar W, et al: Treatment of intraventricular hemorrhage with intraventricular administration of recombinant tissue plasminogen activator a clinical study of 18 cases. Clin Neurol Neurosurg 2006;108:451–455.
47 Kumar K, Demeria DD, Verma A: Recombinant tissue plasminogen activator in the treatment of intraventricular hemorrhage secondary to periventricular arteriovenous malformation before surgery: case report. Neurosurgery 2003;52:964–968.
48 Findlay JM, Weir BK, Stollery DE: Lysis of intraventricular hematoma with tissue plasminogen activator. Case report. J Neurosurg 1991;74:803–807.
49 Wagner KR, Xi G, Hua Y, et al: Ultra-early clot aspiration after lysis with tissue plasminogen activator in a porcine model of intracerebral hemorrhage: edema reduction and blood-brain barrier protection. J Neurosurg 1999;90:491–498.
50 Mayfrank L, Kim Y, Kissler J, et al: Morphological changes following experimental intraventricular haemorrhage and intraventricular fibrinolytic treatment with recombinant tissue plasminogen activator. Acta Neuropathol 2000;100:561–567.
51 Nayan RK, Narayan TM, Katz DA, et al: Lysis of intracranial hematomas with urokinase in a rabbit model. J Neurosurg 1985;62:580–586.
52 Lapointe M, Haines S: Fibrinolytic therapy for intraventricular hemorrhage in adults. Cochrane Database Syst Rev 2002;(3):CD003692.
53 Gaberel T, Magheru C, Parienti JJ, et al: Intraventricular fibrinolysis versus external ventricular drainage alone in intraventricular hemorrhage: a meta-analysis. Stroke 2011;42:2776–2781.
54 Khan NR, Tsivgoulis G, Lee SL, et al: Fibrinolysis for intraventricular hemorrhage: an updated meta-analysis and systematic review of the literature. Stroke 2014;45:2662–2669.
55 Staykov D, Huttner HB, Lunkenheimer J, et al: Single versus bilateral external ventricular drainage for intraventricular fibrinolysis in severe ventricular haemorrhage. J Neurol Neurosurg Psychiatry 2010;81:105–108.

56 Ziai WC, Tuhrim S, Lane K, et al: A multicenter, randomized, double-blinded, placebo-controlled phase III study of Clot Lysis Evaluation of Accelerated Resolution of Intraventricular Hemorrhage (CLEAR III). Int J Stroke 2014;9:536–542.
57 Naff N, Williams M, Keyl PM, et al: Low-dose rt-PA enhances clot resolution in brain hemorrhage: the intraventricular hemorrhage thrombolysis trial. Stroke 2011;42:3009–3016.
58 Ziai WC, McBee N, Butcher K, et al: Safety endpoints for the first 250 patients enrolled in the Clot Lysis: Evaluation of Accelerated Resolution of Intraventricular Hemorrhage trial (CLEAR III) (abstract 5589). 2014 International Stroke Conference (ISC), San Diego, CA, 2014.
59 Ziai WC, Ullman N, Thompson C, et al: Stabilizing bleeding prior to acute therapies for spontaneous intracerebral hemorrhage. (abstract 3215). 2014 International Stroke Conference (ISC), San Diego, CA, 2014.
60 Lyke KE, Obasanjo OO, Williams MA, et al: Ventriculitis complicating use of intraventricular catheters in adult neurosurgical patients. Clin Infect Dis 2001;33:2028–2033.
61 Korinek AM, Reina M, Boch AL, et al: Prevention of external ventricular drain-related ventriculitis. Acta Neurochir (Wien) 2005;147:39–45.
62 Wada R, Aviv RI, Fox AJ, et al: CT angiography 'spot sign' predicts hematoma expansion in acute intracerebral hemorrhage. Stroke 2007;38:1257–1262.
63 Chutinet A, Rost NS: White matter disease as a biomarker for long-term cerebrovascular disease and dementia. Curr Treat Options Cardiovasc Med 2014;16:292.
64 Lou M, Al-Hazzani A, Goddeau RP Jr, et al: Relationship between white-matter hyperintensities and hematoma volume and growth in patients with intracerebral hemorrhage. Stroke 2010;41:34–40.
65 Greenberg CH, Frosch MP, Goldstein JN, et al: Modeling intracerebral hemorrhage growth and response to anticoagulation. PLoS One 2012;7:e48458.
66 Kim BJ, Lee SH, Ryu WS, et al: Extents of white matter lesions and increased intraventricular extension of intracerebral hemorrhage. Crit Care Med 2013;41:1325–1331.
67 Caprio FZ, Maas MB, Rosenberg NF, et al: Leukoaraiosis on magnetic resonance imaging correlates with worse outcomes after spontaneous intracerebral hemorrhage. Stroke 2013;44:642–646.
68 Biffi A, Anderson CD, Jagiella JM, et al: APOE genotype and extent of bleeding and outcome in lobar intracerebral haemorrhage: a genetic association study. Lancet Neurol 2011;10:702–709.
69 Brouwers HB, Biffi A, Ayres AM, et al: Apolipoprotein E genotype predicts hematoma expansion in lobar intracerebral hemorrhage. Stroke 2012;43:1490–1495.
70 Goldenstein H, Levy NS, Levy AP: Haptoglobin genotype and its role in determining heme-iron mediated vascular disease. Pharmacol Res 2012;66:1–6.
71 Zhao X, Song S, Sun G, et al: Cytoprotective role of haptoglobin in brain after experimental intracerebral hemorrhage. Acta Neurochir Suppl 2011;111:107–112.
72 Zhao X, Song S, Sun G, et al: Neuroprotective role of haptoglobin after intracerebral hemorrhage. J Neurosci 2009;29:15819–15827.
73 Murthy SB, Levy AP, Duckworth J, et al: Presence of haptoglobin-2 allele is associated with worse functional outcomes following spontaneous intracerebral hemorrhage. World Neurosurg 2015;83:583–587.
74 Naff NJ, Hanley DF, Keyl PM, et al: Intraventricular thrombolysis speeds blood clot resolution: results of a pilot, prospective, randomized, double-blind, controlled trial. Neurosurgery 2004;54:577–583.
75 Staykov D, Wagner I, Volbers B, et al: Dose effect of intraventricular fibrinolysis in ventricular hemorrhage. Stroke 2011;42:2061–2064.
76 Webb AJ, Ullman NL, Mann S, et al: Resolution of intraventricular hemorrhage varies by ventricular region and dose of intraventricular thrombolytic: the Clot Lysis: Evaluating Accelerated Resolution of IVH (CLEAR IVH) program. Stroke 2012;43:1666–1668.
77 Wang YC, Lin CW, Shen CC, et al: Tissue plasminogen activator for the treatment of intraventricular hematoma: the dose-effect relationship. J Neurol Sci 2002;202:35–41.
78 Syrovets T, Tippler B, Rieks M, et al: Plasmin is a potent and specific chemoattractant for human peripheral monocytes acting via a cyclic guanosine monophosphate-dependent pathway. Blood 1997;89:4574–4583.
79 Gross TJ, Leavell KJ, Peterson MW: CD11b/CD18 mediates the neutrophil chemotactic activity of fibrin degradation product D domain. Thromb Haemost 1997;77:894–900.
80 Montrucchio G, Lupia E, De Martino A, et al: Plasmin promotes an endothelium-dependent adhesion of neutrophils. Involvement of platelet activating factor and P-selectin. Circulation 1996;93:2152–2160.
81 Nagy Z, Kolev K, Csonka E, et al: Perturbation of the integrity of the blood – brain barrier by fibrinolytic enzymes. Blood Coagul Fibrinolysis 1998;9:471–478.
82 Stanimirovic D, Satoh K: Inflammatory mediators of cerebral endothelium: a role in ischemic brain inflammation. Brain Pathol 2000;10:113–126.
83 Volbers B, Wagner I, Willfarth W, et al: Intraventricular fibrinolysis does not increase perihemorrhagic edema after intracerebral hemorrhage. Stroke 2013;44:362–366.

84 Ziai WC, Moullaali T, Nekoovaght-Tak S, et al: No Exacerbation of perihematomal edema with intraventricular tissue plasminogen activator in patients with spontaneous intraventricular hemorrhage. Neurocrit Care 2013;18:354–361.
85 Gulba DC, Bode C, Runge MS, et al: Thrombolytic agents – an overview. Ann Hematol 1996;73:S9–S27.
86 Werner RG, Bassarab S, Hoffmann H, et al: Quality aspects of fibrinolytic agents based on biochemical characterization. Drug Res 1991;41:1196–1200.
87 Gaberel T, Montagne A, Lesept F, et al: Urokinase versus Alteplase for intraventricular hemorrhage fibrinolysis. Neuropharmacology 2014;85:158–165.
88 Keep RF, Hua Y, Xi G: Intracerebral haemorrhage: mechanisms of injury and therapeutic targets. Lancet Neurol 2012;11:720–731.
89 Parcq J, Goulay R, Gaberel T, et al: Is optimized tissue plasminogen activator (optPA) the future of intracerebral haemorrhage treatment? (abstract 771.13). Society for Neuroscience Meeting, Lille, 2014.
90 Jaffe J, Melnychuk E, Muschelli J, et al: Ventricular catheter location and the clearance of intraventricular hemorrhage. Neurosurgery 2012;70:1258–1263; discussion 1263–1264.
91 Jackson DA, Patel AV, Darracott RM, et al: Safety of intraventricular hemorrhage (IVH) thrombolysis based on CT localization of external ventricular drain (EVD) fenestrations and analysis of EVD tract hemorrhage. Neurocrit Care 2013;19:103–110.
92 Wiesmann M, Mayer TE: Intracranial bleeding rates associated with two methods of external ventricular drainage. J Clin Neurosci 2001;8:126–128.
93 Ehtisham A, Taylor S, Bayless L, et al: Placement of external ventricular drains and intracranial pressure monitors by neurointensivists. Neurocrit Care 2009; 10:241–247.
94 Hinson HE, Melnychuk E, Muschelli J, et al: Drainage efficiency with dual versus single catheters in severe intraventricular hemorrhage. Neurocrit Care 2012;16:399–405.
95 Longatti PL, Martinuzzi A, Fiorindi A, et al: Neuroendoscopic management of intraventricular hemorrhage. Stroke 2004;35:e35–e38.
96 Longatti P, Fiorindi A, Martinuzzi A: Neuroendoscopic aspiration of hematocephalus totalis: technical note. Neurosurgery 2005;57(suppl 4):E409.
97 Yadav YR, Mukerji G, Shenoy R, et al: Endoscopic management of hypertensive intraventricular haemorrhage with obstructive hydrocephalus. BMC Neurol 2007;7:1.
98 Zhang Z, Li X, Liu Y, et al: Application of neuroendoscopy in the treatment of intraventricular hemorrhage. Cerebrovasc Dis 2007;24:91–96.
99 Hamada H, Hayashi N, Kurimoto M, et al: Neuroendoscopic removal of intraventricular hemorrhage combined with hydrocephalus. Minim Invasive Neurosurg 2008;51:345–349.
100 Basaldella L, Marton E, Fiorindi A, et al: External ventricular drainage alone versus endoscopic surgery for severe intraventricular hemorrhage: a comparative retrospective analysis on outcome and shunt dependency. Neurosurg Focus 2012;32:E4.
101 Chen CC, Liu CL, Tung YN, et al: Endoscopic surgery for intraventricular hemorrhage (IVH) caused by thalamic hemorrhage: comparisons of endoscopic surgery and external ventricular drainage (EVD) surgery. World Neurosurg 2011;75:264–268.
102 Li Y, Zhang H, Wang X, et al: Neuroendoscopic surgery versus external ventricular drainage alone or with intraventricular fibrinolysis for intraventricular hemorrhage secondary to spontaneous supratentorial hemorrhage: a systematic review and meta-analysis. PLoS One 2013;8:e80599.
103 Trnovec S, Halatsch ME, Putz M, et al: Irrigation can cause prolonged intracranial pressure elevations during endoscopic treatment of intraventricular haematomas. Br J Neurosurg 2012;26:247–251.
104 Huttner HB, Schwab S, Bardutzky J: Lumbar drainage for communicating hydrocephalus after ICH with ventricular hemorrhage. Neurocrit Care 2006; 5:193–196.
105 Staykov D, Huttner HB, Struffert T, et al: Intraventricular fibrinolysis and lumbar drainage for ventricular hemorrhage. Stroke 2009;40:3275–3280.
106 Nwachuku EL, Puccio AM, Fetzick A, et al: Intermittent versus continuous cerebrospinal fluid drainage management in adult severe traumatic brain injury: assessment of intracranial pressure burden. Neurocrit Care 2014;20:49–53.

Prof. Daniel F. Hanley
Department of Neurology, Divisions of Brain Injury Outcomes and Neurocritical Care
The Johns Hopkins University School of Medicine
600 North Wolfe Street, Baltimore, MD 21287 (USA)
E-Mail dhanley@jhmi.edu

Toyoda K, Anderson CS, Mayer SA (eds): New Insights in Intracerebral Hemorrhage.
Front Neurol Neurosci. Basel, Karger, 2016, vol 37, pp 148–154 (DOI: 10.1159/000437119)

Surgical Craniotomy for Intracerebral Haemorrhage

A. David Mendelow

Institute of Neuroscience, Neurosurgical Trials Group, Newcastle University, Newcastle upon Tyne, UK

Abstract

Craniotomy is probably indicated for patients with superficial spontaneous lobar supratentorial intracerebral haemorrhage (ICH) when the level of consciousness drops below 13 within the first 8 h of the onset of the haemorrhage. Once the level drops below 9, it is probably too late to consider craniotomy for these patients, so clinical vigilance is paramount. While this statement is only backed up by evidence that is moderately strong, meta-analysis of available data suggests that it is true in the rather limited number of patients with ICH. Meta-analyses like this can often predict the results of future prospective randomised controlled trials a decade or more before the trials are completed and published. Countless such examples exist in the literature, as is the case for thrombolysis in patients with myocardial infarction in the last millennium: meta-analysis determined the efficacy more than a decade BEFORE the last trial (ISIS-2) confirmed the benefit of thrombolysis for myocardial infarction. Careful examination of the meta-analysis' Forest plots in this chapter will demonstrate why this statement is made at the outset. Other meta-analyses of surgery for ICH have also indicated that minimal interventional techniques using topical thrombolysis or endoscopy via burrholes or even twist drill aspiration may be particularly successful for the treatment of supratentorial ICH, especially when the clot is deep seated. Ongoing clinical trials (CLEAR III and MISTIE III) should confirm this in the fullness of time. There are 2 exceptions to these generalisations. First, based on trial evidence, aneurysmal ICH is best treated with surgery. Second, cerebellar ICH represents a special case because of the development of hydrocephalus, which may require expeditious drainage as the intracranial pressure rises. The cerebellar clot will then require evacuation, usually via posterior fossa craniectomy, rather than craniotomy. Technical advances suggest that image-guided surgery may improve the completeness of surgical evacuation and outcomes, regardless of which surgical technique is employed.

© 2016 S. Karger AG, Basel

Introduction

Surgical treatment for intracerebral haemorrhage (ICH) remains controversial. Craniotomy has been the mainstay of surgical treatment for over a century, but in addition to craniotomy, ICH can be removed through a burrhole, albeit often only partially. This attempt at removal can be performed with an endoscope or via a catheter (with or without topical thrombolysis). Burrhole evacuation of liquid from chronic subdural haematomas is commonplace and effective. However, a solid clot (intracerebral or subdural) cannot be removed effectively through a catheter, so topical thrombolysis has more recently been used to liquefy the clot, with encouraging results. Craniotomy has the advantage of being ubiquitous. Every neurosurgery unit in the world can perform craniotomies. What is not ubiquitous is the aftercare, or nursing and rehabilitation. Given infinite resources, disability can be conquered, and patients who survive an ICH can be re-integrated into their communities. For these reasons, craniotomy for ICH can be undertaken anywhere, but the resulting disability and the costs of rehabilitation vary around the world. Most countries cannot afford this type of rehabilitation because of the very high cost per quality-adjusted life year of craniotomy for ICH. They also cannot afford decompressive craniectomy as a variant of craniotomy for ICH or as decompression for infarction. All of these factors are fuelling controversy about the role of surgery in ICH.

However, there are some situations in ICH for which there is no controversy about the role of surgery. Most neurosurgeons who encounter a post-operative clot after elective neurosurgery would remove it. The whole neurocritical care environment is geared towards the early detection and treatment of such post-operative complications. Similarly, a patient who was initially well after an ICH but who later deteriorated would have the clot urgently removed by the majority of neurosurgeons. The problem with and the dilemma in surgical treatment arise when the patient presents with disturbed consciousness ab initio. If the patient is in a deep coma and has a very large clot, most neurosurgeons will make a treatment-limiting decision and will not operate, particularly if the patient is elderly or is already impaired by a pre-existing disability. However, many patients have intermediate levels of disturbed consciousness, and it is this group of patients with ICH that has been the main cause of the controversy about the role of craniotomy. Having said that, there are some types of patients with ICH for whom clear evidence has emerged about the benefit of craniotomy. For example, in a prospective randomised controlled trial (PRCT), Heiskanen et al. [1] showed that patients with aneurysmal ICH had much better outcomes with surgery than with conservative treatment. Mortality was only 27% in the patients who had surgery to remove the ICH and to clip the aneurysm. By contrast, mortality in the conservatively treated group of patients was 80%. Additionally, patients with cerebellar haemorrhage have to be considered separately. This is because the haematoma may obstruct the outflow of cerebrospinal fluid from the IVth ventricle and may thereby cause obstructive hydrocephalus. The hydrocephalus needs to be treated in its own right. Unfortunately, no PRCTs on cerebellar ICH have been conducted. Nevertheless, Mathew and Teasdale [2] have published a very useful algorithm for the management of cerebellar ICH.

Pathophysiological Considerations

The pathophysiology of supratentorial ICH is well documented, and spontaneous and traumatic ICH often have much in common. Various experimental models have been developed to study these processes [3–5]. These models include the concept of a penumbra, the destruction of large white-matter tracts as a form of axonal damage, clot expansion and rebleeding. Clinical imaging in patients has confirmed the existence of a penumbra and infarction in some cases [6, 7]. These may be the very patients for whom surgical evacuation may provide the greatest benefit. Another imaging finding that can help with understanding of the pathophysiology of ICH is the identification of ongoing bleeding. Ongoing bleeding is a poor prognostic sign and can be identified based on the spot sign [8]. It may be that these too are the patients who are most likely to benefit from craniotomy because during craniotomy, precise and pinpointed haemostasis can be achieved. Intracranial pressure (ICP) monitoring can be useful in determining the cerebral perfusion pressure because lowering the blood pressure may adversely affect the cerebral perfusion pressure if the ICP is high. In such cases, surgical lowering of the ICP is likely to be of value. By contrast, if the ICP is low, then lowering the blood pressure may limit further bleeding, as has been suggested in the INTERACT II trial [9]. For all of these reasons, clinical intuition must remain an integral part of the management of patients with ICH. Evidence for efficacy from clinical trials influences such intuition and will be discussed later in this chapter.

Technique of Craniotomy

Traditional craniotomy consists of an inverted U-shaped skin flap that preserves the blood supply to the skin. However, the skin incision can also be linear. The skin flap is usually placed over the part of the clot that is nearest to the surface but avoids access through eloquent areas. Image-guiding surgery (IGS) is often used for more accurate placement over the most superficial part of the clot. IGS thus limits the cortical damage that might otherwise occur in the process of getting to the clot. An alternative is to create a slightly larger craniotomy and to use intra-operative ultrasound for real-time image guidance. The BrainLAB Image Guidance System can also utilise intra-operative 3D ultrasound to update the position of the original clot or any residual clot once the surgeon feels that the whole clot has been removed. Using these IGS techniques, total clot removal with very little damage to the surrounding brain can be achieved. Sometimes, the ICP is high, and the brain immediately starts to herniate through the first dural incision. If that happens, the ICH can be partially aspirated with a Dandy cannula, which will reduce the pressure and make dural opening safer, even if only a few millilitres of clot are removed. When the clot is solid in the acute phase, it is unlikely that much can be immediately aspirated, but just a few millilitres may move the pathophysiology down the pressure-volume curve and facilitate the opening of the dura. Retractors can be used once the clot has been entered. These take various forms, from hand-held to rigid, fixed systems. Recently, a disposable plastic speculum has been used to minimise the size of the cortical incision. This speculum can be attached to rigid retractors to avoid movement of the corticotomy. Suction is used to evacuate the clot under vision, often using the operating microscope. Bleeding vessels are coagulated with bipolar coagulation using non-stick forceps. Again, several different types are available. Haemostatic agents should be avoided until all vessels have been coagulated because the placement of topical haemostats allows more clots to accumulate beneath them. This can happen regardless of the material that is used. Then, a new peri-cavity haematoma may form. Therefore, good coagulation of all vessels is the preferred method of haemostasis. This is best achieved using the operating microscope because of the better lighting and magnification that this microscope provides. If there is clot tucked away under the eloquent cortex, then an endoscope can be utilised. There are different types of angled endoscopes that can be safely deployed in the cavity while the microscope remains in situ. This can be achieved with a pneumatic robotic arm (Storz) that holds the endoscope absolutely rigid within the operating microscope's field. Once good haemostasis has been accomplished, then haemostatic materials can be used to line the cavity to prevent later re-haemorrhage, as, for example, can take place if there is a surge in blood pressure during emergence from anaesthesia or post-operatively. There is a wide variety of topical haemostatic materials that can be applied to the lining of the evacuated clot cavity after careful coagulation of all bleeding vessels, but these materials are not a substitute for careful and meticulous haemostasis with bipolar coagulation. When used after such meticulous coagulation, they then add to the value of craniotomy because haemostats cannot be used in the catheter-based techniques of clot removal.

Evidence from Clinical Trials

The Oxford Centre for Evidence-Based Medicine puts systematic reviews of randomised clinical trials at the top of the list of treatment benefits [10]. Such a systematic review was undertaken by the European Stroke Organisation, which published their guidelines for the management of ICH in 2014 [11, 12]. These guidelines state that 'There is no evidence to support surgical intervention on a routine basis to improve outcome after supratentorial ICH in comparison with conservative management, but early surgery may be of value for patients with a GCS score 9–12'. These recommendations were classified as weak and were based on moderate evidence. There have been 15 PRCTs on surgery in patents with spontaneous ICH. The largest trial was the Surgical Trial in Intracerebral Haemorrhage (STICH) [13], which revealed that there was a trend towards improved outcomes with early surgery within 72 h of the onset of ictus, particularly for superficial lobar haematomas. This finding led to the STICH II trial for this subgroup of patients. STICH II also revealed a trend towards improved outcomes, particularly in those patients whose Glasgow Coma Score (GCS) was between 9 and 12 initially [14]. This same trend was evident in the Surgical Trial

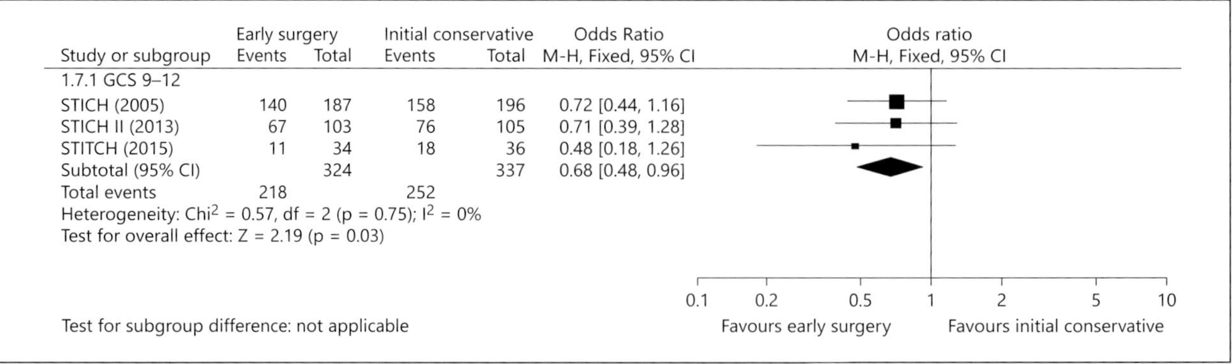

Study or subgroup	Early surgery Events	Early surgery Total	Initial conservative Events	Initial conservative Total	Odds Ratio M-H, Fixed, 95% CI
1.7.1 GCS 9–12					
STICH (2005)	140	187	158	196	0.72 [0.44, 1.16]
STICH II (2013)	67	103	76	105	0.71 [0.39, 1.28]
STITCH (2015)	11	34	18	36	0.48 [0.18, 1.26]
Subtotal (95% CI)		324		337	0.68 [0.48, 0.96]
Total events	218		252		

Heterogeneity: $Chi^2 = 0.57$, df = 2 (p = 0.75); $I^2 = 0\%$
Test for overall effect: Z = 2.19 (p = 0.03)

Test for subgroup difference: not applicable

Fig. 1. Meta-analysis of the 3 STICH trials with patients who presented with a Glasgow Coma Score of 9–12. Courtesy of Dr. Barbara A. Gregson, Newcastle University.

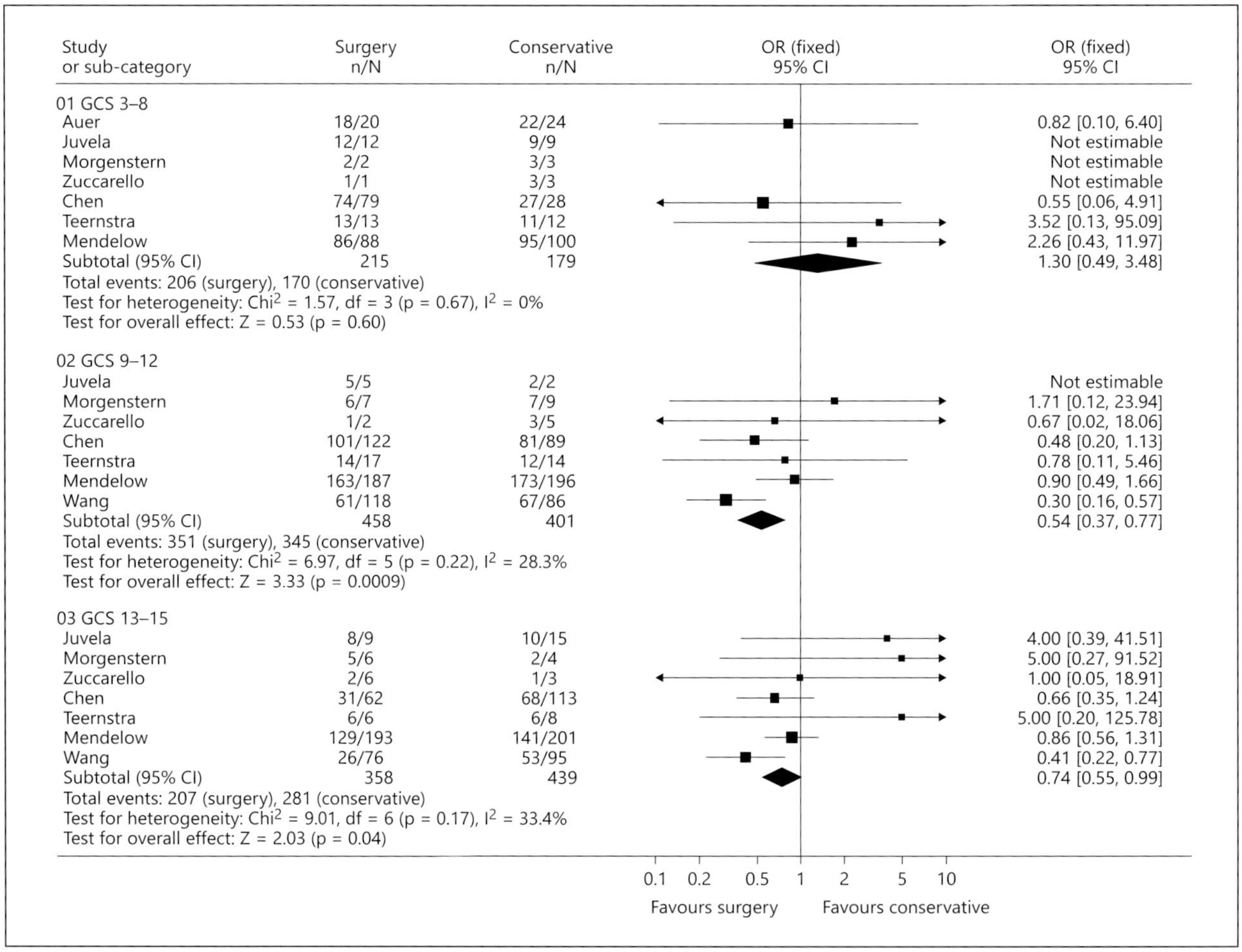

Study or sub-category	Surgery n/N	Conservative n/N	OR (fixed) 95% CI
01 GCS 3–8			
Auer	18/20	22/24	0.82 [0.10, 6.40]
Juvela	12/12	9/9	Not estimable
Morgenstern	2/2	3/3	Not estimable
Zuccarello	1/1	3/3	Not estimable
Chen	74/79	27/28	0.55 [0.06, 4.91]
Teernstra	13/13	11/12	3.52 [0.13, 95.09]
Mendelow	86/88	95/100	2.26 [0.43, 11.97]
Subtotal (95% CI)	215	179	1.30 [0.49, 3.48]
Total events: 206 (surgery), 170 (conservative)			
Test for heterogeneity: $Chi^2 = 1.57$, df = 3 (p = 0.67), $I^2 = 0\%$			
Test for overall effect: Z = 0.53 (p = 0.60)			
02 GCS 9–12			
Juvela	5/5	2/2	Not estimable
Morgenstern	6/7	7/9	1.71 [0.12, 23.94]
Zuccarello	1/2	3/5	0.67 [0.02, 18.06]
Chen	101/122	81/89	0.48 [0.20, 1.13]
Teernstra	14/17	12/14	0.78 [0.11, 5.46]
Mendelow	163/187	173/196	0.90 [0.49, 1.66]
Wang	61/118	67/86	0.30 [0.16, 0.57]
Subtotal (95% CI)	458	401	0.54 [0.37, 0.77]
Total events: 351 (surgery), 345 (conservative)			
Test for heterogeneity: $Chi^2 = 6.97$, df = 5 (p = 0.22), $I^2 = 28.3\%$			
Test for overall effect: Z = 3.33 (p = 0.0009)			
03 GCS 13–15			
Juvela	8/9	10/15	4.00 [0.39, 41.51]
Morgenstern	5/6	2/4	5.00 [0.27, 91.52]
Zuccarello	2/6	1/3	1.00 [0.05, 18.91]
Chen	31/62	68/113	0.66 [0.35, 1.24]
Teernstra	6/6	6/8	5.00 [0.20, 125.78]
Mendelow	129/193	141/201	0.86 [0.56, 1.31]
Wang	26/76	53/95	0.41 [0.22, 0.77]
Subtotal (95% CI)	358	439	0.74 [0.55, 0.99]
Total events: 207 (surgery), 281 (conservative)			
Test for heterogeneity: $Chi^2 = 9.01$, df = 6 (p = 0.17), $I^2 = 33.4\%$			
Test for overall effect: Z = 2.03 (p = 0.04)			

OR (fixed) 95% CI
0.1 0.2 0.5 1 2 5 10
Favours surgery   Favours conservative

Fig. 2. Independent patient data meta-analysis of surgery for spontaneous supratentorial intracerebral haemorrhage and a Glasgow Coma Score of 9–12 [16] (reproduced with permission). In this published meta-analysis, the STICH II and STITCH TRAUMA trial results were not included.

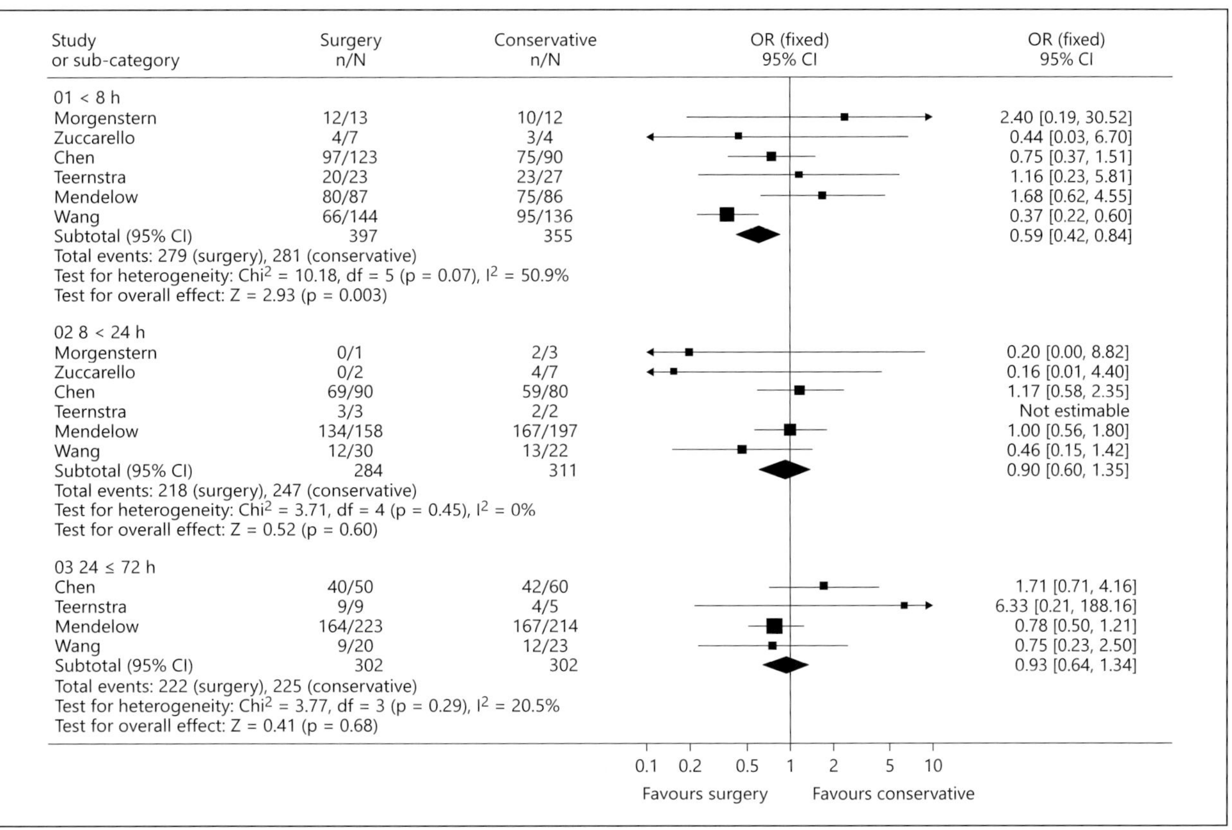

Fig. 3. Independent patient data meta-analysis of patients with spontaneous supratentorial intracerebral haemorrhage, showing that surgery within 8 h was best. Reproduced with permission from [16].

in Traumatic ICH (STITCH TRAUMA) [15]. Meta-analysis of these 3 trials, in which craniotomy was the main method of clot evacuation, shows that patients whose GCS at the outset is between 9 and 12 are best treated surgically (fig. 1). An individual patient data meta-analysis has already shown that patients with a GCS of 9–12 are most likely to benefit from early surgery and that the earlier the intervention is, the better (fig. 2) [16]. This meta-analysis therefore provides strong evidence for early surgery in patients who present with intermediate levels of depressed consciousness (GCS of 9–12). Additionally, the individual patient data meta-analysis suggests that intervention within the first 8 h is more likely than later surgery to improve the outcome (fig. 3).

Cerebellar ICH is a special case because of the progressive onset of hydrocephalus. The pathophysiology is also different because of the small size of the posterior fossa, the strategic importance of the brainstem and the early obstruction of the IVth ventricle. There have been no clinical trials on surgery or its timing in cerebellar ICH to date. However, the Mathew algorithm does make sense [2].

Aneurysmal ICH is also a special case because of the clear and dramatic evidence of efficacy from the Heiskanen trial [1].

Conclusion

Clinical observation of the patient is of paramount importance, and the GCS is well established for this. A GCS of 9–12 should alert the clinician to the need for early surgery. Evidence from clinical trials suggests that in these patients, craniotomy is indicated for lobar ICH because the clot reaches the surface of the brain and because access is easy and safe. Meanwhile, external ventricular drains and catheters may be better for patients with deep ICH. These principles do not apply to aneurysmal or cerebellar ICH.

References

1 Heiskanen O, Poranen A, Kuurne T, et al: Acute surgery for intracerebral haemotomas caused by rupture of an intracranial arterial aneurysm: a prospective randomized study. Acta Neurochir (Wein) 1988;90:81–83.

2 Mathew P, Teasdale G, Bannan A, et al: Neurosurgical management of cerebellar haematoma and infarct. J Neurol Neurosurg Psychiatry 1995;59:287–292.

3 Liu Y, Ao LJ, Lu G, et al: Quantitative gait analysis of long-term locomotion deficits in classical unilateral striatal intracerebral hemorrhage rat model. Behav Brain Res 2013;257:166–177.

4 Mendelow AD: Mechanisms of ischaemic brain damage with intracerebral haemorrhage. Stroke 1993;24(12 suppl):I115–I117; discussion I118–I119.

5 Keep RF, Xi G, Hua Y, et al: The deleterious or beneficial effects of different agents in intracerebral hemorrhage: think big, think small, or is hematoma size important? Stroke 2005;36:1594–1596.

6 Siddique MS, Fernandes HM, Wooldridge TD, et al: Reversible ischemia around intracerebral hemorrhage: a single-photon emission computerized tomography study. J Neurosurg 2002;96:736–741.

7 Kidwell CS, Heiss W-D: Advances in stroke: imaging. Stroke 2012;43:302–304.

8 Brouwers H, Chang Y, Falcone, GJ, et al: Predicting hematoma expansion after primary intracerebral hemorrhage. JAMA Neurol 2014;71:158–164.

9 Anderson CS, Heeley E, Huang Y, et al: Rapid blood-pressure lowering in patients with acute intracerebral hemorrhage. New Engl J Med 2013;368:2355–2365.

10 OCEBM Levels of Evidence Working Group: The Oxford 2011 levels of evidence. Oxford Centre for Evidence-Based Medicine, 2011. http://www.cebm.net/index.aspx?o=5653 (accessed February 11, 2015).

11 Steiner T, Al-Shahi Salman R, Beer R, et al: European Stroke Organisation (ESO) guidelines for the management of spontaneous intracerebral hemorrhage. Int J Stroke 2014;9:840–855.

12 Steiner T, Al-Shahi Salman R, Ntaios G: The European Stroke Organisation (ESO) guidelines. Int J Stroke 2014;9:838–839.

13 Mendelow AD, Gregson BA, Fernandes HM, et al: Early surgery versus initial conservative treatment in patients with spontaneous supratentorial intracerebral haematomas in the International Surgical Trial in Intracerebral Haemorrhage (STICH): a randomised trial. Lancet 2005;365:387–397.

14 Mendelow AD, Gregson BA, Rowan EN, et al: Early surgery versus initial conservative treament in patients with spontaneous supratentorial intracerebral haematomas (STICH II): a randomised trial. Lancet 2013;382:396.

15 Mendelow AD, Gregson BA, Rowan EN, et al: Early surgery versus initial conservative treatment in patients with traumatic intracerebral hemorrhage (STITCH[Trauma]): the first randomized trial. J Neurotrauma DOI: 10.1089/neu.2014.3644 .

16 Gregson BA, Broderick JP, Auer LM, et al: Individual patient data subgroup meta-analysis of surgery for spontaneous supratentorial intracerebral hemorrhage. Stroke 2012;43:1496–1504.

Prof. A. David Mendelow
Institute of Neuroscience, Neurosurgical Trials Group, Newcastle University
Wolfson Research Centre, Campus for Ageing and Vitality, Westgate Road
Newcastle upon Tyne, NE4 5PL (UK)
E-Mail david.mendelow@newcastle.ac.uk

Toyoda K, Anderson CS, Mayer SA (eds): New Insights in Intracerebral Hemorrhage.
Front Neurol Neurosci. Basel, Karger, 2016, vol 37, pp 155–165 (DOI: 10.1159/000437120)

New Insights in Minimally Invasive Surgery for Intracerebral Hemorrhage

Wei-Min Wang · Che Jiang · Hong-Min Bai

Department of Neurosurgery, Liuhuaqiao Hospital, Guangzhou, China

Abstract

The poor clinical outcome of acute intracerebral hemorrhage (ICH) relates closely to the bleeding amount per unit of time and the hematoma position in the brain. Removal of an intracerebral hematoma in time can effectively improve clinical prognosis. Minimally invasive surgery (MIS) for the treatment of ICH is the main clinical method that is currently used, despite the lack of large-scale, clinical, multi-center, randomized controlled trials. This article comprehensively reviews the history and development of MIS for ICH and analyzes various roles of MIS in ICH treatment. General CT image-guided surgery with the local use of thrombolysis techniques is a major MIS method used in current ICH treatment.

© 2016 S. Karger AG, Basel

Poor prognosis of intracerebral hemorrhage (ICH) is closely related to the rate, amount and sites of bleeding in the brain. Clearing away an intracerebral hematoma in time can effectively reduce intracranial pressure (ICP), improve cerebral perfusion, reduce structural brain damage and improve survival and prognosis. Before the computed tomography (CT) era, minimally invasive surgery (MIS) was hardly performed, and temporal craniectomy for evacuation of clots and decompression of bone flaps was widely adopted. However, the high levels of surgical invasion and stress caused by craniectomy not only increase the difficulty of postoperative treatment but also easily lead to rebleeding and other complications, with extended hospital stays and high costs. A randomized trial has shown no advantages of open surgery over medical treatment [1]. In the 1980s when CT was introduced into the clinical setting, MIS gradually became the major ICH treatment method.

Principles of Minimally Invasive Surgical Treatment of Intracerebral Hemorrhage

Acute cerebral hemorrhage causes direct laceration of brain tissue. Mechanical compression by hematoma on brain tissue and dramatically increased ICP result in a decrease in brain perfusion [2]. In addition, 1–2 days after ICH, hematomas release large amounts of biochemically harmful factors, leading to secondary damage and ending in irreversible neurological dysfunction. Therefore, removal of a hematoma timely and with minimal surgical injury can not only effectively eliminate various harmful effects of the hematoma on brain tissue but can also improve the cerebral and systemic physiological environments, saving patients' lives and reducing the disability incidence.

Advanced modern neuroimaging techniques (CT/CT angiography, MRI/MR angiography/MR venography/spatially modulated illumination, and digital subtraction angiography) are available for doctors to find out bleeding causes, to accurately locate intracerebral hematomas and to select the appropriate treatment for ICH at an early stage. Advances in stereotactic techniques and neuronavigation have greatly improved surgeons' abilities to locate an ICH in a timely manner and to perform accurate operation. Continuous advances in microsurgical and neuroendoscopic techniques and pharmacology make it possible to remove cerebral hematomas in a minimally invasive way. However, MIS has shortcomings: it cannot remove a hematoma or handle bleeding caused by intracranial aneurysm/arteriovenous malformation/Moyamoya disease/a tumor simultaneously, and it cannot completely remove a large hematomas in one session. In addition, it may give rise to intracerebral thrombolytic rebleeding and drainage infection.

Historical Overview of Minimally Invasive Surgery of Intracerebral Hemorrhage

Currently, MIS for the treatment of ICH generally includes the following procedures: (1) CT-guided keyhole craniotomy, which is performed for intracerebral hematoma clearance under microscopy or for emptying it using a device/neuroendoscope; and (2) stereotactic needle aspiration for intracerebral hematoma removal or its combination with injection of a thrombolytic agent into the hematoma and soft catheter draining under CT guidance.

In 1964, Bene [3] reported the treatment of typical ICH by stereotactic surgical aspiration, and it was the first report of MIS of cerebral hemorrhage based on skull X-ray and anatomical landmarks. In 1978, Backlund et al. [4] reported the use of stereotactic equipment combined with an Archimedes device to clear away ICH. In 1985, Kandel et al. [5] reported MIS with improvements in surgical equipment under CT guidance, achieving good results in 32 cases, with the completely safe removal of the hematoma. In 1989, Auer [6] first reported a randomized controlled trial (RCT) comparing MIS with medical treatment only, showing that MIS with endoscopy improved functional recovery and reduced mortality. The surgical equipment limitations may be the reason that these procedures are not currently widely performed in the clinical setting. At the same time, Matsumoto et al. [7] introduced the thrombolytic agent urokinase (UK), which was injected into the hematoma cavity after stereotactic hematoma aspiration to dissolve a clot, receiving a more satisfactory result. Thereafter, in 1995, Schaller et al. [8] reported application of recombinant tissue plasminogen activator (rt-PA) in MIS to treat ICH. Compared with the mechanical methods of hematoma removal, application of agents to dissolve clots is safer, simpler and more effective in MIS and is currently the most widely used method for the treatment of ICH. Ramanan et al. reviewed previous studies, evaluating differences between MIS, medical treatment and craniotomy. Their review included 1,717 patients from 11 studies and showed that MIS was associated with the lowest mortality rate among the three groups [9]. Zhou et al. [10] conducted meta-analysis and further discovered that MIS resulted in a better outcome than other therapeutic options for treating spontaneous supratentorial ICH. The patients most likely to benefit from MIS include those of both genders who are 30–80 years old, have a superficial hematoma, a Glasgow Coma Scale score of ≥9, a hematoma volume of 25–40 ml, and receive treatment beginning within 72 h after onset. However, there is still a shortage of large-scale and multicenter RCTs of ICH worldwide. A standard ICH treatment protocol is urgently needed currently.

Minimally Invasive Surgery Indications

Until now, there has been no consensus on MIS indications. They have been generally based on the following principles: (1) spontaneous supratentorial ICH of ≥30 ml or cerebellar ICH of ≥15 ml on CT; (2) proven stability of hematoma (at 6 h after the initial volume measurement by CT, the hematoma volume increases by less than 5 ml); (3) MIS suitability for a variety of ICH locations, especially the deep brain, but not for brainstem hemorrhage; (4) neurological dysfunctions, such as disorders of consciousness, hemiplegia, and aphasia, which are aggravating; and (5) hypertension that is well controlled by medicine and is without surgical contraindications. Contraindications of MIS for ICH include the following: (1) a large ICH volume and severe state with brain herniation (acute intracranial hypertension crisis). This item is disputed and regarded as a relative contraindication because some surgeons effectively use MIS to treat herniation before and at the early stage of ICH, especially for patients who cannot receive craniotomy or who are in a very critical condition; (2) a tendency of rebleeding or co-existing hemorrhagic disease; and (3) having a definite cause of cerebral hemorrhage, such as aneurysm/arteriovenous malformation/Moyamoya disease/a tumor.

Minimally Invasive Surgery Timing

The exact timing of surgery is currently still controversial in ICH treatment. However, it is widely believed that it should be performed at an earlier stage rather than at a later stage if the indications are good. According to previous studies, the optimal time window for MIS of ICH may be within 6–12 h after hemorrhage because hypertensive ICH has transient bleeding, but rebleeding is likely to recur within 24 h, usually within 6 h, and especially at 3 h [11–14].

Ultra-Early Surgery
Ultra-early surgery is operation performed within 6 h after ICH [15]. Ultra-early removal of a hematoma is considered to eliminate harmful factors on time and to benefit the patient's clinical condition and neurofunctional recovery. A comparison study of the timing of surgery has shown that patients who undergo ultra-early or early surgery have a significantly better prognosis than those who receive delayed surgery [16]. However, some scholars have argued that premature surgical treatment of an intracranial hematoma can easily lead to postoperative rebleeding due to unstable systemic and intracranial environments, resulting in deterioration. Thus, early timing is not always better [17]. It is generally believed that the coagulation state is unstable around a hematoma within 6 h after ICH. Additionally, BP and vital signs often fluctuate, so the risk of post-surgical rebleeding is often higher at the same stage.

Early Surgery
Early surgery is an operation performed within 6–48 h after brain bleeding [18]. Taking into account the timing of ICH stabilization and secondary neurological damage due to thrombolysis, it is generally recommended that surgery begins after 6 h, when hypertension is controlled and CT shows no rebleeding after stroke. This stage has also been associated with homeostasis, less surgical stress and greater surgical benefits. The rebleeding rate for early surgery is significantly lower than that for ultra-early surgery. Six to twenty-four hours after stroke is regarded as the ideal time window for MIS. However, MIS could also be conducted at less than 6–7 h after ICH in patients with a large hematoma who are in generally good condition.

Delayed Surgery
Surgery performed at 4 days after stroke is generally defined as delayed surgery [18]. With advances in early surgery and MIS techniques, delayed surgery is not commonly performed today. Patients treated with delayed surgery usually have obstinate intracranial hypertension, with obstructive hydrocephalus caused by thalamic hemorrhage or worse, neurodysfunction due to damage caused by the hematoma to crucial structures, such as the internal capsule, during intensive internal medical treatment. Although a hematoma can be aspirated easily with ameliorated intracranial

hypertension through delayed surgery, the neurological prognosis is the poorest compared with early or ultra-early surgery. Hayashi et al. [19] have found that surgery is futile at 40 days after bleeding.

Minimally Invasive Surgery Methods

MIS mainly involves both removal of a hematoma directly under microsurgery or endoscopic surgery with keyhole craniotomy and evacuation by stereotactic or neuronavigational aspiration or soft catheter drainage through a burr hole. Currently, MIS with an Archimedes device and ultrasonic oscillations are rarely used in ICH. CT is considered the main technique for determining ICH location in MIS. Tracking the target by a frame/simple stereotactic method or neuronavigation is critical in surgery of a hematoma, and both mechanical elimination (aspiration, oscillation or endoscopic evacuation) and local thrombolysis (UK/rt-PA) are the main ways to remove an intracerebral hematoma. The principles of MIS trajectory planning for ICH are same as those for other brain surgeries. The closest lesion to the skull should be approached to avoid injuring important brain areas or crucial brain neuron/vascular structures and to facilitate hematoma evacuation. The direction of the maximum diameter of the hematoma is usually chosen as the surgical path direction.

Microsurgery/Endoscopic-Surgery with Keyhole Craniotomy

Microsurgical or neuroendoscope technologies with keyhole (a diameter of less than 3.0 cm) craniotomy have the following advantages for the treatment of ICH: (1) short operative time in the skull; and (2) surgery can be performed to clear away the clots and to stop bleeding under direct vision and thus, clearance of the hematoma is more effective. In recent years, good lighting and high-definition, amplified images provided by endoscopes have been used to aid in surgery; (3) some decompressive effects can be certainly achieved for severe intracranial hypertension; and (4) the incidences of infection and postoperative leakage are less than those for classical craniotomy [20]. However, It is difficult to remove a deep hematoma under a small surgical field of view. Its decompression is weaker than large bone flap craniectomy for huge hemorrhage, it is more surgically invasive and takes a longer time than the MIS drilling method, and it requires special instruments, so its use is limited to emergency situations, such as acute uncontrolled increased ICP with brain herniation or preherniation.

Frame Stereotactic or Neuronavigation Aspiration

Stereotactic aspiration with a head frame can provide precise focus for evacuation of hematomas. Initially, in 1967, stereotactic surgery was performed by coordinating the use of a head frame with anatomical landmarks on X-ray images. Since the beginning of the 1980s, it has been performed under CT scan guidance. To remove residual clots timely and completely, some neurosurgeons recommend using an Archimedes device or ultrasonic oscillation technique to crush and clear away hematomas under stereotaxic aspiration [4, 21]. Teernstra et al. reported a series of 71 cases of supratentorial spontaneous ICH in patients aged 45 years and older with volumes of over than 10 ml. They found that stereotactic hematoma evacuation can result in the effective removal of hematomas and improve prognosis [22]. However, frame stereotactic surgery, which is commonly used in patients at the early stage of ICH, was found to be difficult to perform in severe patients due to the more complex operation with or without CT scan. In recent years, stereotactic MIS has become easier and has been increasingly used by following simple stereotaxic coordinates with CT guidance. A frameless stereotactic technique, neuronavigation-guided MIS, is the major method clinically used for the surgical localization of ICH at present. It has the advantage of accurate localization without a head frame, and it is more convenient than framed surgery for emergency surgical use.

Soft Channel/Catheter Drainage

With the development of the procedure for mechanical evacuation of ICH under stereotaxis with CT scan, another dissolving technique has emerged involving injection of thrombolytic agents (such as rt-PA or UK) into the hematomal cavity for drainage [23]. The soft channel technique involves creation of holes in the skull by both burring and coning under navigation or simple stereotaxis or CT guidance directly, after which a silicone catheter with a guide wire is directly passed through the brain tissue into the target clot. Then, indwelling catheter drainage of the residual hematoma is performed by aspiration combined with injection of thrombolytic agents into the area for a certain period of time. It is the safest, cheapest and most common and effective hematoma evacuation method among the current MIS methods. It is not only suitable for smaller hematomas located deep in the brain but is also quite effectively used to treat large hematomas by placement of multiple catheters for drainage in emergency situations. The MISTIEII study has shown that MIS with catheter drainage results in higher rates of hematoma and cerebral edema elimination compared with medication only in the treatment of ICH [24].

For complete and safe drainage, some neurosurgeons have divided ICH into three surgical types (Types A/B/C), so that trajectory planning is correctly determined according to these different types. Type A is a deep-seated hematoma occupying the anterior third of the basal ganglia, with a typical 'oval' shape (football shape), and a frontal trajectory should be chosen for it; Type B is a deep-seated hematoma occupying the posterior third of the basal ganglia, with a more roundish to elliptical shape, and a temporo-occipital trajectory should be selected; and Type C is a superficial (lobar) hematoma with a variable shape that is most often spherical, and the most superficial trajectory relative to the hematoma should be chosen (fig. 1–3).

The advantages of catheter drainage for ICH are as follows: (1) it can be performed bedside with local anesthesia in case of an emergency and is the most mini-

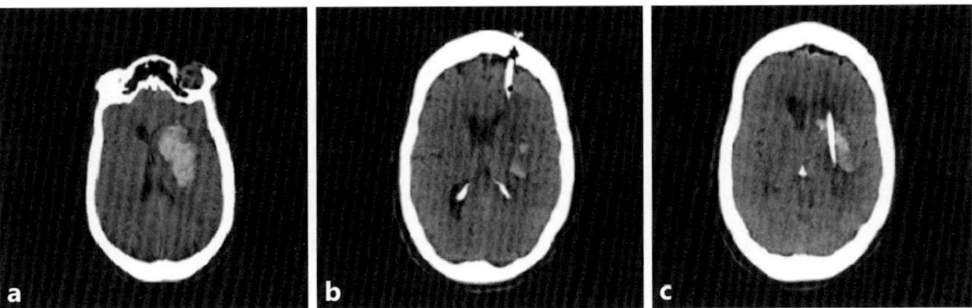

Fig. 1. 'Type A' (anterior basal ganglia): deep-seated, occupying the anterior third of the basal ganglia, with a typical 'oval' shape (football shape). **a** Greatest cross section; **b** entry point; **c** trajectory. With permission from [43, 44].

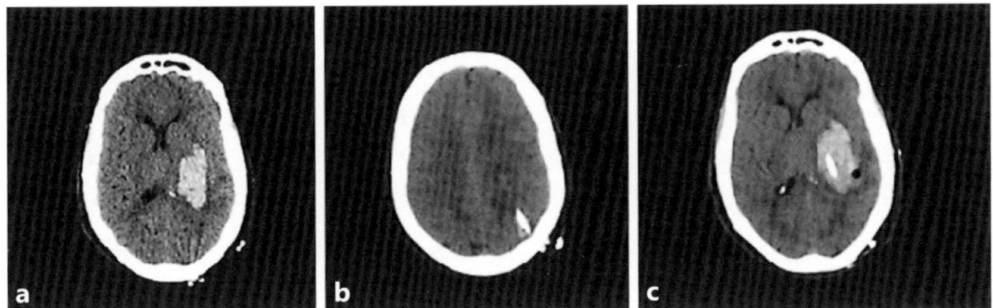

Fig. 2. 'Type B' (posterior basal ganglia): deep-seated, occupying the posterior third of the basal ganglia; the shape can range from more roundish to elliptical. **a** Greatest cross section; **b** entry point; **c** trajectory.

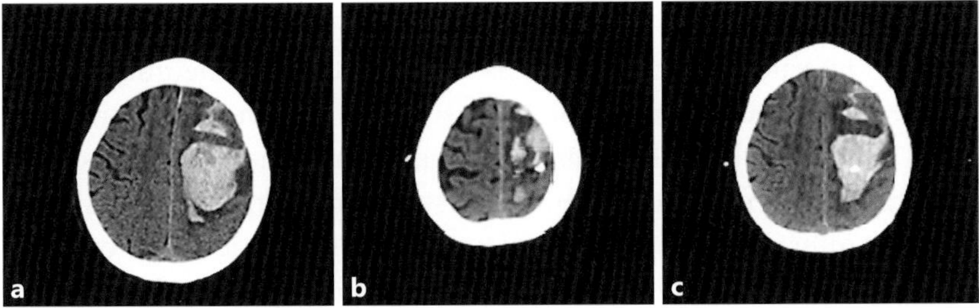

Fig. 3. 'Type C' (lobar and/or superficial): superficial (lobar) with a variable shape, but often more spherical. **a** Greatest cross section; **b** entry point; **c** trajectory.

mally invasive, easiest surgery with the shortest duration; (2) a catheter can be conveniently placed into supratentorial or subtentorial ICH; (3) because of their smooth, round and soft tips, catheters can be used to avoid mechanical injury of intracerebral vascular tissue when they traverse the brain tissue into the hematoma by a gentle swinging and pushing action, and an indwelling catheter placed into a pulsating brain minimizes the risk of rebleeding during the thrombolytic and drainage processes; and (4) it allows for injection of the hematoma with dissolving agents passed through the catheter, which has a large enough inner diameter to redissolve the residual clot and drain the cavity, improving hematoma clearance and surgical safety. Some studies have suggested that CT-guided stereotactic aspiration combined with local thrombolytic agents (such as rt-PA or UK) improve the hematoma clearance rate from 30 to 90%. Furthermore, the average rebleeding rate for a simple aspiration is 5%, while it is 4% after application of thrombolytic agents [25]. This surgical method is particularly suitable for bleeding in deep brain structures and for sufficiently small ICHs. (5) It has lower treatment costs than other types of MIS and is the preferred method for operations when high-cost neurosurgical equipment is unavailable.

However, there are also some limitations; mainly, bleeding cannot be directly stopped by surgery with electrocoagulation and the decompression of critical intracranial hypertension is limited because thorough clearance of hematomas is impractical. Thus, it is not suitable for unstable bleeding or herniation at an ultra-early stage of ICH.

Local Application of Thrombolytic Agents

Urokinase

UK is the first thrombolytic agent used to treat ICH [6]. An animal experiment has shown that injection into the ventricles is safe at a dosage of 40,000 IU/day for 4 consecutive days [26]. Doi et al. [27] first reported injection of UK into a hematoma cavity after stereotactic aspiration in 1982. Since then, some studies have reported the application of UK for treatment of ICH [28, 29]. Their findings have suggested that UK accelerates the resolution of blood clots and is safe. Currently, the use of UK for the treatment of ICH is being increasingly reported in China, Japan and other Asian countries. General use instructions for UK are as follows: it should be injected at a dose of 10,000–50,000 μ/per time with 1–2 ml saline solution into the hematoma cavity, and the catheter should be closed for draining for 1–2 h and then re-drained, and these steps should be repeated once every 12 h. The first thrombolytic injection should be performed at 6–12 h after catheter operation. During thrombolytic treatment, daily CT scans should be performed to detect variations in the brain for making optimal medical decisions. The indication to stop UK treatment is a residual hematoma size of less than 10 ml, and draining should be finished after there is no rebleeding for 24 h without UK.

Recombinant Tissue Plasminogen Activator

Both experimental and clinical studies have indicated that the local application of rt-PA does not aggravate brain edema and that the reduction rate of edema is significantly related to that of blood clots [30–33]. For further understanding of rt-PA application, studies have found that rt-PA effectively increases clot elimination but does not increase rebleeding or perihematomal edema volume complications and that it accelerates the rate of blood clot resolution [16, 33]. The MISTIE II study has confirmed that the 0.3–1 mg/8 h dose is well tolerated and safe. General use instructions for Rt-PA are as follows: administration of 1 mg/8 h, for a total of 9 times. The review time for CT scans and the indications for ending MIS with rt-PA are same as those for UK that are described above.

Minimally Invasive Treatment of Intraventricular Hemorrhage
Intraventricular hemorrhage (IVH) is a common complication of ICH. The amount of clots in the ventricle is an independent predictor of poor outcome [34]. Both animal and clinical studies have shown that UK and rt-PA not only effectively dissolve intraventricular clots but that they also keep ventricular drains unobstructed, which facilitates the control of ICP in acute, serious IVH. In addition, studies have shown that rt-PA is safe and that it does not affect the systemic coagulation state [35, 36]. Naff et al. [37] conducted a randomized, double-blind study with a small number of samples and obtained similar results. Jaffe et al. [38] have shown that blood clots are eliminated faster if a drain is placed on the side closest to the IVH and rt-PA is administered. The results of the RCT CLEAR IVH trial have indicated that with increasing rt-PA dosage, the IVH volume decreases faster [39]. However, the benefit of bilateral drainage is still disputed for injection of thrombolytic agents. Staykov's study have reported that bilateral drainage with rt-PA cannot increase the effective elimination of clots in the ventricles and that it is associated with a high risk of intraventricular infection, so it is not necessary for bilateral drainage after treatment with thrombolytic agents [40]. However, another study has considered that bilateral drainage is suitable for use in cases with intraventricular hematoma of over 40 ml and mass effect [41].

Perioperative Management of Blood Pressure

Hypertension is the major cause of postoperative ICH rebleeding, which directly affects surgical success. Generally, a BP that is slightly higher than normal is regarded as appropriate. Anderson et al. [42] have conducted an RCT (INTERACT) and have found that during the super early stage (within 6 h), strengthening the control of BP (a systolic BP of under 140 mm Hg) limits hemorrhage increase within 72 h more effectively than that achieved using the standard guidelines (a systolic BP of under 180 mm Hg). Intensive BP control is the most critical task in ICH perioperative treatment.

Conclusions

ICH surgical treatment is aimed at rapidly eliminating hematomas, improving cerebral circulation and resolving secondary brain injury to establish maximal convenience for neurofunctional recovery. Compared with conventional craniotomy, MIS can alleviate surgical injury and more quickly promote neurological function and consciousness at the same time. Before performing MIS, correct therapeutic strategies, surgical methods and timing should be chosen based on the etiology of the ICH. In minimally invasive therapy, surgical aspiration with the thrombotic drainage technique is the more safe, convenient and easy to perform ICH treatment. With the development of medical technologies, MIS will become the most common and standard method for the treatment of ICH.

References

1 Mendelow AD, Gregson BA, Fernandes HM, et al: Early surgery versus initial conservative treatment in patients with spontaneous supratentorial intracerebral haematomas in the International Surgical Trial in Intracerebral Haemorrhage (STICH): a randomised trial. Lancet 2005;365:387–397.

2 Barlas O, Karadereler S, Bahar S, et al: Image-guided keyhole evacuation of spontaneous supratentorial intracerebral hemorrhage. Minim Invasive Neurosurg 2009;52:62–68.

3 Benes V, Vladyka V, Zvěrina E: Sterotaxic evacuation of typical brain haemorrhage. Acta Neurochir (Wien) 1965;13:419–426.

4 Backlund EO, von Holst H: Controlled subtotal evacuation of intracerebral haematomas by stereotactic technique. Surg Neurol 1978;9:99–101.

5 Kandel EI, Peresedov VV: Stereotaxic evacuation of spontaneous intracerebral hematomas. J Neurosurg 1985;62:206–213.

6 Auer LM, Deinsberger W, Niederkorn K, et al: Endoscopic surgery versus medical treatment for spontaneous intracerebral hematoma: a randomized study. J Neurosurg 1989;70:530–535.

7 Matsumoto K, Hondo H: CT-guided stereotaxic evacuation of hypertensive intracerebral hematomas. J Neurosurg 1984;61:440–448.

8 Schaller C, Rohde V, Meyer B, et al: Stereotactic puncture and lysis of spontaneous intracerebral hemorrhage using recombinant tissue plasminogen activator. Neurosurgery 1995;36:328–333; discussion 333–335.

9 Ramanan M, Shankar A: Minimally invasive surgery for primary supratentorial intracerebral haemorrhage. J Clin Neurosci 2013;20:1650–1658.

10 Zhou X, Chen J, Li Q, et al: Minimally invasive surgery for spontaneous supratentorial intracerebral hemorrhage: a meta-analysis of randomized controlled trials. Stroke 2012;43:2923–2930.

11 Brott T, Broderick J, Kothari R, et al: Early hemorrhage growth in patients with intracerebral hemorrhage. Stroke 1997;28:1–5.

12 Marinescu, DC. Bajenaru O: Hyperdense artery signs and hypertensive cerebral hemorrhage. Eur J Neurology Suppl 2003;10:58.

13 Wu G, Li S, Wang L, et al: The perihematomal glutamate level is associated with the outcome of patients with basal ganglia hematomas treated by minimally invasive procedures. Neurol Res 2013;35:829–836.

14 Wu G, Wang L, Wang F, et al: Minimally invasive procedures for intracerebral hematoma evacuation in early stages decrease perihematomal glutamate level and improve neurological function in a rabbit model of ICH. Brain Res 2013;1492:140–147.

15 Morgenstern LB, Frankowski RF, Sheddon P: Surgical treatment for intracerebral hemorrhage (stich): a single-center, randomized clinical trial. Neurology 1998;51:1359–1363.

16 Carhuaporna JR, Barrett BJ, Keyl PM, et al: Stereotactic aspiration-thrombolysis of intracerebral hemorrhage and its impact on perihematoma brain edema. Neurocrit Care 2008;8:322–329.

17 Liu W, Ma L, Shen F, et al: Drilling skull plus injection of urokinase in the treatment of epidural haematoma: a preliminary study. Brain Inj 2008;22:199–204.

18 Liu C, Ling F: Cerebro-Spinal Vascular Surgery. Beijing, China Science and Technology Press, 2013.

19 Hayashi M, Hasegawa T, Kobayashi H, et al: [Aspiration of hypertensive intracerebral hematoma by stereotactic technique]. No Shinkei Geka 1981;9:1365–1371.

20 Kaneko M, Koba T, Yokoyama T: Early surgical treatment for hypertensive intracerebral hemorrhage. J Neurosurg 1977;46:579–583.

21 Hondo H, Uno M, Sasaki K, et al: Computed tomography controlled aspiration surgery for hypertensive intracerebral hemorrhage. Experience of more than 400 cases. Stereotact Funct Neurosurg 1990;54–55:432–437.

22 Teernstra OP, Evers SM, Lodder J, et al: Stereotactic treatment of intracerebral hematoma by means of a plasminogen activator: a multicenter randomized controlled trial (SICHPA). Stroke 2003;34:968–974.

23 Niizuma H, Suzuki J: Computed tomography-guided stereotactic aspiration of posterior fossa hematomas: a supine lateral retromastoid approach. Neurosurgery 1987;21:422–427.

24 Hanley DF: MISTIE phase II results: safety, efficacy and surgical performance. International Stroke Conference, New Orleans, LA, 2012.
25 Gebel JM, Broderick JP: Intracerebral hemorrhage. Neurol Clin 2000;18:419–438.
26 Pang D, Sclabassi RJ, Horton JA: Lysis of intraventricular blood clot with urokinase in a canine model: part 2. In vivo safety study of intraventricular urokinase. Neurosurgery 1986;19:547–552.
27 Doi E, Moriwaki H, Komai N, et al: [Stereotactic evacuation of intracerebral hematomas]. Neurol Med Chir (Tokyo) 1982;22:461–467.
28 Mohadjer M, Braus DF, Myers A, et al: CT-stereotactic fibrinolysis of spontaneous intracerebral hematomas. Neurosurg Rev 1992;15:105–110.
29 Montes JM, Wong JH, Fayad PB, et al: Stereotactic computed tomographicguided aspiration and thrombolysis of intracerebral hematoma: protocol and preliminary experience. Stroke 2000;31:834–840.
30 Deinsberger W, Vogel J, Fuchs C, et al: Fibrinolysis and aspiration of experimental intracerebral hematoma reduces the volume of ischemic brain in rats. Neurol Res 1999;21:517–523.
31 Wagner KR, Xi G, Hua Y, et al: Ultra-early clot aspiration after lysis with tissue plasminogen activator in a porcine model of intracerebral hemorrhage: edema reduction and blood-brain barrier protection. J Neurosurg 1999;90:491–498.
32 Rohde V, Rohde I, Thiex R, et al: Fibrinolysis therapy achieved with tissue plasminogen activator and aspiration of the liquefied clot after experimental intracerebral hemorrhage: rapid reduction in hematoma volume but intensification of delayed edema formation. J Neurosurg 2002;97:954–962.
33 Mould WA, Carhuapoma JR, Muschelli J, et al: Minimally invasive surgery plus recombinant tissue-type plasminogen activator for intracerebral hemorrhage evacuation decreases perihematomal edema. Stroke 2013;44:627–634.
34 Hanley DF: Intraventricular hemorrhage: severity factor and treatment target in spontaneous intracerebral hemorrhage. Stroke 2009;40:1533–1538.
35 Pang D, Sclabassi RJ, Horton JA: Lysis of intraventricular blood clot with urokinase in a canine model: part 3. Effects of intraventricular urokinase on clot lysis and posthemorrhagic hydrocephalus. Neurosurgery 1986;19:553–572.
36 Shen PH, Matsuoka Y, Kawajiri K, et al: Treatment of intraventricular hemorrhage using urokinase. Neurol Med Chir (Tokyo) 1990;30:329–333.
37 Naff NJ, Hanley DF, Keyl PM, et al: Intraventricular thrombolysis speeds blood clot resolution: results of a pilot, prospective, randomized, double-blind, controlled trial. Neurosurgery 2004;54:577–583; discussion 583–584.
38 Jaffe J, Melnychuk E, Muschelli J, et al: Ventricular catheter location and the clearance of intraventricular hemorrhage. Neurosurgery 2012;70:1258–1263; discussion 1263–1264.
39 Webb AJ, Ullman NL, Mann S, et al: Resolution of intraventricular hemorrhage varies by ventricular region and dose of intraventricular thrombolytic: the Clot Lysis: Evaluating Accelerated Resolution of IVH (CLEAR IVH) program. Stroke 2012;43:1666–1668.
40 Staykov D, Huttner HB, Lunkenheimer J, et al: Single versus bilateral external ventricular drainage for intraventricular fibrinolysis in severe ventricular haemorrhage. J Neurol Neurosurg Psychiatry 2010; 81:105–108.
41 Hinson HE, Melnychuk E, Muschelli J, et al: Drainage efficiency with dual versus single catheters in severe intraventricular hemorrhage. Neurocrit Care 2012;16:399–405.
42 Anderson CS, Huang Y, Arima H, et al: Effects of early intensive blood pressure-lowering treatment on the growth of hematoma and perihematomal edema in acute intracerebral hemorrhage: the Intensive Blood Pressure Reduction in Acute Cerebral Haemorrhage Trial (INTERACT). Stroke 2010;41:307–312.
43 Mould WA, Carhuapoma JR, Muschelli J, et al: Minimally invasive surgery plus recombinant tissue-type plasminogen activator for intracerebral hemorrhage evacuation decreases perihematomal edema. Stroke 2013;44:627–634.
44 Vespa PM, Martin N, Zuccarello M, et al: Surgical trials in intracerebral hemorrhage. Stroke 2013;44:S79–S82.

Dr. Wei-Min Wang
Department of Neurosurgery, Liuhuaqiao Hospital
111 Liuhua Road
Guangzhou 510010 (China)
E-Mail gzwangwmo@163.com

Toyoda K, Anderson CS, Mayer SA (eds): New Insights in Intracerebral Hemorrhage.
Front Neurol Neurosci. Basel, Karger, 2016, vol 37, pp 166–181 (DOI: 10.1159/000437121)

Surgical Strategies for Acutely Ruptured Arteriovenous Malformations

Jaime L. Martinez • R. Loch Macdonald

Division of Neurosurgery, St. Michael's Hospital, Labatt Family Centre of Excellence in Brain Injury and Trauma Research, Keenan Research Centre for Biomedical Science and The Li Ka Shing Knowledge Institute of St. Michael's Hospital, Department of Surgery, University of Toronto, Ont., Canada

Abstract

Brain arteriovenous malformations (AVMs) are focal neurovascular lesions consisting of abnormal fistulous connections between the arterial and venous systems with no interposed capillaries. This arrangement creates a high-flow circulatory shunt with hemorrhagic risk and hemodynamic abnormalities. While most AVMs are asymptomatic, they may cause severe neurological complications and death. Each AVM carries an annual rupture risk of 2–4%. Intracranial hemorrhage due to AVM rupture is the most common initial manifestation (up to 70% of presentations), and it carries significant morbidity and mortality. This complication is particularly important in the young and otherwise healthy population, in whom AVMs cause up to one-third of all hemorrhagic strokes. A previous rupture is the single most important independent predictor of future hemorrhage. Current treatment modalities for AVM are microsurgery, endovascular embolization, and radiosurgery. In acutely ruptured AVMs, early microsurgical excision is usually avoided. The standard is to wait at least 4 weeks to allow for patient recovery, hematoma liquefaction, and inflammatory reactions to subside. Exceptions to this rule are small, superficial, low-grade AVMs with elucidated angioarchitecture, for which early simultaneous hematoma evacuation and AVM excision is feasible. Emergent hematoma evacuation with delayed AVM excision (unless, as mentioned, the AVM is low grade) is recommended in patients with a decreased level of consciousness due to intracranial hemorrhage, posterior fossa or temporal lobe hematoma of >30 ml, or hemispheric hematoma of >60 ml. The applicability of endovascular techniques for acutely ruptured AVMs is not clear, but feasible options, until a definitive treatment is determined, include occluding intranidal and distal flow-related aneurysms and 'sealing' any rupture site or focal angioarchitectural weakness when one can be clearly identified and safely accessed. Radiosurgery is not performed in acutely ruptured AVMs because its therapeutic effects occur in a delayed fashion.

© 2016 S. Karger AG, Basel

Introduction

Classically, nonneoplastic cerebrovascular malformations have been classified into four histopathologic categories [1], namely capillary telangiectasias, developmental venous anomalies (venous angiomas), cavernous malformations, and arteriovenous malformations, with a possible fifth being direct arteriovenous fistulae. Brain arteriovenous malformations (AVMs) are focal vascular lesions consisting of arrangements of tangled blood vessels (niduses) that result from pathologic fistulous connections between arteries and veins with no intervening capillary bed. Although most AVMs lie asymptomatically within neural tissue, they can cause serious neurologic complications and death. AVMs are responsible for 3% of strokes in young patients, 9% of all subarachnoid hemorrhages, and 4% of all intracerebral hemorrhages (ICHs) [2]. ICH resulting from AVM rupture is the most serious and, unfortunately, the most common complication, with annual rupture rates ranging from 2 to 4%. AVM is the leading cause of ICH in the young and healthy population, comprising almost one-third of all cases, with each carrying up to 10% mortality and up to 50% morbidity. Other less common presentations result from intracranial hemodynamic changes, especially changes in the surrounding brain that could manifest as seizures, which is the initial presentation in about 15–40% of AVM patients [2–4], or neurological deficits, by means of the vascular 'steal' phenomenon.

AVMs can be treated with open microsurgery, radiosurgery, endovascular techniques, or a combination of these modalities. Most treatments can be rendered electively, except in cases of major intracranial hemorrhage. Low-grade AVMs may not present major management dilemmas, whereas controversy and difficulty arise in cases of hemorrhage associated with complex AVMs. In this chapter, we will discuss the role of early open microsurgery in acutely ruptured brain AVMs.

Epidemiology

Brain AVMs are relatively uncommon lesions, with an incidence of approximately 1 in 100,000 person-years [5, 6] and an estimated prevalence of less than 10.3 in 100,000 individuals in the population [6], which is 10–15-fold lower than the prevalence of intracranial aneurysms [5]. A large number of patients remain asymptomatic. Autopsy studies have found an overall frequency of detection of 4.3% [7] and have reported that only 12% of all AVMs manifest clinically at some point during patients' lives [8].

Pathology and Pathogenesis

AVMs appear grossly like a 'bag of worms' and are typically wedge-shaped, with the base toward the leptomeninges and the apex toward the ventricles, and they can develop anywhere in the central nervous system, but larger pathologies are encountered in the region of the middle cerebral arteries [1]. The overlying leptomeninges are often thickened and opacified [1], which can serve as a landmark surgically. Nearly all brain AVMs are single focal lesions, but 2% are multiple lesions. AVMs have three components: (1) feeding artery(ies); (2) a nidus of tangled blood vessels where arterial-to-venous shunts occur; and (3) arterialized draining vein(s), which are often tortuous and with aneurysmal dilations. Despite hypertrophic changes, the intranidal vessels have preserved wall integrity. On the other hand, ultrastructural studies have demonstrated interesting abnormalities of the perinidal capillaries using electron microscopy [9, 10]. These abnormalities consist of exaggerated perinidal capillary dilations, blood-brain barrier disruption secondary to a lack of endothelial gap junctions, and endothelial cell differentiation and proliferation. They may explain the excessive intraoperative and postoperative hemorrhage and edema associated with AVM surgery, even with minimal nidus manipulation. Additionally, the presence of endothelial proliferation [11] and case reports of postoperative recurrence [9, 12], *de novo* formation [13], and even AVM regression [14] without treatment, suggest that AVMs are not static but are actively and continuously evolving lesions.

The true etiology of brain AVMs is not clear, but it is most likely multifactorial, involving genetic susceptibility and mechanical and environmental triggering factors [13]. The strong association of AVMs with some genetic disorders, such as ataxia-telangiectasia and Osler-Weber-Rendu, Wyburn-Mason, and Sturge-Weber syndromes [15] imply a genetic influence in some cases. Traditionally, AVMs have been thought to be congenital in nature. According to Mullan et al. [16], AVMs originate from aberrations in the absorption of numerous pial-to-dural veins during the 40–80 mm stage of human embryologic development, with persistent growth thereafter. Lasjaunias [17] has argued that AVMs originate from alterations in vascular remodeling at the junctions between capillaries and veins and that the earlier the insult, the larger the lesion. Another theory postulates that AVMs originate from embryologic venous anomalies and microvascular thrombosis, causing tissue hypoxia and thus activating the release of neovascular growth factors, such as hypoxia-inducible factors [18]. Downstream from hypoxia-inducible factor 1, vascular endothelial growth factor may initiate focal angiogenesis. Other important AVM angiogenesis factors include angiopoietins (Ang-1 and Ang-2) and their receptor Tie-2 and matrix metalloproteinases (MMP-2 and MMP-9), which degrade the extracellular matrix, facilitating angiogenesis.

Clinical Presentation and Natural History

The initial clinical presentation of brain AVMs may include hemorrhage, seizures, focal neurological deficits, or headaches. Hemorrhage is the most common presenting symptom, occurring in 38–71% of patients [3] and manifesting in the following forms:

ICH in 60%, ICH with an intraventricular component in 26%, intraventricular hemorrhage (IVH) alone in 8%, subarachnoid hemorrhage in 4% and subdural hemorrhage in 2%. Any sudden loss of consciousness or neurological deficit in a young patient without risk factors for stroke or primary ICH should always raise suspicion of a ruptured vascular malformation [19].

Management is based on balancing the lesion-specific natural history with the treatment-related risks. Regarding lesion-specific prognosis, the AVM-related annual mortality rate is approximately 1.0% but ranges from 0.7 to 3.4% [5, 20, 21], with combined rates of major morbidity and mortality of 2.7% per year [21]. A study conduced in Finland has demonstrated that patients with AVMs have a 51% increase in mortality compared with the general population [5]. Each AVM has an overall annual hemorrhage rate of between 2 and 4%, and this rate is higher for ruptured (4.8%) compared to unruptured AVMs (1–3%) [22, 23]. A lifetime rupture risk (%) can be estimated using the following formula, which supports more aggressive treatment in younger patients: 105 – age in years [24]. A hemorrhagic presentation is the most important independent predictor of future hemorrhage (hazard ratio = 2.15, $p < 0.01$) [3], with reported annual rebleeding risks of approximately 9.65% during the first year and 3.67% after 5 years [3]. Every hemorrhage carries a mortality rate of approximately 18% [25], ranging from 10 to 30% [26], and 40–50% of survivors have a neurological deficit thereafter [4, 25, 27], with one-fifth of patients losing their independence [27]. These data suggest that ruptured AVMs pose significant rebleeding risks and that each hemorrhage leads to an increasingly worse outcome. Therefore, a more earnest effort towards a definitive cure is indicated for previously ruptured lesions. Incomplete interventions, such as partial embolization, have not resulted in a reduction in the risk of future hemorrhage [3].

Pathoanatomical characteristics that have been associated with an increased risk of rupture include the following: (1) venous outflow restriction, which is associated with lesions with a small nidus (<2.5 cm) and a single long draining vein that is prone to stenosis or spontaneous obliteration, perhaps due to nonphysiological venous flow rates [28, 29]; (2) exclusive deep venous drainage (i.e. the periventricular, Galenic or cerebellar system) [3, 30]; (3) distal flow-related and intranidal AVM-associated aneurysms; (4) a deep hemispheric location; and (5) an infratentorial location [3, 31]. Additionally, increasing age has been associated with an increased risk of hemorrhage. Combinations of these risk factors have additive effects, further increasing the hemorrhage risk.

In a previously reported case series of early microsurgery in acutely ruptured AVMs, the patient demographics, including age and gender, were fairly similar. Almost universally, the patients presented in a poor clinical condition with sudden neurological deterioration manifested by decreased mentation, coma (Glasgow Coma Scale score of 8 or less), and decerebrate posturing [32–35]. Jafar et al. [32] divided patients into the following 2 groups: those presenting initially with an ICH secondary to AVM rupture and those with an ICH following endovascular intervention in a previously unruptured AVM. In the endovascular cohort, ICH manifested as a seizure in 75%, which is much higher than the already established 15–40% in patients who did not receive endovascular intervention; however, the sample size was small.

Neuroimaging

The initial neuroimaging assessment of patients with ruptured brain AVMs is conducted using computed tomography (CT). Magnetic resonance imaging (MRI) and other imaging may be performed if the clinical condition of the patient permits. If CT discloses spontaneous intracranial hemorrhage, we obtain immediate CT angiography (CTA) in almost all cases. CTA helps to determine if there is an underlying lesion, such as an AVM or an aneurysm, and shows the enhancing nidus and some prominent feeding arteries and draining veins. However, it cannot be used to assess temporal flow-related changes, and small AVMs are difficult to detect [36].

Unless a patient requires emergency surgery for intracranial hemorrhage, additional imaging is indicated. MRI is useful for evaluating the surrounding brain and involvement of eloquent cerebral cortex [36]. AVM components are represented as flow voids. Susceptibility-weighted imaging, like gradient echo sequences, help to detect evidence of prior hemorrhage with high sensitivity and also help to differentiate arteries from veins, which is often difficult to achieve with other techniques. Hyperintensity on T2 and fluid attenuated inversion recovery sequences indicates perinidal gliosis secondary to the vascular ischemic 'steal' phenomenon. Diffusion-tensor imaging defines the white matter tracts in relation to the AVM and can be useful in preoperative planning for AVMs affecting eloquent hemispheric or brainstem areas. Functional MRI relies on blood flow changes elicited by brain tissue activation and can be performed, but it may be difficult to interpret areas adjacent to AVMs where there is already abnormal blood flow.

Catheter digital subtraction cerebral angiography with 3-dimensional reconstruction is the gold standard neuroimaging modality and should be performed in all cases, except when emergency ICH evacuation is needed [19]. It allows for identification of important elements for surgical planning, such as arterial feeder anatomy, nidus location and morphology, drainage patterns, venous varices, associated aneurysms, and venous outflow obstruction [30, 36]. The excellent temporal and spatial resolution allows for a better determination of the nidus size prior to venous filling [36] and furthermore, it allows for identification of venous drainage [30], which facilitates preservation and protection of the area until later stages of surgical resection. While cerebral angiography is very sensitive, 'angiographically occult' AVMs can develop following hemorrhage. In ruptured AVMs, the hematoma may compress the nidus and impair visualization of small lesions [36]. Therefore, repeat imaging, usually catheter angiography, is recommended weeks after hemorrhages for which no etiology is found. Patients with ICH in whom the risk of angiography outweighs its benefit include those with systemic hypertension who are older and have ICH in the thalamus, putamen or cerebellum typical of hypertension [37]. Also, if surgery is not performed acutely for a ruptured AVM, repeat delayed angiography is important after the hematoma has resolved to better assess the AVM anatomy and angioarchitecture.

Management

After any intracranial hemorrhage, the patient is first resuscitated, and a noncontrast CT is obtained, which will dictate, along with clinical examination, if further interventions, such as intubation, medical management for increased intracranial pressure, insertion of a ventricular drain or emergency craniotomy to evacuate the hematoma, are indicated. Then, noninvasive vascular neuroimaging assessments (CTA or magnetic resonance angiography) are performed, which help to determine the etiology of the hemorrhage. Finally, catheter cerebral angiography is performed unless the patient requires emergency craniotomy for clot evacuation.

Following initial stabilization and admission to a neurointensive care unit, the general medical management of a ruptured AVM is very similar to that of spontaneous primary ICH [38, 39]. Oral anticoagulation and antiplatelet agents are discontinued, and any bleeding abnormality is corrected immediately to minimize hematoma expansion, to lessen the severity of a rebleed and to prepare the patient for a possible neurosurgical intervention. At some time (hours to days) after hematoma stabilization, it is recommended that anticoagulation therapy with subcutaneous heparin or low-molecular-weight heparin is started, accompanied by mobilization or pneumatic compression if the patient is paralyzed to prevent deep vein thrombosis and pulmonary embolism [19, 26]. Strict blood pressure control is encouraged, preferably to a systolic blood pressure of <140 mm Hg [40] while maintaining the cerebral perfusion pressure within 60–80 mm Hg, theoretically because it prevents hematoma growth and could be associated with better clinical outcome [19, 26, 38]. Any cause of fever should be treated, and hyperthermia should be corrected with antipyretics. Insulin administration is recommended when glucose levels are >185 mg/dl [19, 26, 38] to prevent the neurological complications of hyperglycemia. Seizures occur in 10.6% of hemorrhagic strokes [41]. Acute-phase antiepileptic treatment is often initiated immediately and maintained for an extended period of time in patients with lobar or cortical hemorrhage [26]. Continuous electroencephalogram monitoring is often recommended for unresponsive patients. Some experts advocate seizure prophylaxis in all patients with cortical hemorrhage [19].

Microsurgical Treatment

Microsurgery is the gold standard for the definitive treatment of brain AVMs. It provides an immediate angiographic cure once the results are confirmed by postoperative imaging, in addition to virtually permanent protection from recurrent hemorrhage and hemodynamic consequences. On the other hand, surgery is not without risks. In 1986, Spetzler and Martin [42] introduced a simple grading system to classify AVMs and to help estimate surgical risks based on the following 3 features: size, the presence of deep venous drainage, and involvement of eloquent cortex. High Spetzler-Martin grades (SMGs) are associated with high surgical risks. More recently, Spetzler and Ponce recommended reducing this grading system to a 3-tier system with the following classifications: SMGs I–II (Spetzler-Ponce Class A), SMG III (Spetzler-Ponce Class B), and SMGs IV–V (Spetzler-Ponce Class C). Accordingly, SMG I–II (Class A) lesions are low-risk lesions that can be safely treated with microsurgery [43, 44], with favorable outcomes attained in 92–100% of patients [42, 45]. There is disagreement regarding the best treatment strategies for intermediate-risk lesions (SMG III); however, these lesions may be initially embolized and then resected [19]. SMG IV–V (Class C) lesions are high-risk lesions that are preferably managed medically because microsurgery is associated with poor outcome in 14.3% and mortality in 4.3% [45]. To further help in estimating surgical risk, Lawton et al. [46] introduced a 'supplementary' grading scale with 5 extra points, which showed better accuracy at predicting AVM surgical outcome than the SMG alone [47]. This supplementary scale is based on patient age (<20 = 1 point; 20–40 = 2 points; >40 = 3 points), hemorrhagic presentation (1 point), and nidus morphology (diffuse and no well-defined margins = 1 point). Adding the results of both scales yields a total of 10 points, which can be used to stratify surgical candidates into low-risk (1–3 points), intermediate-risk (4–6 points), and high-risk (7–10 points) groups. An SM-supplementary grade of 6 is the cutoff or boundary for AVM operability.

Early surgical intervention in acutely ruptured AVMs is generally avoided. Overall, the risk of early rebleeding associated with AVM hemorrhage is relatively low, averaging about 6% over the first 6 months [26, 32, 48, 49]. Additionally, early microsurgery on a swollen, acutely injured brain could increase the risk of permanent neurological deficits [19, 35, 50]. These deficits can be obscured or difficult to detect because most patients improve neurologically after hemorrhage from an AVM; however, failure to do so could be due the hemorrhage itself or to surgery. Moreover, the hematoma may compress and obscure the AVM nidus, making it difficult to visualize its true angiographic architecture, which is essential for surgical planning, and it also may increase the chance of incomplete resection. Therefore, surgery is usually delayed for weeks to allow for patient recovery, brain edema resolution, hematoma liquefaction, and perinidal gliosis and encephalomalacia formation. This delay simplifies surgery, which can be performed under controlled conditions during elective hours, with better delineation of the AVM (perinidal

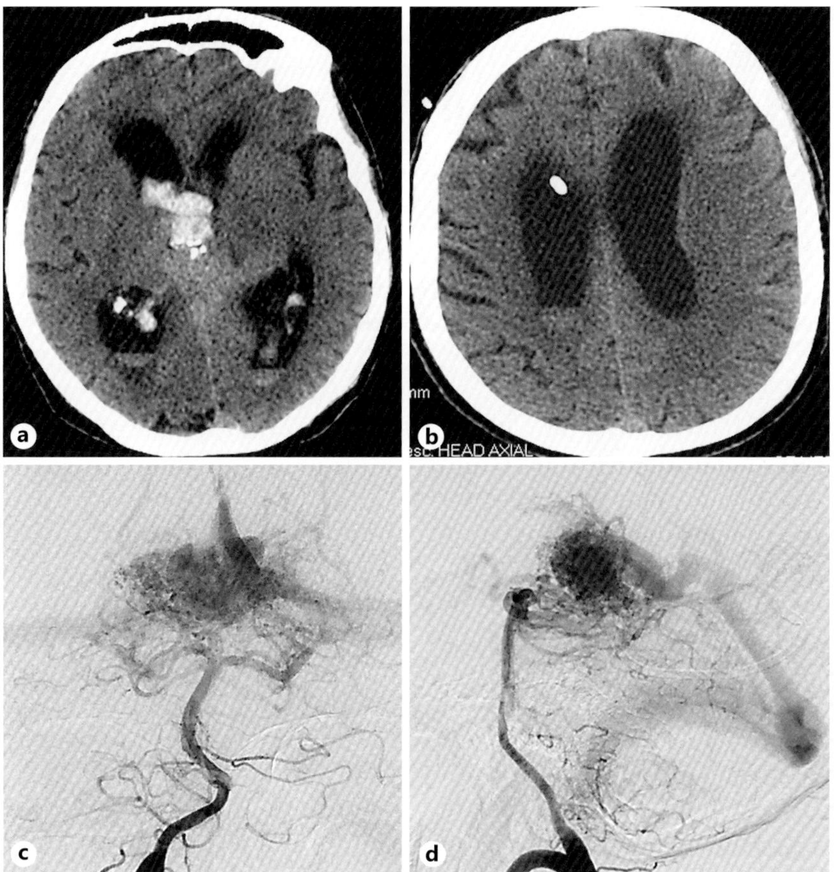

Fig. 1. External ventricular drain placement in acute hydrocephalus associated with intraventricular hemorrhage from an arteriovenous malformation (AVM). This 76-year-old man presented with a sudden decreased level of consciousness. CT scan of the head (**a**) showed an intraventricular hemorrhage associated hydrocephalus and a thalamic/midbrain lesion suggestive of an AVM. CT angiogram was performed, and a ventricular drain was inserted, resulting in neurological improvement (**b**). Anteroposterior and lateral vertebral cerebral angiography (**c**, **d**) revealed a high-grade (Spetzler-Martin grade 5 or 6), essentially inoperable diencephalic AVM with deep venous drainage. Associated intranidal and distal flow-related microaneurysms were identified; however, they were not amenable for endovascular repair. After removal of the ventricular drain, hydrocephalus and cognitive dysfunction persisted, and a programmable ventriculoperitoneal shunt was inserted. Follow-up assessments showed very good functional recovery so that he was living at home with minimal assistance with daily living activities due to poor short-term memory.

gliosis) and with creation of a dissection plane between the AVM and the surrounding brain (the combined effects of the hematoma cavity and encephalomalacia) [32, 51].

Other than hematoma evacuation, the other emergency surgical treatment is placement of a ventricular drain, which can be necessary if there is acute hydrocephalus associated with IVH from an AVM (fig. 1).

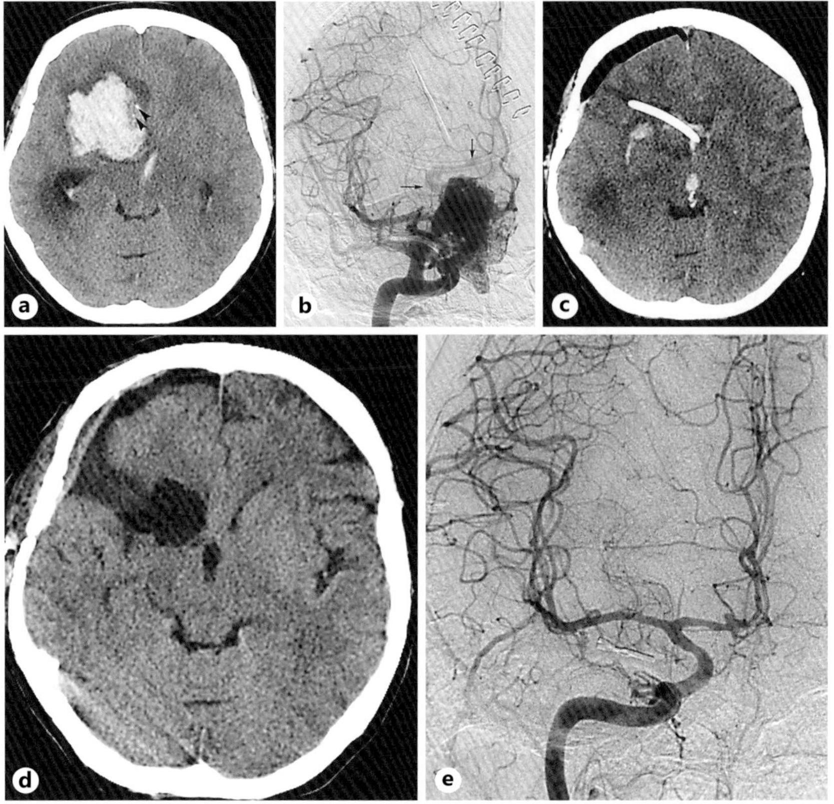

Fig. 2. Early hematoma evacuation and delayed AVM excision. This 57-year-old woman was found unconscious at home and was brought to a hospital by paramedics with a Glasgow Coma Scale score of 5. Upon arrival, she was rapidly intubated and medically stabilized. CT scan of the head (**a**) showed a large, right, frontal intracranial hemorrhage extending into the ventricles and causing hydrocephalus. Because of the location of the hematoma and presence of minute calcifications adjacent to it (arrowheads), a secondary vascular abnormality was suspected. CT angiogram was performed preoperatively, in addition to cerebral angiography only after intracranial hemorrhage evacuation (**b**), which revealed a Spetzler-Martin grade 3 orbitofrontal AVM fed by anterior and middle cerebral artery branches and drained mainly by a large vein coursing to the superior sagittal sinus (arrows), as well as deep venous drainage. The coma, substantial mass effect with a 14 mm midline shift and hydrocephalus prompted acute surgical intervention with hematoma evacuation and external ventricular drain placement after CT and CT angiogram (**c**). At this point in time, the AVM was left alone. Three months later, craniotomy was reopened, and the AVM was excised. An unremarkable postoperative course ensued. Follow-up CT (**d**) and cerebral angiography (**e**) demonstrated complete removal of the AVM. The patient's cognition and overall function improved so that she was independent at home with no assistance and walked independently without aid, but she did not return to work.

Hematoma Removal versus Hematoma Plus Arteriovenous Malformation Resection

In some instances, however, acute ICH evacuation is necessary and lifesaving. Hematomas causing mass effects or neurological deficits should be evacuated urgently through craniotomy (fig. 2). Decompressive craniectomy may be required. An emerging management strategy for primary ICH is to perform decompressive craniectomy and leave the ICH alone. This strategy has not been well studied for AVM ruptures. In general, we operate emergently on ICH associated with AVM rupture under the following conditions:

1. Decreased level of consciousness due to an ICH, with or without a focal deficit, including but not limited to hemiparesis or pupillary dilation.

2. Hematomas of larger than 30 ml in the temporal lobe or cerebellum or 60 ml in other parts of the hemispheres, with or without a midline shift of more than several millimeters.

We do not attempt resection of AVMs other than small AVMs of SMG 2 or less with straightforward anatomy or clearly elucidated angioarchitecture (fig. 3). Castel et al. [52] have reported an operative morbidity of 8.6% and mortality of 3.3%, which increase with increasing SMG and are related to AVM location. Small lesions of <3 cm are associated with 4.6% morbidity and 0% mortality. The rationale for early craniotomy with hematoma evacuation and AVM resection is threefold: first, it quickly relieves intracranial hypertension; second, it removes potentially neurotoxic blood degradation products [26]; and third, resection of surrounding gliotic and hemosiderin-stained tissue improves seizure control [53]. Steudel et al. [33] reported good outcomes of 6 comatose patients who underwent acute AVM and hematoma removal, providing another justification for intervention in severely disabled patients. Additionally, Jafar et al. [32] have advocated prompt hematoma evacuation with simultaneous AVM excision in patients with profound neurological deterioration and have stated that early surgery accompanied by perioperative intracranial pressure control with mannitol and barbiturates yields good-to-excellent outcomes. In addition, Kuhmonen et al. [35] operated on 45 patients with ruptured AVM with early hematoma evacuation and AVM extirpation within 4 days from presentation and obtained good outcomes in 55% of the cases, although 2/3 of the patients were in poor clinical condition on admission (Hunt and Hess grades 4–5). Good outcome is significantly negatively correlated with the Hunt and Hess grade, age, and the presence of IVH ($p < 0.006$) but not with the SMG, location, or hematoma size. The authors concluded that acute surgery is lifesaving and accelerates rehabilitation compared with delayed surgery and AVM's natural course. Lastly, Pavesi et al. [34] have reported that early surgery in ruptured SMG I and II AVMs is a safe and definitive treatment for immediate cerebral decompression, rebleeding prevention, and hospital stay reduction and that it allows for faster rehabilitation.

In conclusion, early microsurgery of ruptured AVMs is generally avoided for those that are SMG 3 and higher. A recovery period of usually more than 4 weeks facilitates resection. Simultaneous hematoma evacuation and AVM excision is sometimes amenable in small, superficial AVMs with elucidated angioarchitecture. Craniotomy or craniectomy with hematoma evacuation is performed in patients with large clots causing neurological compromise or uncontrollable intracranial hypertension.

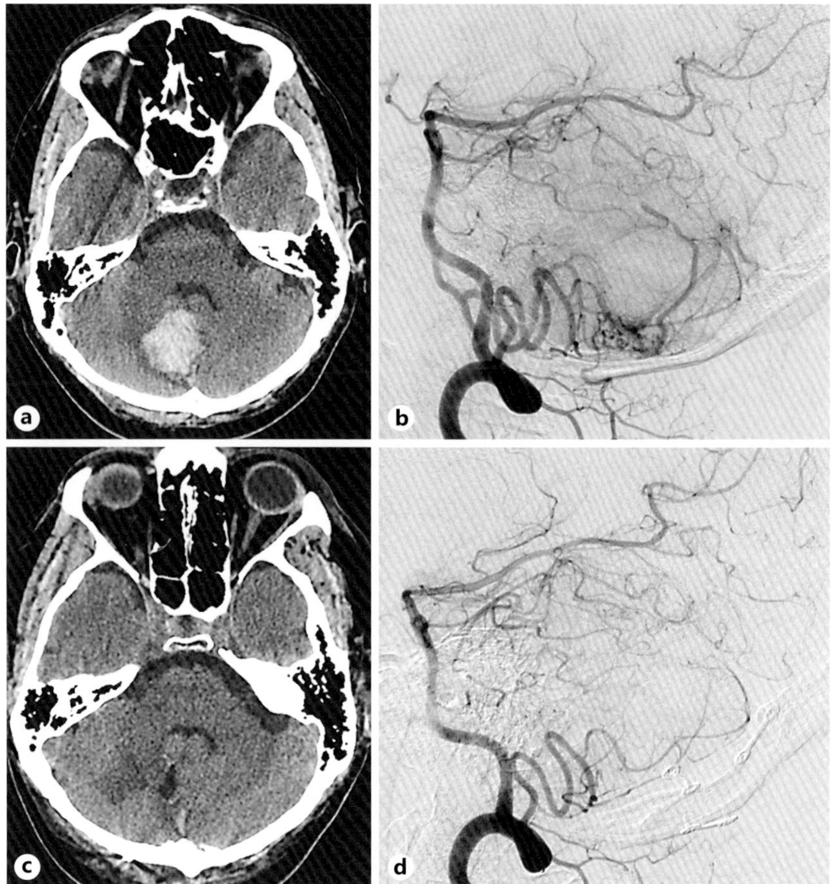

Fig. 3. Early simultaneous AVM excision and hematoma evacuation. This 58-year-old man presented with a sudden onset of headache, nausea and vomiting without loss of consciousness. He was on warfarin because of prior deep vein thrombosis that developed after liver transplantation for hepatitis C, all occurring 6 months previously. CT scan of the head showed a right cerebellar hemispheric hemorrhage extending into the vermis (**a**). Cerebral angiography (**b**) revealed a Spetzler-Martin grade 1 AVM within the right inferior cerebellar hemisphere fed by right posterior inferior cerebellar artery branches and drained by superficial bilateral cerebellar hemispheric veins and a vermian vein. Because of the hematoma location in the posterior fossa and the AVM size, accessibility, and straightforward anatomy, suboccipital craniotomy with simultaneous AVM excision and hematoma evacuation was performed at 48 hours after hemorrhage, when anticoagulation was reversed. The patient's symptoms improved, and follow-up neuroimaging assessments (**c** and **d**) revealed complete removal of the AVM. He recovered fully and remained off of warfarin since 6 months after the venous thromboembolism.

Intraoperative Management

General principles apply to craniotomy for ruptured AVM. Blood pressure should be controlled and should not be allowed to fluctuate. Anesthesia should be induced with this in mind, as well as consideration that the patient likely has increased intracranial pressure. We generally use a radiolucent head holder so that intraoperative angiography can be performed either through the superficial temporal artery [54] or transfemorally [55]. Peripheral vascular access should be adequate in the case of massive blood loss in all but the smallest AVMs.

A generous craniotomy is usually advisable, with consideration as to whether decompressive hemicraniectomy may be required at initial surgery or in a delayed fashion. Intraoperative neuronavigation facilitates craniotomy planning and hematoma localization. Once the dura is opened, the hematoma cavity can be entered at the point at which it is the closest to the brain surface. If the AVM is not going to be resected, then the hematoma should be evacuated under microscopic vision without disturbing the AVM. If the AVM is to be resected, then the principles of AVM resection apply. These include perinidal dissection without entering the nidus, early identification and control of feeding arteries, preservation of draining veins until late in resection, and meticulous circumferential dissection.

Intraoperative angiography is useful to confirm resection. We perform this procedure through the superficial temporal artery in cases of unilateral AVMs fed by only anterior circulation. Otherwise, transfemoral angiography is required but may not be feasible under emergency conditions.

Endovascular Treatment

While classically, endovascular techniques have been reserved only as adjuvants to microsurgery or radiosurgery, currently, thanks to innovations in this arena, they play significant roles in AVM management, with the following 5 main uses [56]: (1) preoperative blood flow reduction and embolization of deep, surgically inaccessible, feeder arteries; (2) preradiosurgical AVM volume reduction; (3) targeting of specific angioarchitectural features, such as intranidal aneurysms; (4) palliative flow reduction in large, high-flow, AVMs causing venous congestion or the arterial steal phenomenon; and possibly, (5) complete curative occlusion, with reported occlusion rates of 60–100% [56], in selected lesions. However, the ideal targets for embolization are also ideal for microsurgery, namely AVMs in noneloquent cortex that are SMG II or less and have the following feeder characteristics: <3 in number [57–59], large diameters (defined as twice the normal diameter) [60], and a superficial (cortical) arterial supply [60]. This endovascular armamentarium could be an alternative for poor surgical candidates and for patients in whom the latency period between treatment and thrombosis, inherent to radiosurgical intervention, carries a high hemorrhagic risk [56].

Early curative endovascular embolization is generally not recommended for acutely ruptured AVMs. Stemer et al. [61] reported 21 Onyx embolizations in ruptured AVMs, attaining complete occlusion in 52%, of which only 33% were cured with a single procedure, and the procedural complication rate was 10%. It has been documented that partial embolization does not reduce the risk of future hemorrhage [3] and that pursuing a second endovascular procedure is associated with worse neurological outcome [62]. In addition to incomplete obliteration, other disadvantages of endovascular therapy of AVMs include embolization of unintended vessels (early occlusion of draining veins), hemorrhage, and normal perfusion pressure breakthrough, with further hemorrhage and edema [63, 64].

A more accepted option is a strategic targeted partial embolization to 'seal' the AVM rupture site or focal angioarchitectural weakness – when this site can be clearly identified and safely accessed – to potentially prevent early rebleeding until a definitive intervention is undertaken and also to enhance surgical safety [59, 65–68]. These focal angioarchitectural weaknesses associated with a high hemorrhagic risk include distal flow-related aneurysms and intranidal aneurysms.

Early radiosurgery is not generally performed in the setting of acute AVM rupture because its therapeutic effects, both positive and negative, occur in a delayed fashion. Therefore, this modality is not recommended in severely unstable patients or those with a high rebleeding risk. Furthermore, in acutely ruptured AVMs, hemorrhage and edema obscures the boundaries of the nidus, thus decreasing the accuracy of targeting the lesion [69, 70]. Additionally, hemosiderin could cause postradiosurgical adverse reactions by potentially radiosensitizing the surrounding normal brain [71]. For this reason, some clinicians have advocated waiting from 6 to 12 weeks before treating ruptured AVMs with radiosurgery [70].

References

1 McCormick WF: The pathology of vascular ('arteriovenous') malformations. J Neurosurg 1966;24: 807–816.

2 Al-Shahi R, Warlow C: A systematic review of the frequency and prognosis of arteriovenous malformations of the brain in adults. Brain 2001;124(Pt 10):1900–1926.

3 da Costa L, Wallace MC, Ter Brugge KG, et al: The natural history and predictive features of hemorrhage from brain arteriovenous malformations. Stroke 2009;40:100–105.

4 Crawford PM, West CR, Chadwick DW, et al: Arteriovenous malformations of the brain: natural history in unoperated patients. J Neurol Neurosurg Psychiatry 1986;49:1–10.

5 Laakso A, Hernesniemi J: Arteriovenous malformations: epidemiology and clinical presentation. Neurosurg Clin N Am 2012;23:1–6.

6 Berman MF, Sciacca RR, Pile-Spellman J, et al: The epidemiology of brain arteriovenous malformations. Neurosurgery 2000;47:389–396; discussion 397.

7 Michelsen WJ: Natural history and pathophysiology of arteriovenous malformations. Clin Neurosurg 1978;26:307–313.

8 Friedlander RM: Clinical practice. Arteriovenous malformations of the brain. N Engl J Med 2007;356: 2704–2712.

9 Tu J, Stoodley MA, Morgan MK, et al: Ultrastructure of perinidal capillaries in cerebral arteriovenous malformations. Neurosurgery 2006;58:961–970; discussion 961–970.

10 Wong JH, Awad IA, Kim JH: Ultrastructural pathological features of cerebrovascular malformations: a preliminary report. Neurosurgery 2000;46:1454–1459.

11 Hatva E, Jääskeläinen J, Hirvonen H, et al: Tie endothelial cell-specific receptor tyrosine kinase is upregulated in the vasculature of arteriovenous malformations. J Neuropathol Exp Neurol 1996;55:1124–1133.

12 Kader A, Goodrich JT, Sonstein WJ, et al: Recurrent cerebral arteriovenous malformations after negative postoperative angiograms. J Neurosurg 1996;85:14–18.

13 Morales-Valero SF, Bortolotti C, Sturiale CL, et al: Are parenchymal AVMs congenital lesions? Neurosurg Focus 2014;37:E2.
14 Lee SK, Vilela P, Willinsky R, et al: Spontaneous regression of cerebral arteriovenous malformations: clinical and angiographic analysis with review of the literature. Neuroradiology 2002;44:11–16.
15 Moftakhar P, Hauptman JS, Malkasian D, et al: Cerebral arteriovenous malformations. Part 1: cellular and molecular biology. Neurosurg Focus 2009;26:E10.
16 Mullan S, Mojtahedi S, Johnson DL, et al: Embryological basis of some aspects of cerebral vascular fistulas and malformations. J Neurosurg 1996;85:1–8.
17 Lasjaunias P: A revised concept of the congenital nature of cerebral arteriovenous malformations. Interv Neuroradiol 1997;3:275–281.
18 Moftakhar P, Hauptman JS, Malkasian D, et al: Cerebral arteriovenous malformations. Part 2: physiology. Neurosurg Focus 2009;26:E11.
19 Zacharia BE, Vaughan KA, Jacoby A, et al: Management of ruptured brain arteriovenous malformations. Curr Atheroscler Rep 2012;14:335–342.
20 ApSimon HT, Reef H, Phadke RV, et al: A population-based study of brain arteriovenous malformation: long-term treatment outcomes. Stroke 2002;33:2794–2800.
21 Ondra SL, Troupp H, George ED, et al: The natural history of symptomatic arteriovenous malformations of the brain: a 24-year follow-up assessment. J Neurosurg 1990;73:387–391.
22 Kim H, Al-Shahi Salman R, McCulloch CE, et al: Untreated brain arteriovenous malformation: patient-level meta-analysis of hemorrhage predictors. Neurology 2014;83:590–597.
23 Gross BA, Du R: Natural history of cerebral arteriovenous malformations: a meta-analysis. J Neurosurg 2013;118:437–443.
24 Kondziolka D, McLaughlin MR, Kestle JR: Simple risk predictions for arteriovenous malformation hemorrhage. Neurosurgery 1995;37:851–855.
25 Brown RD Jr, Wiebers DO, Torner JC, et al: Incidence and prevalence of intracranial vascular malformations in Olmsted County, Minnesota, 1965 to 1992. Neurology 1996;46:949–952.
26 Aoun SG, Bendok BR, Batjer HH: Acute management of ruptured arteriovenous malformations and dural arteriovenous fistulas. Neurosurg Clin N Am 2012;23:87–103.
27 Duong DH, Young WL, Vang MC, et al: Feeding artery pressure and venous drainage pattern are primary determinants of hemorrhage from cerebral arteriovenous malformations. Stroke 1998;29:1167–1176.
28 Abdulrauf SI, Malik GM, Awad IA: Spontaneous angiographic obliteration of cerebral arteriovenous malformations. Neurosurgery 1999;44:280–287; discussion 287–288.
29 Patel MC, Hodgson TJ, Kemeny AA, et al: Spontaneous obliteration of pial arteriovenous malformations: a review of 27 cases. AJNR Am J Neuroradiol 2001;22:531–536.
30 Ajiboye N, Chalouhi N, Starke RM, et al: Cerebral arteriovenous malformations: evaluation and management. ScientificWorldJournal 2014;2014:649036.
31 Hernesniemi JA, Dashti R, Juvela S, et al: Natural history of brain arteriovenous malformations: a long-term follow-up study of risk of hemorrhage in 238 patients. Neurosurgery 2008;63:823–829; discussion 829–831.
32 Jafar JJ, Rezai AR: Acute surgical management of intracranial arteriovenous malformations. Neurosurgery 1994;34:8–12; discussion 12–13.
33 Steudel WI, Lorenz R, Berkefeld J: Acute operation on arteriovenous malformation with hematomas–report on six cases. Neurochirurgia (Stuttg) 1992;35:26–30.
34 Pavesi G, Rustemi O, Berlucchi S, et al: Acute surgical removal of low-grade (Spetzler-Martin I-II) bleeding arteriovenous malformations. Surg Neurol 2009;72:662–667.
35 Kuhmonen J, Piippo A, Väärt K, et al: Early surgery for ruptured cerebral arteriovenous malformations. Acta Neurochir Suppl 2005;94:111–114.
36 Mossa-Basha M, Chen J, Gandhi D: Imaging of cerebral arteriovenous malformations and dural arteriovenous fistulas. Neurosurg Clin N Am 2012;23:27–42.
37 Zhu XL, Chan MS, Poon WS: Spontaneous intracranial hemorrhage: which patients need diagnostic cerebral angiography? A prospective study of 206 cases and review of the literature. Stroke 1997;28:1406–1409.
38 Broderick J, Connolly S, Feldmann E,et al: Guidelines for the management of spontaneous intracerebral hemorrhage in adults: 2007 update: a guideline from the American Heart Association/American Stroke Association Stroke Council, High Blood Pressure Research Council, and the Quality of Care and Outcomes in Research Interdisciplinary Working Group. Circulation 2007;116:e391–e413.
39 Morgenstern LB, Hemphill JC 3rd, Anderson C, et al: Guidelines for the management of spontaneous intracerebral hemorrhage: a guideline for healthcare professionals from the American Heart Association/American Stroke Association. Stroke 2010;41:2108–2129.

40 Anderson CS, Huang Y, Arima H, et al: Effects of early intensive blood pressure-lowering treatment on the growth of hematoma and perihematomal edema in acute intracerebral hemorrhage: the Intensive Blood Pressure Reduction in Acute Cerebral Haemorrhage Trial (INTERACT). Stroke 2010;41:307–312.
41 Bladin CF, Alexandrov AV, Bellavance A, et al: Seizures after stroke: a prospective multicenter study. Arch Neurol 2000;57:1617–1622.
42 Spetzler RF, Martin NA: A proposed grading system for arteriovenous malformations. J Neurosurg 1986; 65:476–483.
43 Potts MB, Lau D, Abla AA, et al: Current surgical results with low-grade brain arteriovenous malformations. J Neurosurg 2015;122:912–920.
44 Bervini D, Morgan MK, Ritson EA, et al: Surgery for unruptured arteriovenous malformations of the brain is better than conservative management for selected cases: a prospective cohort study. J Neurosurg 2014;121:878–890.
45 Heros RC, Korosue K, Diebold PM: Surgical excision of cerebral arteriovenous malformations: late results. Neurosurgery 1990;26:570–577; discussion 577–578.
46 Lawton MT, Kim H, McCulloch CE, et al: A supplementary grading scale for selecting patients with brain arteriovenous malformations for surgery. Neurosurgery 2010;66:702–713; discussion 713.
47 Kim H, Abla AA, Nelson J, et al: Validation of the supplemented Spetzler-Martin grading system for brain arteriovenous malformations in a multicenter cohort of 1,009 surgical patients. Neurosurgery 2015; 76:25–31; discussion 31–32; quiz 32–33.
48 Hartmann A, Mast H, Mohr JP, et al: Morbidity of intracranial hemorrhage in patients with cerebral arteriovenous malformation. Stroke 1998;29:931–934.
49 Ashley WW Jr, Charbel FT, Amin-Hanjani S: Surgical management of acute intracranial hemorrhage, surgical aneurysmal and arteriovenous malformation ablation, and other surgical principles. Neurol Clin 2008;26:987–1005, ix.
50 Ogilvy CS, Stieg PE, Awad I, et al: AHA Scientific Statement: recommendations for the management of intracranial arteriovenous malformations: a statement for healthcare professionals from a special writing group of the Stroke Council, American Stroke Association. Stroke 2001;32:1458–1471.
51 Lawton MT, Du R, Tran MN, et al: Effect of presenting hemorrhage on outcome after microsurgical resection of brain arteriovenous malformations. Neurosurgery 2005;56:485–493; discussion 485–493.
52 Castel JP, Kantor G: [Postoperative morbidity and mortality after microsurgical exclusion of cerebral arteriovenous malformations. Current data and analysis of recent literature]. Neurochirurgie 2001; 47(2–3 Pt 2):369–383.
53 Barr JC, Ogilvy CS: Selection of treatment modalities or observation of arteriovenous malformations. Neurosurg Clin N Am 2012;23:63–75.
54 Lee MC, Macdonald RL: Intraoperative cerebral angiography: superficial temporal artery method and results. Neurosurgery 2003;53:1067–1074; discussion 1074–1075.
55 Munshi I, Macdonald RL, Weir BK: Intraoperative angiography of brain arteriovenous malformations. Neurosurgery 1999;45:491–497; discussion 497–499.
56 Potts MB, Zumofen DW, Raz E, et al: Curing arteriovenous malformations using embolization. Neurosurg Focus 2014;37:E19.
57 Fournier D, TerBrugge KG, Willinsky R, et al: Endovascular treatment of intracerebral arteriovenous malformations: experience in 49 cases. J Neurosurg 1991;75:228–233.
58 Yu SC, Chan MS, Lam JM, et al: Complete obliteration of intracranial arteriovenous malformation with endovascular cyanoacrylate embolization: initial success and rate of permanent cure. AJNR Am J Neuroradiol 2004;25:1139–1143.
59 Sahlein DH, Mora P, Becske T, et al: Nidal embolization of brain arteriovenous malformations: rates of cure, partial embolization, and clinical outcome. J Neurosurg 2012;117:65–77.
60 Strauss I, Frolov V, Buchbut D, et al: Critical appraisal of endovascular treatment of brain arteriovenous malformation using Onyx in a series of 92 consecutive patients. Acta Neurochir (Wien) 2013;155:611–617.
61 Stemer AB, Bank WO, Armonda RA, et al: Acute embolization of ruptured brain arteriovenous malformations. J Neurointerv Surg 2013;5:196–200.
62 Starke RM, Komotar RJ, Otten ML, et al: Adjuvant embolization with N-butyl cyanoacrylate in the treatment of cerebral arteriovenous malformations: outcomes, complications, and predictors of neurologic deficits. Stroke 2009;40:2783–2790.
63 Spetzler RF, Wilson CB, Weinstein P, et al: Normal perfusion pressure breakthrough theory. Clin Neurosurg 1978;25:651–672.
64 Rangel-Castilla L, Spetzler RF, Nakaji P: Normal perfusion pressure breakthrough theory: a reappraisal after 35 years. Neurosurg Rev 2015;38:399–405.
65 Bendok BR, El Tecle NE, El Ahmadieh TY, et al: Advances and innovations in brain arteriovenous malformation surgery. Neurosurgery 2014;74(suppl 1): S60–S73.
66 Pollock GA, Shaibani A, Awad I, et al: Intraventricular hemorrhage secondary to intranidal aneurysm rupture-successful management by arteriovenous malformation embolization followed by intraventricular tissue plasminogen activator: case report. Neurosurgery 2011;68:E581–E586; discussion E586.

67 van Rooij WJ, Jacobs S, Sluzewski M, et al: Endovascular treatment of ruptured brain AVMs in the acute phase of hemorrhage. AJNR Am J Neuroradiol 2012; 33:1162–1166.
68 Marks MP, Lane B, Steinberg GK, et al: Intranidal aneurysms in cerebral arteriovenous malformations: evaluation and endovascular treatment. Radiology 1992;183:355–360.
69 Rubin BA, Brunswick A, Riina H, et al: Advances in radiosurgery for arteriovenous malformations of the brain. Neurosurgery 2014;74(suppl 1):S50–S59.
70 Ding D, Yen CP, Starke RM, et al: Radiosurgery for ruptured intracranial arteriovenous malformations. J Neurosurg 2014;121:470–481.
71 St George EJ, Perks J, Plowman PN: Stereotactic radiosurgery XIV: The role of the haemosiderin 'ring' in the development of adverse reactions following radiosurgery for intracranial cavernous malformations: a sustainable hypothesis. Br J Neurosurg 2002; 16:385–391.

Prof. R. Loch Macdonald
Division of Neurosurgery
St. Michael's Hospital, University of Toronto
30 Bond Street, Toronto, ON M5B 1W8 (Canada)
E-Mail macdonaldlo@smh.ca

Toyoda K, Anderson CS, Mayer SA (eds): New Insights in Intracerebral Hemorrhage.
Front Neurol Neurosci. Basel, Karger, 2016, vol 37, pp 182–192 (DOI: 10.1159/000437122)

Prognosis and Outcome of Intracerebral Haemorrhage

Solène Moulin · Charlotte Cordonnier

Inserm U 1171 – University of Lille, Department of Neurology and Stroke Unit, Roger Salengro Hospital, Lille, France

Abstract

Spontaneous intracerebral haemorrhage (ICH) accounts for approximately 15% of all strokes and is a leading cause of disability, with a one-month mortality rate of 40%. Whereas factors predicting short-term mortality are well known, data regarding long-term outcome are scarce and imprecise. The two main underlying vasculopathies responsible for ICH, i.e. deep perforating vasculopathy and cerebral amyloid angiopathy, might have an impact on the overall prognosis of ICH survivors. ICH survivors are at high risk of epileptic seizures, depression and cognitive impairment, which may influence their functional outcome. Lobar location of an ICH, frequently due to cerebral amyloid angiopathy, partly determines the long-term risk of recurrent haemorrhage. Because of common vascular risk factors, patients with ICH are also at considerable risk of serious ischaemic events. Risks of future ischaemic events may be as high as that of recurrent ICH, raising the relevance of antithrombotic treatment in ICH survivors. Future studies of long-term follow-up after ICH are needed to determine predictors of outcome, including biomarkers of the underlying vasculopathies, to tailor preventive strategies to survivors.
© 2016 S. Karger AG, Basel

Introduction

Spontaneous intracerebral haemorrhage (ICH) accounts for approximately 15% of all strokes among the Western population. Although huge progress has been made in the management of ischaemia, ICH remains a major cause of morbidity and mortality worldwide. The case fatality rate of ICH at 1 month is around 40%, and less than one survivor out of two is independent at 1 year [1]. The overall case-fatality rate has remained unchanged for several decades, but data regarding long-term outcome are scarce. Despite the apparent stability in the overall incidence, important changes have occurred in the profiles of patients with ICH. A recent population-based study has shown an 80% increase in the incidence of ICH among people aged 75 years and over [2], while a 50% decrease was found among patients younger than 60 years old. These data suggest changes in the weights of the two main underlying vasculopathies, including a decrease in deep perforating vasculopathy due to better treatment of arterial hypertension and an increase in the incidence of lobar ICH, which is often associated with underlying cerebral amyloid angiopathy, probably triggered by an increasing use of antithrombotic drugs among elderly people. The evolution of the underlying vasculopathies leading to ICH may influence the overall prognoses of those patients, who deserve more attention in the near future.

Short- and Long-Term Mortality after Spontaneous Intracerebral Haemorrhage

ICH is a dynamic phenomenon, and all action must be taken to fight against haematoma expansion. Indeed, over 20% of patients experience a decrease in the Glasgow Coma Scale (GCS) score between pre-hospital assessment and admission to hospital [3]. Approximately one-third of patients demonstrate significant haematoma expansion within the first 24 h of onset, explaining their early neurological deterioration, which further aggravates outcome [4]. The initial haematoma volume remains the strongest predictor of 30-day mortality and functional outcome [5]. The hazard ratio of mortality goes up by 5% with every 10% increase in ICH volume [6]. A systematic review has found that the 1-month case-fatality rate has remained stable at around 40% for several decades [1]. The ICH location is another variable influencing both short- and long-term prognoses. Despite the larger volume with subarachnoid or subdural extension in lobar ICH, a recent population-based study has shown that the 1-year case-fatality rate is lower in patients with lobar ICH compared with those with deep ICH [7]. One explanation for this finding may be that the smaller volume in deep ICH is counterbalanced by the frequent extension into the ventricular system, a well-known radiological factor of poor outcome. Regarding infratentorial ICH, cerebellar ICH has a better prognosis than brainstem ICH. However, dichotomizing haemorrhages as supratentorial versus infratentorial or lobar versus deep might be too simplistic.

The most widely used and externally validated score for evaluating 1-month prognosis is the ICH score [8], which includes age, GCS score at admission, ICH volume, ICH location and intraventricular extension. These five prognostic factors may help to assess the risk of death within 1 month (table 1). With regard to imaging, computed tomography angiography is being increasingly used for the prognostication of ICH. First, it may assist with visualization of underlying intracranial vascular malformations, such as aneurysms and arteriovenous malformations, which may require

Table 1. Scoring system to assess 30-day case fatality* after intracerebral haemorrhage

Component	Score
Glasgow Coma Scale (at initial presentation or after resuscitation)	
3–4	2
5–12	1
13–15	0
Intracerebral haemorrhage volume, ml	
≥30	1
<30	0
Any intraventricular haemorrhage on initial computed tomography	
Yes	1
No	0
Infratentorial origin of intracerebral haemorrhage	
Yes	1
No	0
Patient age	
≥80	1
<80	0

(Adapted from Hemphill et al. [8].) * Thirty-day case fatality as a percentage (95% CI), as indicated by scores: Score 1: 13 (5–28); Score 2: 26 (13–45); Score 3: 72 (55–84); Score 4: 97 (83–99); Score 5: 100 (61–100). There were no patients with a score of 6.

further specific interventional treatment. Second, it enables visualization of contrast extravasation within the haematoma, also called a 'spot sign', which is predictive of further haematoma expansion [9]. Additional factors that are harder to quantify, such as withdrawal of care and 'do not resuscitate' orders, may have important impacts on prognosis [10].

Whereas short-term mortality following ICH is known to be high, the pattern of long-term mortality following ICH has not been well documented. Previous studies have analysed some aspects of this problem but have been limited by a small sample size, a retrospective design [11–13], or the absence of important known predictors of outcome in analysis [11–13]. A recent systematic review and meta-analysis of 122 longitudinal cohort studies reporting long-term (>30 days) outcome after spontaneous ICH has reported a 1-year survival rate of 46% (95% CI 43.4–48.6) and a 5-year survival rate of 29.2% (95% CI 25.7–32.8) in population-based studies [14]. These long-term survival rates do not appear to have changed over time. Interestingly, the most frequently studied predictors of long-term mortality are the principal components of the ICH score, i.e. increasing age, decreasing GCS score, increasing ICH volume, presence of intraventricular haemorrhage and deep/infratentorial ICH location [14]. However, a recent population-based study of 1-year ICH survivors has shown that the classical risk factors affecting short-term survival are less important when focusing on long-term prognosis [15]. The authors have found that independent risk factors for death among 1-year survivors are age, diabetes mellitus at baseline and anticoagulant therapy at ICH onset. Lastly, recent meta-analysis of randomized controlled trials has shown that stroke unit care appears to be a major prognostic factor because patients with ICH seem to benefit at least as much as those with ischaemic stroke from this type of care for the prevention of death or dependency [16].

Functional Outcome

Meta-analysis that included population-based studies of ICH conducted from 1980 to 2008 identified six studies reporting functional outcomes at various time points after ICH [1]. The proportion of patients leading an independent life after ICH varied from 12% at 12 months in Estonian patients [17] to 39% at the last follow-up visit in young Italian adults (mean follow-up period of 50 months, range of 19–79 months) [18]. No conclusion could be drawn from these data because of the heterogeneity of the methodologies and the variability of the time of assessment. More recently, Poon et al. [14] conducted meta-analysis that was restricted to the four population-based studies published between 2004 and 2011, finding independence (modified Rankin Scale score of 0–2) at 6 months among 33–42% of all ICH patients (i.e. 54–84% of survivors) [19, 20] and independence at 1 year among 17–25% of all ICH patients (i.e. 54–57% of survivors) [17, 21]. However, there were many methodological flaws in those previous studies, highlighting the small amount of data available on this topic.

Early and Late Seizures in Intracerebral Haemorrhage

Seizures are a common complication of ICH and can even be the presenting symptom [22]. Seizures can be delayed but most frequently occur at the onset of ICH. The reported incidence of seizures after ICH has varied widely depending on the study design, diagnostic criteria, duration of follow-up and the studied population.

Early Seizures

According to the International League Against Epilepsy guidelines [23], early seizures are defined as those occurring within 7 days of stroke. About 50–70% of seizures occur within the first 24 h, and 90% occur within the first 72 h [24, 25], with an overall risk of seizures of about 8% within 1 month of symptom onset [22]. A prospective hospital-based study with good external validity has found early clinical seizures in 14% (95% CI 11–17) of patients with ICH, with half of the early seizures occurring at ICH onset [26]. Lobar location is an independent predictor of early seizures due to an increased probability of cortical involvement in lobar versus deep ICH [22, 26]. Regarding the influence of early seizures on outcome and mortality, studies have shown conflicting results. However, the results mainly suggest that early seizures do not influence in-hospital mortality or short-term functional outcome [22, 26]. This finding raises the issue of preventive antiepileptic treatment in spontaneous ICH patients, which cannot be recommended because early seizures do not worsen prognosis [27].

Late Seizures

Late seizures are defined as those occurring 7 days or more after stroke [23]. The incidence of late seizures is around 4 new cases/100 person-years, with a median delay between ICH and late seizures of 9 months (interquartile range, 3–23) [28]. The only factor independently associated with the occurrence of late seizures is cortical involvement of the ICH. Among MRI biomarkers, the presence of lobar brain microbleeds, as well as their number, has been associated with the occurrence of late seizures during long-term follow-up, which might suggest a link to the underlying vasculopathy (cerebral amyloid angiopathy) [28]. The risk of developing late seizures cannot be predicted by the occurrence of early seizures. In contrast with early seizures, the occurrence of late seizures has been associated with worse functional outcome (modified Rankin Scale score of ≥3) after 3 years of follow-up [28]. This finding suggests that late seizures may either have a direct influence on outcome or may simply be symptomatic of the underlying disease.

Status Epilepticus

The reported frequency of status epilepticus post-ICH varies from 0.3 to 21.4% [29, 30]. In a previous study that included 1,402 patients with ICH, status epilepticus occurred in 11 (17%) of 64 patients with seizures and was the initial presentation of ICH in 6 of these 64 patients.

Subclinical Seizures

As subclinical seizures can be detected through the use of continuous electroencephalographic (EEG) monitoring only, the true incidence of seizures might be underestimated. The overall incidence of subclinical seizures after ICH is 29–31%. In a small cohort of 63 patients with ICH, continuous EEG monitoring showed that 28% of patients had predominantly non-convulsive seizures within the first 3 days after admission [24]. The factors independently associated with seizures were increased midline brain shift on head CT scans at follow-up, neurological worsening and poorer outcome [24]. In a retrospective study of 102 consecutive patients with ICH who underwent continuous EEG monitoring, the authors reported a prevalence of clinical seizures of 31% before monitoring [25]. Eighteen per cent of patients had electrographic seizures, and only one of them had clinical seizures that were recorded during continuous EEG monitoring. After adjustments for demographic and clinical predictors, electrographic seizures were found to be associated with haematoma expansion and poor outcome [25].

Futures prospective studies of larger cohorts that include EEG monitoring are needed to determine the influence of post-ICH seizures on long-term outcome, not only regarding the risk of epilepsy post-ICH, but also regarding functional and cognitive outcomes.

Depression Post-Intracerebral Haemorrhage

Stroke and depression are closely related. Depression occurs frequently after stroke and has a negative impact on functional outcome. Post-stroke depression reduces the capacity for functional recovery and is associated with a higher mortality rate. Its prevalence is estimated to be 33%, and it has remained stable over time [31]. Predictive factors for post-stroke depression that have been identified in the literature are the severity of stroke, disability in daily living activities after stroke, pre-existing cognitive decline, a history of depression and social factors [31]. However, all data on post-stroke depression have been obtained using cohorts of ischaemic stroke patients or mixed cohorts of stroke patients and few ICH patients. Very limited data are available on the prevalence, predictive factors and other associated factors for depression after ICH [32]. The poorer functional prognosis of ICH compared to that of ischaemic stroke suggests that it carries a higher risk of developing depression.

Cognitive Decline and Dementia Post-Intracerebral Haemorrhage

About 10% of patients have dementia before their first stroke, 10% develop new-onset dementia after their first-ever stroke, and more than 30% develop dementia after a recurrent stroke [33]. Moreover, stroke and dementia share similar risk factors, and each increases the risk of the other [34]. Most of the knowledge about post-stroke dementia has been obtained using cohorts that included solely or mostly ischaemic stroke patients. Only a few ICH patients have been included in the cohorts, and dedicated ICH cohorts have rarely been published. Associated factors for post-stroke dementia that have been identified in the literature are history of asymptomatic or symptomatic stroke detected on imaging, recurrent ischaemic or haemorrhagic stroke, several stroke lesions, aphasia, the severity and volume of stroke and the location of stroke (increased risk with left hemisphere location and decreased risk with brainstem location) [33]. Complications of stroke, such as seizures and confusion, are also predictive of post-stroke dementia, although the extent to which these are related to stroke severity rather than being independent factors is unclear. Interestingly, several predictors of post-stroke dementia that are not directly related to the characteristics of stroke itself, such as age, a low education level, the female sex, atrial fibrillation, diabetes, leukoaraiosis and global and medial temporal lobe atrophy, have also been associated with Alzheimer's dementia [33]. These findings suggest that stroke might trigger the expression of an underlying silent neurodegenerative process [35].

Table 2. Prevalence of post-stroke dementia and characteristics of studies including ICH patients

Author, publication, year	Duration after stroke, months	Number of patients (IS/ICH)	Diagnosis of dementia	Exclusion of pre-stroke dementia	Prevalence of dementia in IS	Prevalence of dementia in ICH
Barba et al., 2000 [38]	3	222/29	DSM-4	no	30 (24–36)	28 (15–46)
Madureira et al., 2001 [40]	3	165/55	DSM-4	yes, interview	6 (3–11)	5 (2–15)
Hénon et al., 2001 [39]	36	150/19	ICD-10	yes, IQCODE	23 (17–30)	10 (3–31)
Tang et al., 2004 [42]	3	257/22	DSM-4	no	20 (15–25)	18 (2–33)
Altieri et al., 2004 [41]	68	170/4	ICD-10	yes	22 (17–29)	25 (5–70)
De Koning et al., 2005 [43]	9	77/19	DSM-4	no	35 (25–46)	42 (23–64)
Ihle-Hansen et al., 2011 [44]	12	159/16	ICD-10	yes, IQCODE	17 (11–23)	44 (19–68)

Adapted from Murao et al. [45]. IS = Ischaemic stroke; ICH = intracerebral haemorrhage; DSM-4 = the diagnostic and statistical manual of mental disorders, fourth edition; ICD 10 = 10th revision of the international classification of diseases; IQCODE = informant questionnaire on cognitive decline in the elderly.

Similarly, the relationship between ICH and dementia might be of interest because the most frequent underlying vasculopathies in ICH are cerebral amyloid angiopathy and deep perforating vasculopathy, both of which have been associated with cognitive impairment of either the vascular [36] or Alzheimer's [37] type. Among studies of post-stroke dementia, data on ICH are scarce and have only been reported in seven studies, which assessed a total of 164 ICH patients and found incidences of post-ICH dementia ranging from 5 to 44% [38–44]. These studies have been hampered by many methodological limitations, such as the use of a small sample size and retrospective design, inclusion of pre-ICH cognitive impairment, and the use of different timing for diagnosis of post-ICH dementia (from 3 to 68 months after ICH) (table 2) [45]. A recent prospective population-based study including 1,618 patients described cognitive impairment after stroke. Among 169 patients (10%) with ICH, 68 (40%; 95% CI: 34–48%) developed post-ICH cognitive impairment, as detected by Mini-Mental State Examination or by the Abbreviated Mental Test, at 3 months after stroke [46]. Because they did not specifically focus on ICH, all of these previous studies were not designed to identify predictors of ICH prognosis, such as ICH location or volume. Only one published study addressed this topic using a single-centre ICH cohort that included 78 ICH survivors [47]. Among 48 patients with ICH (62%) who underwent neuropsychological assessment, 37 (77%; 95% CI 65–89%) had cognitive impairment without dementia, and 18 (23%; 95% CI 13–32%) were diagnosed as demented after a mean follow-up of 41 months. Possible risk factors identified for post-ICH dementia were the severity of ICH, large volume and discharge to a nursing home. However, the results remain questionable because of the retrospective design of the study. Furthermore, MRI biomarkers of both vascular and neurodegenerative natures, including markers of atrophy and brain microbleeds, were not included in analysis. A recent consensus has highlighted the importance of these biomarkers in future studies [48].

Until now, the incidence, nature and predictors of post-ICH cognitive impairment or dementia remain unknown. The nature of the underlying vessel disease (deep perforating vasculopathy or cerebral amyloid angiopathy) should be carefully studied because it may have an impact on the post-ICH cognitive profile.

Risks of Future Recurrent Intracerebral Haemorrhage and Ischaemic Events

Ischaemic and haemorrhagic strokes share common risk factors for potential ischaemic events (heart or brain) in patients who have suffered from spontaneous ICH. Indeed, ICH patients often exhibit arterial hypertension (60%) and diabetes mellitus (15%) and are smokers (16%) [2, 49]. These risk factors also contribute to the occurrence of other diseases prior to ICH, such as ischaemic stroke (14–23%), ischaemic heart disease (8–21%), and atrial fibrillation (11–14%). As a result, ICH survivors are at a high risk of serious vascular events. Indeed, this population presents, on one hand, a considerable risk of ICH recurrence, and on the other hand, a major risk of vaso-occlusive disease, raising questions about the relevance of antithrombotic drug treatment after ICH. Recent meta-analysis showed that the annual rate of ICH recurrence was 2.0–2.4% in five studies and that the long-term rate of recurrence for early survivors in mostly hospital-based studies varied from 1.3 to 7.4% per year (with durations ranging from 1 to 7 years) [14]. Focusing on ICH location, lobar ICH carries a higher risk of recurrent haemorrhage compared with non-lobar ICH, which is more likely to be recurrent lobar ICH [50]. The higher rate of ICH recurrence after lobar ICH than after non-lobar ICH is possibly due to the nature of the underlying vessel disease because a high proportion of patients have cerebral amyloid angiopathy [51, 52]. Additional risk factors that have been described for lobar ICH recurrence include the baseline numbers of symptomatic and asymptomatic haemorrhages [52] and the apolipoprotein E genotype [53]. Recent meta-analysis conducted by Poon et al. [14] has demonstrated that the risk of ischaemic stroke is at least as frequent as that of recurrent ICH. Therefore, the risks of all ischaemic events (including those occurring in veins, arteries, and all organs) may be at least as high as the risk of recurrent ICH. In light of these considerations, randomized controlled trials (e.g. http://www.RESTARTtrial.org, ISRCTN71907627) are needed to guide the resumption or not of antithrombotic drugs after ICH.

Conclusions

The overall poor prognosis of ICH makes this disease a major public health issue for which there is a desperate need for effective therapies. The short-term outcome of ICH seems to have remained stable over time, considering the stability of the 1-month case-fatality rate [1]. Haematoma expansion appears to be the only modifiable predictor of short-term outcome compared to the ICH volume at admission and location, which are both determined upon presentation. The high early case-fatality rate in ICH explains the paucity of long-term follow-up data and the need to pool data from different population-based studies that have used consistent methodologies. The quality of studies that have focused on ICH predictors is limited by the absence of important predictors in analyses (such as covariates of the ICH score) [14]. Recent reporting guidelines for prognostic studies may improve study quality in the near future [54]. Huge uncertainties remain concerning predictors of functional outcome, the risk of haemorrhagic or ischaemic events after ICH and, more broadly, the influence of antithrombotic therapy on outcome. Similarly, the influence of biomarkers of the underlying cause of ICH on the risk of ICH recurrence, such as the location of ICH or the presence and anatomical distribution of brain microbleeds, should be investigated [48]. Further studies of long-term prognosis are needed to optimise care and to tailor preventive strategies to survivors.

References

1 van Asch CJ, Luitse MJ, Rinkel GJ, van der Tweel I, Algra A, Klijn CJ: Incidence, case fatality, and functional outcome of intracerebral haemorrhage over time, according to age, sex, and ethnic origin: a systematic review and meta-analysis. Lancet Neurol 2010;9:167–176.

2 Béjot Y, Cordonnier C, Durier J, Aboa-Eboule C, Rouaud O, Giroud M: Intracerebral haemorrhage profiles are changing: results from the Dijon population-based study. Brain 2013;136:658–664.

3 Moon J-S, Janjua N, Ahmed S, Kirmani JF, Harris-Lane P, Jacob M, Ezzeddine MA, Qureshi AI: Prehospital neurologic deterioration in patients with intracerebral hemorrhage. Crit Care Med 2008;36:172–175.

4 Dowlatshahi D, Demchuk AM, Flaherty ML, Ali M, Lyden PL, Smith EE, VISTA Collaboration: Defining hematoma expansion in intracerebral hemorrhage: relationship with patient outcomes. Neurology 2011;76:1238–1244.

5 Broderick JP, Brott TG, Duldner JE, Tomsick T, Huster G: Volume of intracerebral hemorrhage. A powerful and easy-to-use predictor of 30-day mortality. Stroke 1993;24:987–993.

6 Davis SM, Broderick J, Hennerici M, Brun NC, Diringer MN, Mayer SA, Begtrup K, Steiner T, Recombinant Activated Factor VII Intracerebral Hemorrhage Trial Investigators: Hematoma growth is a determinant of mortality and poor outcome after intracerebral hemorrhage. Neurology 2006;66:1175–1181.

7 Samarasekera N, Fonville A, Lerpiniere C, Farrall AJ, Wardlaw JM, White PM, Smith C, Al-Shahi Salman R, Lothian Audit of the Treatment of Cerebral Haemorrhage Collaborators: Influence of intracerebral hemorrhage location on incidence, characteristics, and outcome: population-based study. Stroke 2015;46:361–368.

8 Hemphill JC, Bonovich DC, Besmertis L, Manley GT, Johnston SC: The ICH score: a simple, reliable grading scale for intracerebral hemorrhage. Stroke 2001;32:891–897.

9 Demchuk AM, Dowlatshahi D, Rodriguez-Luna D, Molina CA, Blas YS, Dzialowski I, Kobayashi A, Boulanger J-M, Lum C, Gubitz G, Padma V, Roy J, Kase CS, Kosior J, Bhatia R, Tymchuk S, Subramaniam S, Gladstone DJ, Hill MD, Aviv RI, PREDICT/Sunnybrook ICH CTA study group: Prediction of haematoma growth and outcome in patients with intracerebral haemorrhage using the CT-angiography spot sign (PREDICT): a prospective observational study. Lancet Neurol 2012;11:307–314.

10 Hemphill JC, Newman J, Zhao S, Johnston SC: Hospital usage of early do-not-resuscitate orders and outcome after intracerebral hemorrhage. Stroke 2004;35:1130–1134.

11 Vermeer SES, Algra AA, Franke CLC, Koudstaal PJP, Rinkel GJEG: Long-term prognosis after recovery from primary intracerebral hemorrhage. Neurology 2002;59:205–209.

12 Fogelholm R: Long term survival after primary intracerebral haemorrhage: a retrospective population based study. J Neurol Neurosurg Psychiatry 2005;76:1534–1538.

13 Flaherty ML, Haverbusch M, Sekar P, Kissela B, Kleindorfer D, Moomaw CJ, Sauerbeck L, Schneider A, Broderick JP, Woo D: Long-term mortality after intracerebral hemorrhage. Neurology 2006;66: 1182–1186.
14 Poon MTC, Fonville AF, Salman RA-S: Long-term prognosis after intracerebral haemorrhage: systematic review and meta-analysis. J Neurol Neurosurg Psychiatry 2014;85:660–667.
15 Hansen BM, Nilsson OG, Anderson H, Norrving B, Säveland H, Lindgren A: Long term (13 years) prognosis after primary intracerebral haemorrhage: a prospective population based study of long term mortality, prognostic factors and causes of death. J Neurol Neurosurg Psychiatry 2013;84:1150–1155.
16 Langhorne P, Fearon P, Ronning OM, Kaste M, Palomaki H, Vemmos K, Kalra L, Indredavik B, Blomstrand C, Rodgers H, Dennis MS, Al-Shahi Salman R, Stroke Unit Trialists' Collaboration: Stroke unit care benefits patients with intracerebral hemorrhage: systematic review and meta-analysis. Stroke 2013;44:3044–3049.
17 Vibo R, Kõrv J, Roose M: One-year outcome after first-ever stroke according to stroke subtype, severity, risk factors and pre-stroke treatment. A population-based study from Tartu, Estonia. Eur J Neurol 2007;14:435–439.
18 Marini C, Totaro R, De Santis F, Ciancarelli I, Baldassarre M, Carolei A: Stroke in young adults in the community-based L'Aquila registry: incidence and prognosis. Stroke 2001;32:52–56.
19 Lavados PM, Sacks C, Prina L, Escobar A, Tossi C, Araya F, Feuerhake W, Galvez M, Salinas R, Alvarez G: Incidence, 30-day case-fatality rate, and prognosis of stroke in Iquique, Chile: a 2-year community-based prospective study (PISCIS project). Lancet 2005;365:2206–2215.
20 Cabral NL, Gonçalves ARR, Longo AL, Moro CHC, Costa G, Amaral CH, Fonseca LAM, Eluf-Neto J: Incidence of stroke subtypes, prognosis and prevalence of risk factors in Joinville, Brazil: a 2 year community based study. J Neurol Neurosurg Psychiatry 2009;80:755–761.
21 Bailey RD, Hart RG, Benavente O, Pearce LA: Recurrent brain hemorrhage is more frequent than ischemic stroke after intracranial hemorrhage. Neurology 2001;56:773–777.
22 Passero S, Rocchi R, Rossi S, Ulivelli M, Vatti G: Seizures after spontaneous supratentorial intracerebral hemorrhage. Epilepsia 2002;43:1175–1180.
23 Guidelines for epidemiologic studies on epilepsy. Commission on Epidemiology and Prognosis, International League Against Epilepsy. Epilepsia 1993;34: 592–596.
24 Vespa PM, O'Phelan K, Shah M, Mirabelli J, Starkman S, Kidwell C, Saver J, Nuwer MR, Frazee JG, McArthur DA, Martin NA: Acute seizures after intracerebral hemorrhage: a factor in progressive midline shift and outcome. Neurology 2003;60:1441–1446.
25 Claassen J, Jetté N, Chum F, Green R, Schmidt M, Choi H, Jirsch J, Frontera JA, Connolly ES, Emerson RG, Mayer SA, Hirsch LJ: Electrographic seizures and periodic discharges after intracerebral hemorrhage. Neurology 2007;69:1356–1365.
26 De Herdt V, Dumont F, Henon H, Derambure P, Vonck K, Leys D, Cordonnier C: Early seizures in intracerebral hemorrhage: incidence, associated factors, and outcome. Neurology 2011;77:1794–1800.
27 Steiner T, Al-Shahi Salman R, Beer R, Christensen H, Cordonnier C, Csiba L, Forsting M, Harnof S, Klijn CJM, Krieger D, Mendelow AD, Molina C, Montaner J, Overgaard K, Petersson J, Roine RO, Schmutzhard E, Schwerdtfeger K, Stapf C, Tatlisumak T, Thomas BM, Toni D, Unterberg A, Wagner M: European Stroke Organisation (ESO) guidelines for the management of spontaneous intracerebral hemorrhage. Int J Stroke 2014;9:840–855.
28 Rossi C, De Herdt V, Dequatre-Ponchelle N, Hénon H, Leys D, Cordonnier C: Incidence and predictors of late seizures in intracerebral hemorrhages. Stroke 2013;44:1723–1725.
29 Bateman BT, Claassen J, Willey JZ, Hirsch LJ, Mayer SA, Sacco RL, Schumacher HC: Convulsive status epilepticus after ischemic stroke and intracerebral hemorrhage: frequency, predictors, and impact on outcome in a large administrative dataset. Neurocrit Care 2007;7:187–193.
30 De Reuck J, Hemelsoet D, Van Maele G: Seizures and epilepsy in patients with a spontaneous intracerebral haematoma. Clin Neurol Neurosurg 2007;109:501–504.
31 Hackett ML, Anderson CS, Auckland Regional Community Stroke (ARCOS) Study Group: Frequency, management, and predictors of abnormal mood after stroke: the Auckland Regional Community Stroke (ARCOS) study, 2002 to 2003. Stroke 2006;37:2123–2128.
32 Christensen MC, Mayer SA, Ferran J-M, Kissela B: Depressed mood after intracerebral hemorrhage: the FAST trial. Cerebrovasc Dis 2009;27:353–360.
33 Pendlebury ST, Rothwell PM: Prevalence, incidence, and factors associated with pre-stroke and post-stroke dementia: a systematic review and meta-analysis. Lancet Neurol 2009;8:1006–1018.
34 Imfeld P, Bodmer M, Schuerch M, Jick SS, Meier CR: Risk of incident stroke in patients with Alzheimer disease or vascular dementia. Neurology 2013;81: 910–919.

35 Pasquier F, Leys D: Why are stroke patients prone to develop dementia? J Neurol 1997;244:135–142.
36 Gorelick PB, Bowler JV: Advances in vascular cognitive impairment 2007. Stroke 2008;39:279–282.
37 Jellinger KA, Attems J: Incidence of cerebrovascular lesions in Alzheimer's disease: a postmortem study. Acta Neuropathol 2003;105:14–17.
38 Barba R, Martínez-Espinosa S, Rodríguez-García E, Pondal M, Vivancos J, Del Ser T: Poststroke dementia: clinical features and risk factors. Stroke 2000;31:1494–1501.
39 Henon H, Durieu I, Guerouaou D, Lebert F, Pasquier F, Leys D: Poststroke dementia: incidence and relationship to prestroke cognitive decline. Neurology 2001;57:1216–1222.
40 Madureira S, Guerreiro M, Ferro JM: Dementia and cognitive impairment three months after stroke. Eur J Neurol 2001;8:621–627.
41 Altieri M, Di Piero V, Pasquini M, Gasparini M, Vanacore N, Vicenzini E, Lenzi GL: Delayed poststroke dementia: a 4-year follow-up study. Neurology 2004;62:2193–2197.
42 Tang WK, Chan SSM, Chiu HFK, Ungvari GS, Wong KS, Kwok TCY, Mok V, Wong KT, Richards PS, Ahuja AT: Frequency and determinants of poststroke dementia in Chinese. Stroke 2004;35:930–935.
43 de Koning I, van Kooten F, Koudstaal PJ, Dippel DWJ: Diagnostic value of the Rotterdam-CAMCOG in post-stroke dementia. J Neurol Neurosurg Psychiatry 2005;76:263–265.
44 Ihle-Hansen H, Thommessen B, Wyller TB, Engedal K, Øksengård AR, Stenset V, Løken K, Aaberg M, Fure B: Incidence and subtypes of MCI and dementia 1 year after first-ever stroke in patients without pre-existing cognitive impairment. Dement Geriatr Cogn Disord 2011;32:401–407.
45 Murao K, Rossi C, Cordonnier C: Intracerebral haemorrhage and cognitive decline. Rev Neurol (Paris) 2013;169:772–778.
46 Douiri A, Rudd AG, Wolfe CDA: Prevalence of poststroke cognitive impairment: South London Stroke Register 1995–2010. Stroke 2013;44:138–145.
47 Garcia PY, Roussel M, Bugnicourt JM, Lamy C, Canaple S, Peltier J, Loas G, Deramond H, Godefroy O: Cognitive impairment and dementia after intracerebral hemorrhage: a cross-sectional study of a hospital-based series. J Stroke Cerebrovasc Dis 2013;22:80–86.
48 Wardlaw JM, Smith EE, Biessels GJ, Cordonnier C, Fazekas F, Frayne R, Lindley RI, O'Brien JT, Barkhof F, Benavente OR, Black SE, Brayne C, Breteler M, Chabriat H, DeCarli C, de Leeuw F-E, Doubal F, Duering M, Fox NC, Greenberg S, Hachinski V, Kilimann I, Mok V, Oostenbrugge RV, Pantoni L, Speck O, Stephan BCM, Teipel S, Viswanathan A, Werring D, Chen C, Smith C, van Buchem M, Norrving B, Gorelick PB, Dichgans M: STandards for ReportIng Vascular changes on nEuroimaging (STRIVE v1). Neuroimaging standards for research into small vessel disease and its contribution to ageing and neurodegeneration. Lancet Neurol 2013;12:822–838.
49 Lovelock CE, Molyneux AJ, Rothwell PM: Change in incidence and aetiology of intracerebral haemorrhage in Oxfordshire, UK, between 1981 and 2006: a population-based study. Lancet Neurol 2007;6:487–493.
50 Neau JP, Ingrand P, Couderq C, Rosier MP, Bailbe M, Dumas P, Vandermarcq P, Gil R: Recurrent intracerebral hemorrhage. Neurology 1997;49:106–113.
51 Knudsen KA, Rosand J, Karluk D, Greenberg SM: Clinical diagnosis of cerebral amyloid angiopathy: validation of the Boston criteria. Neurology 2001;56:537–539.
52 Greenberg SM, Eng JA, Ning M, Smith EE, Rosand J: Hemorrhage burden predicts recurrent intracerebral hemorrhage after lobar hemorrhage. Stroke 2004;35:1415–1420.
53 O'Donnell HC, Rosand J, Knudsen KA, Furie KL, Segal AZ, Chiu RI, Ikeda D, Greenberg SM: Apolipoprotein E genotype and the risk of recurrent lobar intracerebral hemorrhage. N Engl J Med 2000;342:240–245.
54 Hemingway H, Croft P, Perel P, Hayden JA, Abrams K, Timmis A, Briggs A, Udumyan R, Moons KGM, Steyerberg EW, Roberts I, Schroter S, Altman DG, Riley RD, PROGRESS Group: Prognosis research strategy (PROGRESS) 1:a framework for researching clinical outcomes. BMJ 2013;346:e5595.

Prof. Charlotte Cordonnier
Inserm U 1171 – University of Lille, Department of Neurology and Stroke Unit
Roger Salengro Hospital
rue Emile Laine, FR–59037 Lille (France)
E-Mail charlotte.cordonnier@chru-lille.fr

Author Index

Alobeidi, F. 13
Al-Shahi Salman, R. 1
Anderson, C.S. VII
Aviv, R.I. 13

Bai, H.-M. 155
Bell, S.M. 1

Cordonnier, C. 182

Hanley, D.F. 130
Hayakawa, M. 62

Jiang, C. 155

Küppers-Tiedt, L. 27

Levi, M. 51

Macdonald, R.L. 166
Manning, L.S. 35
Martinez, J.L. 166
Mayer, S.A. VII, 107
Mendelow, A.D. 148
Moulin, S. 182

Nyquist, P.A. 130

Poon, M.T.C. 1

Robinson, T.G. 35

Steiner, T. 27

Toyoda, K. VII

Wang, W.-M. 155
Wartenberg, K.E. 107

Yakushiji, Y. 78
Yasaka, M. 93

Ziai, W.C. 130

Subject Index

Age-related macular degeneration (AMD), intracranial hemorrhage association 8, 9
Alzheimer's disease
  cerebral microbleeds 86
  intracranial hemorrhage patients 188
AMD, *see* Age-related macular degeneration
Aminocaproic acid, hemostatic therapy 121
Andexanet alfa, oral anticoagulant reversal 103
Apixaban
  intracranial hemorrhage risks 96
  reversal 98–100
APOE, alleles and intracranial hemorrhage risk 7, 8
Aprotinin, hemostatic therapy 121, 122
Arteriovenous malformation (AVM)
  classification 167
  clinical presentation 168–170
  endovascular embolization 177, 178
  epidemiology 167
  imaging 170, 171
  intracranial hemorrhage incidence 5, 6, 167
  pathogenesis 167, 168
  rupture management
    hematoma removal 174, 175
    intraoperative management 176, 177
    microsurgery 172, 173
    overview 171
Aspirin, reversal 52, 57
AVM, *see* Arteriovenous malformation

Blood pressure, *see* Hypertension
BRAIN score, hematoma expansion prediction 119
Brain distribution
  cerebral microbleeds 82
  intracranial hemorrhage 5, 6

CADASIL, cerebral microbleeds 86
Cangrelor, reversal 52, 58
Cerebral cavernous malformation (CCM), intracranial hemorrhage incidence 5, 6
Cerebral microbleed (CMB)
  Alzheimer's disease 86
  antithrombotic drug-related intracerebral hemorrhage risks 89
  CADASIL 86
  detection
    magnetic resonance imaging 79–81
    mimics 80, 81
  distribution 82
  Moyamoya disease 86, 87
  neurological dysfunction
    cognitive impairment 87, 88
    gait disturbance 88
  overview 78, 79
  pathology
    blood breakdown products 79
    vascular burden 82, 83
  prevalence 81
  risk factors 82
  small vessel disease markers 83–85
  spontaneous intracerebral hemorrhage 85, 86
  stroke
    cerebral microbleed following stroke 85
    cerebral microbleed leading to stroke 88, 89
  thrombolytic therapy intracerebral hemorrhage risks 89
Charcoal, oral anticoagulant reversal 98, 99
Clevidipine, hypertension control in intracranial hemorrhage 47
Clopidogrel, reversal 52, 58
CMB, *see* Cerebral microbleed

Cognition
cerebral microbleeds and impairment 87, 88
intracranial hemorrhage patients 187–189
Computed tomography (CT), intracranial hemorrhage
angiography 14–16, 18, 19, 21, 24, 110–119
arteriovenous malformation 170, 171
emergency imaging 21, 22
hematoma growth 108
overview 14
prospects for study 22
reperfusion-related intracranial hemorrhage 68–70
screening for secondary hemorrhage 17–19
spot sign and hematoma expansion 19–21, 110–119
Coumadin, *see* Warfarin
Craniotomy, intracranial hemorrhage
clinical trials 151–153
indications 149, 154
minimally invasive surgery, *see* Minimally invasive surgery, intracranial hemorrhage
overview 148, 149
pathophysiological considerations 150
technique 150, 151
Critical care, intracranial hemorrhage
blood glucose control 29
deep venous thrombosis prophylaxis 30
electrolyte disturbances 29
fever reduction 28, 29
hemostatic therapy 30
hypertension control 28
intracranial pressure management 29, 30
neurosurgery 31, 32
seizure control 30
CT, *see* Computed tomography

Dabigatran
intracranial hemorrhage risks 94, 95
reversal 56, 98–100, 102, 103
Deep venous thrombosis (DVT), prophylaxis in intracranial hemorrhage critical care 30
Dementia, intracranial hemorrhage patients 187–189
Depression, intracranial hemorrhage patients 187
Diabetes, intracranial hemorrhage risks 8
DVT, *see* Deep venous thrombosis

Edoxaban, reversal 98–100
Emergency care, *see* Critical care, intracranial hemorrhage
Endovascular therapy, *see* Arteriovenous malformation; Reperfusion-related intracranial hemorrhage
Epilepsy, *see* Seizure

Factor VII
hemostatic therapy 122–124
oral anticoagulant reversal 100, 101
FFP, *see* Fresh frozen plasma
Fresh frozen plasma (FFP), oral anticoagulant reversal 101
Functional outcome, intracranial hemorrhage patients 185

Geographic distribution, intracranial hemorrhage 4

Hematoma
early growth pathophysiology 119, 120
growth characteristics 107–109
hemostatic agents
aminocaproic acid 121
aprotinin 121, 122
factor VII 122–124
tranexamic acid 122
hypertension control effects on growth 44, 45
prediction score for expansion 118, 119
risk factors for growth 109
spot sign and hematoma expansion 19–21, 110–119
Hemodialysis, oral anticoagulant reversal 98, 99
Hemorrhagic stroke, types 2, 3
Heparin, reversal 52, 55
Hypercholesterolemia, intracranial hemorrhage risks 8
Hyperglycemia, control in intracranial hemorrhage critical care 29
Hypertension
control in intracranial hemorrhage
blood pressure variability effect on outcomes 45, 46
clevidipine 47
clinical guidelines 39
critical care 28
hematoma growth response 44, 45
impact on outcomes 41–44

incidence and pathophysiology 36
labetalol 46, 47
nicardipine 47
nitroglycerine 47
safety and feasibility 46, 47
sodium nitroprusside 47
urapidil 47
intracranial hemorrhage risks 6, 7
minimally invasive surgery perioperative hypertension management 163
pathophysiological effects in intracranial hemorrhage 37
prognostic significance in intracranial hemorrhage 36–38

ICP, *see* Intracranial pressure
Idarucizumab, oral anticoagulant reversal 102
Incidence, intracranial hemorrhage
overview 1, 2, 27, 182, 183
seasonal effect 5
secular trends 3, 4
sex differences 5
Intracranial pressure (ICP), management in intracranial hemorrhage critical care 29, 30
Intravenous thrombolysis, *see* Cerebral microbleed; Reperfusion-related intracranial hemorrhage
Intraventricular hemorrhage (IVH)
differential diagnosis 132
epidemiology 130, 131
management
external ventricular drain 134–136
mechanical removal 142, 143
thrombolytic agent injection to enhance drainage
delivery 139–142
drain management during thrombolysis 143
outcomes 135–137
predictors of safety and outcome 139
safety 137, 138
minimally invasive surgery 163
pathophysiology 131
prognosis 132–134
scoring 132, 133

Labetalol, hypertension control in intracranial hemorrhage 46, 47

Magnetic resonance imaging (MRI), intracranial hemorrhage diagnosis
arteriovenous malformation 170, 171
cerebral microbleed 79–81
emergency imaging 22
overview 14
prospects for study 23
reperfusion-related intracranial hemorrhage 68–70
Microbleed, *see* Cerebral microbleed
Minimally invasive surgery, intracranial hemorrhage
historical perspective 156, 157
indications 157
intraventricular hemorrhage 163
local thrombolytic agents
tissue plasminogen activator 162, 163
urokinase 162
perioperative hypertension management 163
principles 156
prospects 163, 164
techniques
microsurgery/endoscopic surgery with keyhole craniotomy 159
soft channel/catheter drainage 160–162
stereotactic or neuronavigation aspiration 159, 160
timing 157, 158
Mortality, intracranial hemorrhage
early case fatality rate 2, 3
short- and long-term rates 183–185
Moyamoya disease, cerebral microbleeds 86, 87
MRI, *see* Magnetic resonance imaging

Nicardipine, hypertension control in intracranial hemorrhage 47
Nitroglycerine, hypertension control in intracranial hemorrhage 47

Obesity, intracranial hemorrhage risks 8

PCC, *see* Prothrombin complex concentrate
PER977, oral anticoagulant reversal 103, 104
Prasugrel, reversal 52, 58
Prothrombin complex concentrate (PCC), oral anticoagulant reversal 99, 100

Recurrent intracranial hemorrhage, risks 189
Reperfusion-related intracranial hemorrhage
imaging 68–70
management 73, 74

pathophysiology 63, 64
prevention 73
risk factors
endovascular therapy 70–72
intravenous thrombolysis therapy 66, 67
symptomatic intracranial hemorrhage
definition and frequency 64–66
tissue plasminogen activator dose effects 67
Risk factors, intracranial hemorrhage
APOE alleles 7, 8
diabetes 8
hypercholesterolemia 8
hypertension 6, 7
obesity 8
recurrent intracranial hemorrhage 189
Rivaroxaban
intracranial hemorrhage risks 94, 95, 98–100
reversal 98–100, 103

Seizure
control in critical care 30
outcomes after intracranial hemorrhage
early seizures 185, 186
late seizures 186
status epilepticus 186
subclinical seizures 186, 187
Selective serotonin reuptake inhibitors (SSRIs), intracranial hemorrhage risks 9
Sex differences, intracranial hemorrhage incidence 5
Sodium nitroprusside, hypertension control in intracranial hemorrhage 47
SSRIs, *see* Selective serotonin reuptake inhibitors
Surgery, *see* Arteriovenous malformation; Craniotomy, intracranial hemorrhage; Minimally invasive surgery, intracranial hemorrhage

Tissue plasminogen activator, *see* Intraventricular hemorrhage; Reperfusion-related intracranial hemorrhage; Minimally invasive surgery, intracranial hemorrhage
Tranexamic acid, hemostatic therapy 122

Urapidil, hypertension control in intracranial hemorrhage 47
Urokinase, *see* Minimally invasive surgery, intracranial hemorrhage

Warfarin
hematoma features 96
intracranial hemorrhage risks 53, 54, 94–97
reversal 52, 54, 101